Handbook of Epilepsy Treatment

Simon D. Shorvon MA, MD, FRCP

Professor in Clinical Neurology and
Chairman of the Department of Clinical Neurology
Institute of Neurology
University College London
UK

Consultant Neurologist
National Hospital for Neurology and Neurosurgery
Queen Square
London
UK

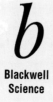

b

Blackwell
Science

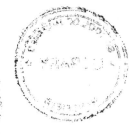

© 2000
Blackwell Science Ltd
Editorial Offices:
Osney Mead, Oxford OX2 0EL
25 John Street, London WC1N 2BL
23 Ainslie Place, Edinburgh EH3 6AJ
350 Main Street, Malden
  MA 02148-5018, USA
54 University Street, Carlton
  Victoria 3053, Australia
10, rue Casimir Delavigne
  75006 Paris, France

Other Editorial Offices:
Blackwell Wissenschafts-Verlag GmbH
Kurfürstendamm 57
10707 Berlin, Germany

Blackwell Science KK
MG Kodenmacho Building
7–10 Kodenmacho Nihombashi
Chuo-ku, Tokyo 104, Japan

First published 2000
Reprinted 2000

Set by Sparks Computer Solutions Ltd,
Oxford, UK
Printed and bound in Great Britain
at the Alden Press Ltd, Oxford and
Northampton

The Blackwell Science logo is a
trade mark of Blackwell Science Ltd,
registered at the United Kingdom
Trade Marks Registry

A catalogue record for this title
is available from the British Library

ISBN 0-632-04849-2

Library of Congress
Cataloging-in-publication Data

Shorvon, S.D. (Simon D.)
  Handbook of epilepsy treatment/
  Simon D. Shorvon.
    p. cm
  Includes index.
  ISBN 0-632-04849-2
  1 Epilepsy—Handbooks, manuals, etc.
  2 Anticonvulsants–Handbooks,
  manuals, etc.
  [DNLM: 1. Epilepsy–therapy–Handbooks.
  WL 39 S5589h 2000]
  RC372.S528 2000
  616.8'53—dc21

DISTRIBUTORS
Marston Book Services Ltd
PO Box 269
Abingdon, Oxon OX14 4YN
(Orders: Tel: 01235 465500
          Fax: 01235 465555)

USA
Blackwell Science, Inc
Commerce Place
350 Main Street
Malden, MA 02148-5018
(Orders: Tel: 800 759 6102
          Tel: 781 388 8250
          Fax: 781 388 8255)

Canada
Login Brothers Book Company
324 Saulteaux Crescent
Winnipeg, Manitoba R3J 3T2
(Orders: Tel: 204 837 2987)

Australia
Blackwell Science Pty Ltd
54 University Street
Carlton, Victoria 3053
(Orders: Tel: 3 9347 0300
          Fax: 3 9347 5001)

For further information on
Blackwell Science, visit our website:
www.blackwell-science.com

Contents

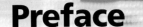

Preface

Sir Edward Henry Sieveking, in 1861 in his book on epilepsy, closed the treatment chapter with these now famous words: 'there is scarcely a substance in the world capable of passing through the gullet of man that has not at one time or other enjoyed the reputation of being an antiepileptic'. Thus was the therapeutic scepticism, the desperation of sufferers and the ineffectiveness of contemporary medicine, paradoxically at a time when epilepsy was taking neurological centre stage. His book closed the pre-modern age of epilepsy treatment, for bromides were just emerging as the first modern drug, and therapy for epilepsy was about to enter an era of unparalleled progress. It is now nearly a century and a half later, and what has changed? We should certainly be less sceptical. Treatment has improved, but there are still no curative medicines, at least none which are universally effective. Desperation still exists, although the stigma of epilepsy has, I am sure, generally greatly diminished. Epilepsy, nevertheless, is still a feared and a common symptom, and many still rummage for explanation and relief in the wilder back cupboards of alternative therapy.

It is the purpose of this book to convey the state of epilepsy treatment as it is now, at the beginning of the 21st century. The clinician has a wide range of options for treatment—medicinal and surgical—yet this greater range of choices makes decisions about treatment more difficult. The book aims to give practical guidance on treatment choice, and to be a manual for the clinician in all circumstances in medical practice where intervention for epilepsy is needed. I have attempted to be evidence-based where this is possible, but many parts of the text reflect my opinions and prejudices. This deserves apology, although our state of incomplete knowledge makes mere opinion inevitable and, until medicine becomes an exact science, medical practice has to fall back on anecdotalism. The text is broadly based on the multiauthored textbook which I had the good fortune to coedit (*The Treatment of Epilepsy*, Blackwell Science, 1996). That book is an authoritative and comprehensive work, which serves as a record and a reference. This book is more of a hands-on practical guide for use in everyday clinical settings and aims to be a rapidly accessed source of clinical information. I am grateful to all the chapter authors for their work, on which this current text rests. A particular debt is owed to my colleagues and friends Professors David Fish and John Duncan and Drs Hartmut Meiorkord and Lina Nashef, from whose contributions in the textbook and other sources, I have particularly drawn upon. I have tried to provide large amounts of information in a succinct and compact form, and to limit discursive discussion. A decision was made early deliberately to restrict citations in the current volume to a few major contributions and reviews—on the basis that minor references impede clarity and add little to understanding—and to emphasize recent publications. I hope in this way that enough citations are included to provide sufficient guidance to the reader interested in following up any point. The book also reflects to a large extent the style of epilepsy treatment practised at the National Hospital for Neurology and Neurosurgery at Queen Square. There are fashions in treatment, and it seemed better to provide the text with a directionality and coherence based on the epilepsy practice with which I am most familiar; I hope this provides a more interesting and distinctive read.

Epilepsy has been the subject, especially in the post-war years, of intense scientific and clinical research. Papers published on the subject are increasing exponentially, with over 17 000 peer-reviewed publications in the last 10 years alone. Impressive though this explosion in printed information is, real advance in the subject has been less spectacular. The great mass of research has been incremental or nonenduring. The really important advances in clinical epilepsy are perhaps in four areas, with varying impact on treatment. First has been the clarification of the electrophysiological basis of epilepsy, and its clinical translation in the form of the electroencephalogram (EEG). The EEG has refined diagnosis and also aided selection of patients for resective surgery. Second has been the advent of magnetic resonance imaging (MRI) which has permitted the *in vivo* demonstration of anatomical changes underpinning epilepsy which were hitherto invisible to other forms of investigation. Therapeutically, MRI has made surgical lesion resection available for patients previously thought to be inoperable. A third advance is the greater understanding of the therapeutic principles underlying drug usage, both in clinical practice and in the assessment of new drugs. This has led to more beneficial drug prescribing. Finally, a raft of new antiepileptic medicines has been introduced, developed by the pharmaceutical industry on the (often shaky) basis of current neurochemical hypotheses. In the text I will broadly concentrate on and emphasize these four particular areas.

There are three components to the treatment of epilepsy from the viewpoint of the practising clinician: medicinal, surgical and non-physical therapy. The first category—the drug treatment of epilepsy—is predominant, and thus occupies the greater part of this book. The characteristics of individual drugs, their clinical therapeutic properties and their place in therapy are described in detail. Surgical treatment for epilepsy has become an option in greater numbers of patients in recent years because MRI can reveal more lesions, although (except for stereotaxy) the technical procedures of epilepsy surgery have hardly changed for 60 years and novel surgical approaches are largely still experimental. The presurgical evaluation has been greatly altered by the advent of EEG telemetry and MRI and this is the major focus of the surgical part of the text. Intuition that non-physical therapies should play an important part in a holistic approach to the alleviation of epilepsy is probably justified, but conclusive evidence is slight. This aspect of therapy is therefore given a smaller part in this book than is perhaps rightful, yet I hope to have covered most salient points. A heavy emphasis has been placed on summary tables and on tabulated information; this is to aid clarity and to allow the reader efficiently to negotiate a way through the mass of available data, especially in the field of drug therapy.

My thanks are offered, as always, to my colleagues at the National Hospital for their advice and opinions which have greatly influenced my own practice over the years, and to my patients from whom I have learnt most. I also thank Mr Douglas Bennett, Chief Executive at the National Society for Epilepsy, for his generosity in allowing me time out to start this book. I am also enormously grateful to Stuart Taylor, senior editor at Blackwell Science, for his encouragement, forbearance and patience during the over-slow gestation of this book. The book is dedicated to Lynne Low and to Matthew, the great interrupter.

Finally, a disclaimer; while every effort has been made in the preparation of this text to ensure that the details are correct (for instance, of drug dosage and pharmacokinetic values) it is possible that errors have been overlooked. The reader is advised to refer to published information from the pharmaceutical companies and regulatory authorities to ensure accuracy.

S.D. Shorvon
London, 2000

Acknowledgements

In the preparation of the text of this book, I am indebted to the following who were the contributors to the *Textbook of Epilepsy*: J. Aicardi; M.J. Aminoff; A. Arzimanoglou; S.A. Baxendale; M.J. Brodie; J. Bruni; G.D. Cascino; O.C. Cockerell; M. Cook; M.A. Dalby; M. Dam; L. De Paula; R.M. Debets; R.J. Delorenzo; A. Draguhn; C. Dravet; F.E. Dreifuss; J.S. Duncan; M.J. Eadie; J. Engel; S.M. Ferguson; D. Fish; R.S. Fisher; G. Franck; J.R. Gates; P. Genton; I.M. Germano; L. Gram; R. Guerrini; W.F. Harkness; Y.M. Hart; U. Heinemann; R.W. Homan; M. Jones-Gotman; J. Kapur; N.D. Kitchen; D. Lamoureux; C. Lehman; I.E. Leppik; D. Lindhout; R.L. Macdonald; A. Malow; P.J. McKee; M. Manford; P.A. Marquet; H. Meierkord; F. Morrell; L. Nashef; G.A. M.R. O'Connell; G. Ojemann; A. Olivier; J.M. Parent; S.L. Parks-Trusz; E. Perucca; C. Polkey; K. Radhakrishnan; A.A. Raymond; M. Rayport; R.A. Reife; J. Roger; H. Rosenberg; A. Sabers; B. Sadzot; J.W.A.S. Sander; S. Sato; J.S. Schweitzer; M. Sillanpaa; S. Sisodiya; M. Smith; D.D. Spencer; S.S. Spencer; R.C. Tallis; W.H. Theodore; D.G. Thomas; P.J. Thompson; M. Trimble; J-G. Villemure; M. Walker; E. Waterhouse; W.W. Whisler; B.J. Wilder; P. Wolf.

I also am grateful for permission to reproduce the illustrations, text and tables from the following sources:

Figures 1.1, 3.6 and 3.7, from articles by Wallace, Tallis and myself in the *Lancet* 1998, **352**, 1971, .

Figure 3.4 from an article by Professor D. Chadwick *et al.* in the *Lancet* 1996, **336**, 1272.

Figures 3.2 and 3.3 from an article by Dr Y. Hart *et al.* in the *Lancet* 1991, **337**, 1175.

Figure 4.17 from the article by the late Dr F. Dreifuss in the *Lancet* 1987, **1**, 47–8.

Figure 4.4 from the article by A. Richens and A. Dunlop 1975, **2**, 247–8, Massachusetts Medical Society.

Table 4.3 from the article by Mattson *et al.* the *New England Journal of Medicine* 1992, **327**, 765–71.

Tables 4.8 and 4.9 from the UCB-pharma database.

Table 4.10, from the Novartis database.

Table 4.7, from the Glaxo-Wellcome database.

Table 1.2, from the article by the Commission of Classification and Terminology of the International League Against Epilepsy in *Epilepsia* 1981, **22**, 489, and for Table 1.5 from the article by Commission of Classification and Terminology of the International League Against Epilepsy in *Epilepsia* 1989, **30**, 389, Lippincott Williams & Wilkins.

Table 4.18, from a chapter by Dr E. Ben-Menarchem and J. French in Engel and T.A. Pedley (eds). *Epilepsy. A Comprehensive Textbook* 1998, Vol 2, p. 1612, Lippincott–Raven, New York, and for figure 4.2 in the chapter by R. Mattson in the same book p. 1497.

Figure 4.1 from the article by Dr H. Kutt in R. Levy, R. Mattson, B.S. Meldrum (eds), *Antiepileptic Drugs* 4th edn, 1995, p. 323, Raven Press, New York, and for table 3.2 from M. Gomez *Tuberose Sclerosis* 2nd Ed 1988, Raven Press, New York.

Tables 4.13–4.15, from an article by Dr E. Ben-Menarchem in *Exp. Opin. Invest. Drugs* 1997, **6**, 1088–9, Ashley publications.

Figure 6.22, the *British Medical Journal* publishing group from the article of Adams *et al.* in the *Journal of Neurology, Neurosurgery and Neuropsychiatry* 1983, **46**, 617–9.

Figure 6.4, The American Academy of Neurology from the article by A. Raymond *et al.* from *Neurology* 1994, **44**, 1841–4.

Figure 5.1, Elsevier Press from the article by the late Dr Lothman *et al.* in *Epilepsy Research* 1990, **6**, 116–8.

Text and tables 5.1, 5.2, and 5.3, from Shorvon S.D. *Status Epilepticus. Its Clinical Features and Treatment in Children and Adults* 1994, Cambridge University Press.

Churchill Livingstone for extensive borrowings of text from J.S. Duncan, D.R. Fish and S.D. Shorvon *Clinical Epilepsy,* and also for the following tables: 1.3, 1.4, 1.6, 1.7, 1.9, 2.7, 3.23, 3.24, 3,27, 3.28.

Butterworth–Heinemann Medical Books for the reproduction of figure 3.1 from the chapter by Profs A.

Richens and E. Perrucca *et al.* in Williams D.C. and Marks V. (eds). *Biochemistry in Clinical Practice*, and for figures 6.24–6.25 from the article by the late the Dr F. Morrell in Andermann F. (ed) *Rasmusssen's chronic Encephalitis and Epilepsy* 1991 pp. 219–234.

I am grateful to Blackwell Science for figure 4.3 from an article by Rupp *et al.* in *British Journal of Clinical Pharmacology* 1979, **7** (suppl. 1), 515–75, and for the opportunity to reproduce the following figures and tables from the *Textbook of Epilepsy*: figure 3.5 from the chapter of Dr P. Genton and Dr C. Dravet, for table 3.38 from the chapter by Dr D. Lindhout, for figures 5.2 and 5.3 from the chapter by Dr M. Walker and myself, for figures 6.5, 6.6, 6.11–6.14, 6.17–6.20 from the chapter by Professor D. Fish, figures 6.1–6.3 from the chapter of M. Cook and S. Sisodiya, figure 6.10 from the chapter of Dr A. Olivier, figures 6.15, 6.16 from the chapter of Mr W. Harkness, figures 6.7–6.9 from the chapter of Drs S. Spencer and D. Lamoureux, figure 6.18 from the chapter of Drs J. Schweitzer and D.D. Spencer, figure 6.21 from Dr J-G. Villemure, figure 6.23 from the chapter of Dr J. Gates and L. De Paola, and figure 6.26 from the chapter of Mr N. Kitchen and Professor D.M.G. Thomas.

I am also grateful to my colleague Mr James Acheson for preparing figure 4.5.

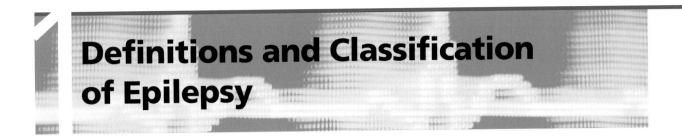

Definitions and Classification of Epilepsy

Epilepsy is a common condition (Fig. 1.1). Its incidence is in the region of 80 cases per 100 000 persons per year, with studies showing rates varying between 50 and 120 per 100 000 per year. Its point prevalence is about 5–10 cases per 1000 persons. An isolated (first and only) seizure occurs in about 20 persons per 100 000 each year. The cumulative incidence of epilepsy—the risk of an individual developing epilepsy in his or her lifetime—is between 3 and 5%. The highest incidence rates are observed in neonates and young children and then with a second peak in old age. In recent times the rate in children seems to be falling and the rate in the elderly rising because of cerebrovascular disease. The prevalence of epilepsy is relatively static after early childhood, but again shows a tendency to rise in old age. Epilepsy is more common in developing countries largely as a result of the poorer standards of nutrition and public hygiene, the prevalence of infectious diseases and the higher proportion of children in a population. Epilepsy is also a very variable condition, both in its severity and its clinical features. Table 1.1 shows an approximate breakdown of epilepsy in a typical population of 1 000 000 persons.

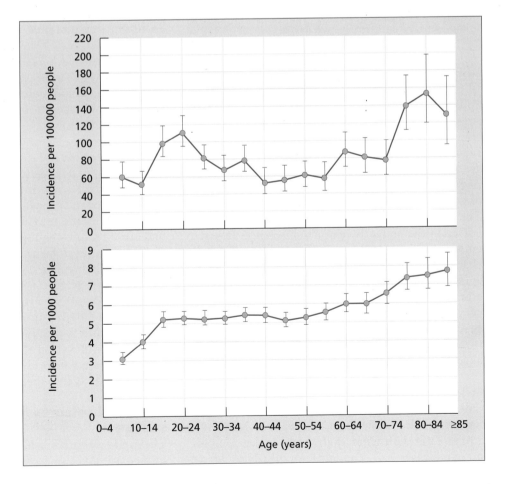

Fig. 1.1 Age-specific prevalence and incidence of treated epilepsy (from age 4 upwards) in a population of 2 052 922 persons in the UK (bars indicate 95% confidence intervals).

Table 1.1 The characteristics of epilepsy in a population of 1 000 000 persons (approximate estimates).

Incident cases (new cases each year)	
Febrile seizures	500
(annual incidence rate 50 per 100 000)	
Single seizures	200
(annual incidence rate 20 per 100 000)	
Epilepsy	500
(annual incidence rate 50 per 100 000)	
Prevalent cases (cases with established epilepsy)	
Active epilepsy (prevalence rate 5 per 1000)	5 000
Epilepsy in remission	15 000
Severity of epilepsy (in active epilepsy)	
More than one seizure a week	15%
Between one seizure a week and one a month	25%
Between one seizure a month and one a year	60%
Type of seizures	
Partial seizures alone	15%
Partial and secondarily generalized	60%
Generalized tonic–clonic alone	20%
Other generalized seizures	5%
Medical care required (in prevalent cases)	
Occasional medical attention	65%
Regular medical attention	30%
Residential or institutional care	5%

DEFINITIONS

Epileptic seizure

An epileptic seizure (fit) is the manifestation of an abnormal and excessive synchronized discharge of a set of cerebral neurones. The clinical manifestations are sudden and transient and can include a wide variety of motor, psychic and sensory phenomena, with or without alteration in consciousness or awareness. The symptoms depend on the part of the brain involved in the epileptic neuronal discharge. In some epileptic seizures there may be only very subtle changes which are apparent only to the patient. Some epileptic discharges detectable on electroencephalogram (EEG) are not accompanied by any evident symptoms or signs and, for most purposes, these subclinical attacks are not considered to be epileptic seizures, although the physiological changes can be identical to overt attacks.

Epilepsy

Epilepsy is defined as a condition in which the sufferer is prone to experience recurrent epileptic seizures. This definition invites uncertainty, as in marginal cases it is often difficult clearly to define

a liability to future attacks. In most practical situations epilepsy is said to be present when two or more attacks have occurred. Even this pragmatic definition is often inadequate: for instance, in patients after a single attack who have a clear liability to further seizures; for patients who have had more than one provoked attack (see below); for those with very infrequent attacks; or for those whose epilepsy has remitted and whose liability for further attacks has lapsed. Furthermore, in physiological terms, the distinction between single and recurrent attacks is often meaningless. It is important to recognize that the diagnosis 'epilepsy' occurs with a wide variety of cerebral pathologies; like 'anaemia' or 'headache' it is, to a large extent, simply a symptomatic definition. Standard definitions are also inadequate in the epileptic states in which physiological changes occur without obvious seizures. In these so-called epileptic encephalopathies deterioration in cognition and other cortical functions occur independently of overt seizures (examples include the Landau–Kleffner syndrome or the childhood epileptic encephalopathies). Patients with subclinical discharges also sometimes have cerebral dysfunction which could be characterized as epileptic in origin (for instance cognitive change in nonconvulsive status). There are also certain non-epileptic conditions where differentiation from epilepsy is problematic. These are sometimes called borderline conditions and include certain psychiatric conditions, some cases of migraine and some forms of movement disorder.

Status epilepticus

Status epilepticus is defined as a condition in which epileptic seizures continue, or are repeated without regaining consciousness, for a period of 30 min or more. This is the maximal expression of epilepsy, and often requires emergency therapy (see Chapter 5). There are physiological and neurochemical changes which distinguish status epilepticus from ordinary epileptic seizures. Recent debate has revolved around the duration of time used to define this condition, with differing suggestions ranging from 10 to 60 min; 30 min is to some extent a compromise. As with the definitions of epilepsy and of epileptic seizures, there are a range of boundary conditions which do not fall easily into the simple clinical definitions.

Provoked seizures (acute symptomatic seizures)

These are seizures which have an obvious and immediate preceding cause (for instance an acute systemic, metabolic or toxic insult), or an acute cerebral event (for instance stroke, trauma, infection). These seizures are often isolated events and do not recur when the cause is removed. Opinions have differed about whether or not these should be included within a definition of epilepsy. The precipitation of seizures is described further on p. 16.

Active epilepsy/epilepsy in remission

A person is said to have active epilepsy when at least one epileptic seizure has occurred in the preceding period (usually 2 or 5 years, depending on definition). Conversely, epilepsy is said to be in remission when no seizures have occurred in this preceding period. The period of time used in these definitions varies in different studies and, furthermore, some definitions of remission require the patient not only to be seizure-free but also off medication. An interesting question, of great importance to those with epilepsy, is after what period of remission can the person claim no longer to have the condition? Logically, the condition has remitted as soon as the last seizure occurred, but this cannot be known except retrospectively. In practice, it is reasonable to consider epilepsy to have ceased in someone off therapy if 2–5 years have passed since the last attack.

CLASSIFICATION OF EPILEPTIC SEIZURES

A classification of epileptic seizures could be based on various criteria, which might include anatomical site of the epilepsy, aetiology, age, neuropsychiatric status or response to treatment. In fact, the commonly used classification, that of the 1981 International League Against Epilepsy (ILAE), uses only two criteria: the clinical form and the EEG abnormality. The 1981 ILAE classification divides seizures into generalized and partial categories (Table 1.2). Generalized seizures are those that arise from large areas of cortex in both hemispheres and consciousness is always lost. Generalized seizures are subdivided into six categories. Partial seizures are those that arise in specific often small loci of cortex in one hemisphere. They are divided into simple partial seizures which occur without alteration of consciousness and complex partial seizures in which consciousness is impaired or lost. A secondarily generalized seizure is a seizure with a partial onset (the aura) which spreads to become a generalized attack. Simple partial seizures may spread to become complex partial seizures and either can spread to become secondarily generalized.

The limitations of a classification based only on clinical and EEG appearance should not be underestimated, and the current classification is inadequate for many clinical and research purposes. The more recent ILAE Classification of the Epilepsies (see below) was devised to be more comprehensive. There have been other criticisms of the ILAE classification. The subdivision of partial seizures on the basis of consciousness is criticized because of the difficulty of deciding, in many cases, whether or not consciousness is altered. Many seizures do not fit well into any of the categories, and treatment can also modify the clinical form. With advances in imaging and neurophysiology, it has become clear that some generalized seizures do in fact have underlying focal brain disorders. Some partial seizures are underpinned by a large neuronal network akin to that of some generalized epilepsies. From the perspective of this book, devoted to therapy, a particular criticism of the classification is that, as a general rule, it does not help in choosing treatment or defining prognosis. There are obvious exceptions (the use of valproate or ethosuximide in generalized absence attacks, for instance) but the lack of treatment specificity for individual categories is striking. The main value of the classification lies in its widespread clinical acceptance and, in spite of all its problems, this classification has become well established in clinical practice.

PARTIAL SEIZURES

Simple partial seizures

Most simple partial seizures last only a few seconds. Their clinical form, and that of the aura of a complex partial or secondarily generalized seizure, depend on the part of the cortex involved in the seizure.

Motor manifestations. The most common are jerking (clonus) or spasm. These usually occur in epilepsies arising in frontal or central regions.

Somatosensory or special sensory manifestations (simple hallucinations). These take the form of tingling or numbness or, less commonly, an electrical shock-like feeling, burning, pain or a feeling of heat. The epileptic focus is usually in the central or parietal region, although similar symptoms occur with spread from epileptic foci in other locations. Simple visual phenomena, such as flashing lights and colours, occur if the calcarine cortex is affected. A ris-

I *Partial (focal) seizures*
A Simple partial seizures
i With motor signs: focal motor with or without march, versive, postural, phonatory
ii With somatosensory or special sensory symptoms: somatosensory, visual, auditory, olfactory, gustatory, vertiginous, simple hallucinations (e.g. tingling, light flashing, buzzing)
iii With autonomic symptoms or signs, including epigastric aura
iv With psychic symptoms (disturbances of higher mental function): dysphasic, dysmnestic, cognitive, affective, illusions, structured hallucinations
B Complex partial seizures
i Simple partial onset followed by impairment of consciousness:
  With simple partial features (Ai–iv) followed by impaired consciousness
  With automatisms
ii With impairment of consciousness at onset
  With impairment of consciousness only
  With automatisms
C Partial seizures evolving to secondarily generalized seizures (tonic–clonic, tonic or clonic)
i Simple partial seizures evolving to generalized seizures
ii Complex partial seizures evolving to generalized seizures
iii Simple partial seizures evolving to complex partial seizures evolving to generalized seizures

II *Generalized seizures (convulsive and non-convulsive)*
A Absence seizures
i With impairment of consciousness only, mild clonic components, atonic components, tonic components, automatisms, autonomic components
ii Atypical absence seizures with changes in tone more pronounced than in Ai and with onset and/or cessation that is not abrupt
B Myoclonic seizures
C Clonic seizures
D Tonic seizures
E Tonic–clonic seizures
F Atonic seizures
  (Combinations may occur, such as myoclonic and atonic seizures or myoclonic and tonic seizures)

III *Unclassified epileptic seizures*

Table 1.2 The International League Against Epilepsy (ILAE) classification of seizure type.

ing epigastric sensation is the most common manifestation of a simple partial seizure arising in the mesial temporal lobe.

Autonomic manifestations. Autonomic symptoms, such as changes in skin colour, blood pressure, heart rate, pupil size and piloerection, are occasionally isolated phenomena in simple partial seizures but, more commonly, are a component of generalized or complex partial seizures of frontal or temporal origin.

Psychic manifestations. Psychic 'auras' can take various forms and are more common in complex partial than in simple partial seizures. They can occur in epilepsy arising from a temporal, frontal or parietal focus. There are six principal categories.

Dysphasic symptoms are prominent if cortical speech areas (frontal or temporoparietal) are affect-ed. Speech usually ceases or is severely reduced and postictal dysphasia is a reliable sign, localizing the seizure discharge to the dominant hemisphere. Repetitive vocalization with formed words may occur in a complex partial seizure originating in the non-dominant temporal lobe. Dysphasia should be distinguished, where possible, from speech arrest which suggests a frontocentral origin.

Dysmnestic symptoms (disturbance of memory) may take the form of flashbacks, *déjà vu, jamais vu* or panoramic experiences (recollections of previous experiences, former life or childhood), and are most common in mesial temporal lobe seizures.

Cognitive symptoms include dreamy states and sensations of unreality or depersonalization and occur primarily in temporal lobe seizures.

Affective symptoms include fear (the most common symptom), depression, anger and irritability.

Elation, erotic thoughts, serenity or exhilaration may occur. Affective symptomatology is most commonly seen with mesial temporal lobe foci. Laughter (without mirth) is a feature of the automatism of seizures which arise in frontal areas and are a consistent feature of the epilepsy associated with hypothalamic harmatomas.

Illusions of size (macropsia, micropsia), shape, weight, distance or sound are usually features of temporal or parieto-occipital epileptic foci.

Structured hallucinations of visual, auditory, gustatory or olfactory forms, which can be crude or elaborate, are usually caused by epileptic discharges in the temporal or parieto-occipital association areas.

Simple partial seizures occur at any age and are caused by focal cerebral disease. Any cortical region may be affected, the most common sites being the frontal and temporal lobes. The symptoms are useful in predicting the anatomical localization of the seizures. The form of the seizures usually has no pathological specificity.

The scalp EEG, both interictally and also during a simple partial seizure, is often normal, presumably because the discharge is too small or too deep to be detected by the scalp electrodes. If an interictal abnormality is present, it will take the form of spikes, sharp waves, focal slow activity or suppression of normal rhythms. Before the seizure the interictal EEG may show a sudden reduction in the frequency of interictal spike or sharp waves. Ictal abnormalities can take the form of rhythmic theta activity, focal spike-wave activity or runs of fast activity (13–30 Hz).

Complex partial seizures

Complex partial seizures, in their complete form, have three components.

Aura. These are equivalent to simple partial seizures and can take any of the forms described above. The aura is usually short-lived, lasting a few seconds or so, although in rare cases a prolonged aura persists for minutes, hours or even days. Many patients experience isolated auras as well as full-blown complex partial seizures.

Altered consciousness. This may follow the aura or evolve simultaneously. The altered consciousness takes the form of an absence and motor arrest, during which the patient is motionless and inaccessible (the 'motionless stare'). There is sometimes no outward sign although usually the patient appears vacant or glazed. There is often associated spasm, posturing or mild tonic jerking.

Automatisms. These are defined as involuntary motor actions which occur during or in the aftermath of epileptic seizures, in a state of unconsciousness. There is total amnesia for the events of the automatism. Sometimes the actions have purposeful elements, are affected by environment and can involve quite complex activity. Automatisms should be distinguished from postictal confusion. Automatisms are most common in temporal and frontal lobe seizures. They are usually divided into:

Oro-alimentary: orofacial movements, such as chewing, lip smacking, swallowing or drooling. These are most common in partial seizures of mesial temporal origin.

Mimicry: including displays of laughter or fear, anger or excitement.

Gestural: fiddling movements with the hands, tapping, patting or rubbing, ordering and tidying movements. Complex actions, such as undressing, are quite common as are genitally directed actions.

Ambulatory automatisms: walking, circling or running.

Verbal automatisms: meaningless sounds, humming, whistling, grunting, words which may be repeated or formed sentences.

Responsive automatisms: quasi-purposeful behaviour, seemingly responsive to environmental stimuli.

Violent behaviour can occur in an automatism and is best considered as a response in an acutely confused person. Such behaviour is especially likely if the patient is restrained. The violent actions of the epileptic automatism are never premeditated, never remembered, never highly coordinated or skilful and seldom goal-directed; these are useful diagnostic features in a forensic context.

Complex partial seizures arise from the temporal lobe in about 60% of cases, and the frontal lobe in about 30%. Complex partial seizures vary considerably in duration. In one series the ictal phase lasted between 3 and 343 s (mean 54 s), the postictal phase 3–767 s and the total seizure duration was 5–998 s (mean 128 s), although longer seizures, sometimes lasting hours, are occasionally encountered. In about 10–30% of seizures the scalp EEG is unchanged and, in the rest, runs of fast activity, localized spike and wave complexes, spikes or sharp waves or slow activity may occur, or the EEG may simply show flattening (desynchronization). The patterns can be focal—indicating the site or origin of the seizure—lateralized, bilateral or diffuse.

Partial seizures evolving to secondarily generalized seizures

Partial seizures (simple, complex or simple evolving to complex) may spread to become generalized. The partial seizure is often experienced as an aura in the seconds before the generalized seizure. The generalized seizure is usually tonic–clonic, tonic or atonic.

GENERALIZED SEIZURES

Consciousness is almost invariably impaired from the onset of the attack, owing to the extensive cortical and subcortical involvement. Motor changes are bilateral and more or less symmetrical, and the EEG patterns are bilateral and grossly synchronous and symmetrical over both hemispheres.

Typical absence seizures (petit mal seizures)

The seizure comprises an abrupt sudden loss of consciousness (absence) and cessation of all motor activity. Tone is usually preserved and there is no fall. The patient is unaware, inaccessible and often appears glazed or vacant. The attack ends as abruptly as it started and previous activity is resumed as if nothing had happened. There is no confusion, but the patient is often unaware that an attack has occurred. Most absence seizures (>80%) last less than 10 s. Other clinical phenomena, including blinking, slight clonic movements, alterations in tone and brief automatisms, can occur, particularly in longer attacks. The attacks can be repeated hundreds of times a day, often cluster and are often worse when the patient is awakening or drifting off to sleep. Absences may be precipitated by fatigue, drowsiness, relaxation, photic stimulation or hyperventilation. Typical absence seizures develop in childhood or adolescence and are encountered almost exclusively in idiopathic generalized epilepsy. Variations from this typical form include the myoclonic absence, absence with perioral myoclonia or with eyelid myoclonia. Whether or not these are distinct entities is controversial (see p. 75).

The EEG during a typical absence is very striking. A regular, symmetric and synchronous 3 Hz spike and wave paroxysm is the classic form, although in longer attacks and in older patients the paroxysms may not be entirely regular and frequencies vary between 2 and 4 Hz. The interictal EEG has normal background activity. Spike and wave paroxysms can frequently be induced by hyperventilation and, less commonly, by photic stimulation.

The features useful in differentiating a complex partial seizure and a typical absence are shown in Table 1.3.

Atypical absence seizures

Atypical absence seizures differ from typical absences in clinical form, EEG, aetiology and clinical context (Table 1.4). Their duration is longer, loss of awareness is often incomplete, associated tone changes are more severe than in typical absence seizures and the onset and cessation of the attacks are not so abrupt. Amnesia may not be complete and

	Typical absence	Complex partial seizure
Age of onset	Childhood or early adult	Any age
Aetiology	Idiopathic generalized epilepsy	Any focal pathology or cryptogenic epilepsy
Underlying focal anatomical lesion	None	Limbic structures, neocortex
Duration of attack	Short (usually < 10 s)	Longer, usually several minutes
Other clinical features	Slight (tone changes or motor phenomena)	Can be prominent; including aura, automatism
Postictal	None	Confusion, headache, emotional disturbances are common
Frequency	May be numerous and cluster	Usually less frequent
Ictal and interictal EEG	3-Hz spike/wave	Variable focal disturbance
Photosensitivity	10–30%	None
Effect of hyperventilation	Often marked increase	None, modest increase

Table 1.3 Differentiation between typical absences and complex partial seizures.

Table 1.4 Clinical features differentiating typical and atypical absence seizures.

	Typical absence	**Atypical absence**
Context	Otherwise no neurological signs or symptoms	Usually in context of learning difficulty and other neurological abnormalities
Consciousness	Totally lost	Often only partially impaired
Focal signs in seizures	Nil	May be present
Onset/offset of seizures	Abrupt	Often gradual
Coexisting seizure types	Sometimes tonic–clonic and myoclonic	Mixed seizure disorder common, all seizure types

the subject may be partially responsive. The patient can wander during the attack and there can be atonic, clonic or tonic phenomena, autonomic disturbance and automatism. The attacks can wax and wane and may be of long duration.

The ictal EEG shows diffuse but often asymmetric and irregular spike and wave bursts at 2–2.5 Hz, and sometimes fast activity or bursts of spikes and sharp waves. The background interictal EEG is abnormal, with continuous slowing, spikes or irregular spike and wave activity. The ictal and interictal EEGs can be very similar. The seizures are often not induced by hyperventilation or photic stimulation.

Atypical absences are usually associated with learning disability, other neurological abnormalities or multiple seizure types. They form part of the Lennox–Gastaut syndrome and manifest at any age.

Myoclonic seizures

A myoclonic seizure is a brief contraction of a muscle, muscle group or several muscle groups caused by a cortical discharge. It can be single or repetitive, varying in severity from an almost imperceptible twitch to a severe jerking, resulting, for instance, in a sudden fall or the propulsion of handheld objects (the 'flying saucer' syndrome). Recovery is immediate, and the patient often maintains that consciousness was not lost. During a myoclonic jerk the electromyogram shows biphasic or polyphasic potentials of 20–120 ms in duration followed by tonic contraction or hypotonia. Myoclonus can be induced by action, noise, startle, photic stimulation or percussion. When part of the syndrome of idiopathic generalized epilepsy, myoclonus occurs on waking or when dropping off to sleep. Myoclonus can develop at any age. It is one of the three seizure types in idiopathic generalized epilepsy, and is also common in the Lennox–Gastaut syndrome and other forms of epilepsy in patients with learning disability. It is the major seizure type in the progressive myoclonic epilepsies.

The ictal EEG usually shows a generalized spike, spike and wave, or polyspike and wave discharge, which is often asymmetrical or irregular and frequently has a frontal predominance. The interictal EEG varies with the cause, being usually normal in idiopathic generalized epilepsy and abnormal in other types of myoclonic epilepsy showing generalized changes.

Clonic seizures

Clonic seizures consist of clonic jerking which is often asymmetrical and irregular. Clonic seizures are most frequent in neonates, infants or young children, and are always symptomatic. The EEG may show fast activity (10 Hz), fast activity mixed with larger amplitude slow waves or, more rarely, polyspike and wave or spike and wave discharges. These should not be confused with bilateral clonic jerking—with or without loss of consciousness, even if involving all four limbs—which can be a form of partial seizure arising in the frontal lobe.

Tonic seizures

Tonic seizures take the form of a tonic muscle contraction with altered consciousness without a clonic phase. The tonic contraction causes extension of the neck; contraction of the facial muscles, with the eyes opening widely; up-turning of the eyeballs; contraction of the muscles of respiration; and spasm of the proximal upper limb muscles, causing the abduction and elevation of the semiflexed arms and the shoulders. If the tonic contractions spread distally, the arms rise up and are held as if defending the head against a blow and the lower limbs become forcibly extended or contracted in triple flexion. There may be a cry followed by apnoea. The spasm may fluctuate during the seizure, causing head nodding or slight alterations in the posture of the extended limbs, and autonomic changes can be marked. Tonic seizures last less than 60 s.

The ictal EEG may show flattening (desynchronization), fast activity (15–25 Hz) with increasing amplitude (to about 100 mV) as the attack progresses, or a rhythmic 10 Hz discharge similar to that seen in the tonic phase of the tonic–clonic seizure. On a scalp recording, however, the ictal EEG changes are often obscured by artefact from muscle activity and movement. The interictal EEG is seldom normal, usually showing generalized changes.

Tonic seizures occur at all ages, occur in the setting of diffuse cerebral damage and learning disability, and are associated with other seizure types. They should be differentiated from partial motor seizures, which can also show predominately tonic features, and from partially treated tonic–clonic seizures.

Tonic–clonic seizures (grand mal seizures)

This is the form of attack usually associated with epilepsy in the public imagination. It has a number of well-defined stages. It is sometimes preceded by a prodromal period during which an attack is anticipated, often by an ill-defined vague feeling or sometimes more specifically, for instance, by the occurrence of increasing myoclonic jerking. If an aura then occurs—in fact a simple or complex partial seizure—in the seconds before the full-blown attack, this indicates that the tonic–clonic seizure is secondarily generalized. The seizure is initiated by loss of consciousness, and sometimes by the epileptic cry. The patient will fall if standing, there is a brief period of tonic flexion and then a longer phase of rigidity and axial extension, with the eyes rolled up, the jaw clamped shut, the limbs stiff, adducted and extended, and the fists either clenched or held in the *main d'accoucheur* position. Respiration ceases and cyanosis is common. This tonic stage lasts on average 10–30 s and is followed by the clonic phase, during which convulsive movements, usually of all four limbs, jaw and facial muscles, occur. Breathing may be stertorous, and saliva, sometimes blood-stained as a result of tongue biting, may froth from the mouth. The convulsive movements decrease in frequency, typically to about four clonic jerks per second, and increase in amplitude as the attack progresses. Autonomic features, such as flushing, changes in blood pressure, changes in pulse rate and increased salivation, are common. The clonic phase lasts between 30 and 60 s and is followed by a further brief tonic contraction of all muscles, sometimes with incontinence. The final phase lasts between 2 and 30 min and is characterized by flaccidity of the muscles. Consciousness is slowly regained. The plantar responses are usually extensor at this time

and the tendon jerks are diminished. Confusion is invariable in the postictal phase, and the patient then often lapses into deep sleep, awakening minutes or hours later with no symptoms other than muscle soreness and headache.

Tonic–clonic seizures can occur at any age and are encountered in many varieties of epilepsy, including idiopathic generalized epilepsy. They have no pathological specificity.

In patients with idiopathic generalized epilepsy, the EEG in the pre-ictal period may show increasing abnormalities with spike and wave or spike paroxysms. The interictal EEG has a variable appearance, depending on the cause of the tonic–clonic seizures. During the tonic phase, the ictal EEG typically shows generalized flattening (desynchronization). This is followed by low-voltage fast activity and then 10 Hz rhythms appear and increase in amplitude (recruiting rhythms). These are followed some seconds later by slow waves increasing in amplitude and decreasing in frequency from 3 to 1 Hz. During the clonic phase, the slow waves are interrupted by bursts of faster activity (at about 10 Hz) corresponding to the clonic jerks and, as the phase progresses, the slow waves widen and these bursts become less frequent. With scalp recordings, however, these EEG patterns will often be obscured by artefact from muscle and movement. As the jerks cease, the EEG becomes silent for several seconds and then slow delta activity develops. This persists for a variable period and the EEG background rhythms then slowly increase in frequency. Minutes or hours may elapse before the EEG activity returns to normal.

Atonic seizures

The most severe form is the classic drop attack (astatic seizure) in which all postural tone is suddenly lost, causing collapse to the ground like a rag doll. The tone change can be more restricted, resulting for instance in nodding of the head, a bowing movement or sagging at the knee. The seizures are short and are followed by immediate recovery. Longer (inhibitory) atonic attacks can develop in a stepwise fashion with progressively increasing nodding, sagging or folding.

The seizures occur at any age and are always associated with diffuse cerebral damage, learning disability and are common in severe symptomatic epilepsies. The ictal EEG shows irregular spike and wave, polyspike and wave, slow wave or low-amplitude fast activity, or a mixture of these, and may be obscured by movement artefact. The interictal EEG usually shows diffuse abnormalities.

Unclassifiable seizures

At least one-third of seizures are unclassifiable using the current ILAE classification scheme, and have forms which do not conform to the typical clinical and EEG patterns described above.

Treatment can markedly modify the form of an epileptic attack. The seizures can be shortened; the aura and the phasic nature of a prolonged seizure can be lost. Tonic–clonic seizures can, for example, be modified and appear more like tonic or atonic attacks.

CLASSIFICATION OF THE EPILEPSIES AND EPILEPSY SYNDROMES (Table 1.5)

In an attempt to encompass a broader range of clinical features than is possible in a classification of seizure type, the ILAE published in 1985, and revised in 1989 a Classification of the Epilepsies and Epileptic Syndromes. An epileptic syndrome is defined as 'an epileptic disorder characterized by a cluster of signs and symptoms customarily occurring together'. The relationship between the epilepsy syndrome and the underlying disease is complex. While some syndromes represent a single disease, others can be the result of many diseases; a good example of the latter is the Lennox–Gastaut syndrome. Furthermore, the same disease can manifest as different epileptic syndromes; an example is tuberous sclerosis. The syndromes are often age-specific and, over time in individual patients, one epileptic syndrome can evolve into another. The advantages of the classification are its flexibility, the potential for change and expansion, and the acknowledgement of the complex interplay of factors underlying epilepsy.

There are, however, serious disadvantages. First, the classification is a complex system with very

Table 1.5 The ILAE Classification of Epilepsies and Epilepsy Syndromes.

1 *Generalized*

Idiopathic generalized epilepsies with age-related onset (in order of age)
  Benign neonatal familial convulsions
  Benign neonatal convulsions
  Benign myoclonic epilepsy in infancy
  Childhood absence epilepsy
  Juvenile absence epilepsy
  Juvenile myoclonic epilepsy
  Epilepsy with generalized tonic–clonic seizures on awakening
  Other generalized idiopathic epilepsies not defined above
  Epilepsies with seizures precipitated by specific modes of activation

Cryptogenic or symptomatic generalized epilepsies (in order of age)
  West syndrome
  Lennox–Gastaut syndrome
  Epilepsy with myoclonic–astatic seizures
  Epilepsy with myoclonic absences

Symptomatic generalized epilepsies
  Non-specific aetiology
  Early myoclonic encephalopathies
  Early infantile encephalopathy with burst suppression
  Other symptomatic epilepsies not defined above
  Specific syndromes
  Epilepsies in other disease states

2 *Localization-related*

Localization-related epilepsies—idiopathic with age-related onset
  Benign epilepsy with centrotemporal spikes
  Childhood epilepsy with occipital paroxysms
  Primary reading epilepsy

Localization-related epilepsies—symptomatic
  Epilepsia partialis continua
  Syndromes characterized by specific modes of precipitation
  Temporal lobe epilepsies

Central region epilepsies
  Frontal lobe epilepsies
  Parietal lobe epilepsies
  Occipital lobe epilepsies

Localization-related epilepsies—cryptogenic

3 *Epilepsies and syndromes undetermined as to whether focal or generalized*

With both generalized and focal seizures
  Neonatal seizures
  Severe myoclonic epilepsy in infancy
  Electrical status epilepticus in slow wave sleep
  Acquired epileptic aphasia

Other undetermined epilepsies (not defined above) with unequivocal generalized or focal features

4 *Special syndromes*

Febrile convulsions
Isolated seizures or isolated status epilepticus
Seizures occurring only when there is an acute metabolic or toxic event caused by factors such as alcohol, drugs, eclampsia, non-ketotic hyperglycinaemia

clumsy terminology and for this reason alone is unlikely ever to gain widespread clinical usage, especially in non-specialist settings. A second problem is the maintenance of the distinction between focal and generalized epilepsies, which in many types of epilepsy is difficult to justify and presumes an unrealistic knowledge of the underlying physiological processes. It is perhaps in recognition of this problem that the third category is introduced, although it might have been better to avoid this distinction altogether. A third problem is that, in the attempt to be all-inclusive, this classification becomes unwieldy. Common syndromes are mixed in with those which are extremely rare and syndromes whose identity is contentious are also included. In normal clinical practice the majority of epilepsy seen (66% in one series) will fall into ill-defined 'non-specific' categories—which undermines the purpose and value of the scheme. Another problem is the arbitrary nature of some categories (notably 3 and 4), results in the grouping of epilepsies which have little else in common. Finally, it is difficult to justify the full sobriquet of 'syndrome' for some of the conditions listed. Some prefer to see the idiopathic generalized epilepsies, for instance, as a 'neurobiological continuum' while others have split the conditions into at least 10 subdivisions.

The categorization is also of limited value from the perspective of therapy. Most of the categories can be treated by most of the available drug therapies (there are exceptions discussed under the relevant sections of this book) and this lack of specificity is disappointing.

Idiopathic generalized epilepsies and syndromes

The idiopathic generalized epilepsies, sometimes called the primary generalized epilepsies, are genetic conditions in which epilepsy is the major clinical feature. Encompassed within this rubric are a variety of age-related syndromes, although to what extent the subdivisions are specific entities is a matter of controversy. These conditions are considered in more detail on p. 72.

Cryptogenic or symptomatic generalized epilepsies

This category includes the epileptic encephalopathies in which epilepsy is a major clinical feature of a diffuse encephalopathic condition. Included in this category are West syndrome (see p. 57), Lennox–Gastaut syndrome (see p. 58) and forms of myoclonic epilepsy. The relative nosological position of these conditions is often unclear, and there is considerable overlap between the core conditions and other symptomatic epileptic encephalopathies. Also included here are the epilepsies caused by malformations, inborn errors of metabolism and hereditary or congenital disorders.

Idiopathic localization-related epilepsies and syndromes

Three conditions are included here, including benign childhood epilepsy with centrotemporal spikes (see p. 59) which is said to account for up to 15% of childhood epilepsies, and two much less common syndromes, childhood epilepsy with occipital paroxysms and primary reading epilepsy. Other genetic and idiopathic syndromes will no doubt be added as knowledge advances, such as the recently described syndrome of dominantly inherited nocturnal frontal lobe epilepsy.

Symptomatic localization-related epilepsies and syndromes

This category includes the large number of epilepsies caused by specific focal cerebral lesions (e.g. tumour, stroke, etc.) in which epilepsy is a variable feature. The epilepsies are divided into anatomical site and these are described below.

Cryptogenic localization-related epilepsies and syndromes

This category has been created to include symptomatic focal epilepsies in which the aetiology is unknown. With increasingly sophisticated neuroimaging techniques, the number of cases falling into this category has become much smaller than when the classification was first proposed.

Undetermined epilepsies and syndromes

The existence of this category is an acknowledgement that the differentiation between focal and generalized epilepsy is not always easy to make. The category is divided into those syndromes with both focal and generalized seizures, and those without unequivocal generalized or focal features. Included in the first subdivision are a rag-bag of 'syndromes' including neonatal seizures, which have a variety of forms which overlap with other categories; infantile myoclonic epilepsy; and electrical status epilepticus during slow wave sleep (ESES) and the Landau–Kleffner syndrome which are epileptic encephalopathies of unknown pathophysiology. In the second subdivision are those epilepsies with tonic–clonic seizures in which clinical and EEG features do not allow categorization into focal or generalized groups.

Special syndromes

This category includes the 'situational-related syndromes' (reflex epilepsy, see p. 17), febrile seizures (see p. 55), isolated seizures—including single seizures and isolated status epilepticus—and the epilepsies precipitated by acute toxic or metabolic events.

PARTIAL EPILEPSY ARISING IN DIFFERENT ANATOMICAL REGIONS

From the point of view of epilepsy surgery, it is clearly imperative to have a classification based on anatomical localization. This requirement is accommodated within the ILAE Classification of Epilepsies and Epilepsy Syndromes.

Partial seizures arising in different anatomical locations take different forms. About 60% of complex partial seizures have their origin in the temporal lobe and about 40% are extratemporal; simple partial seizures probably have a similar disposition. Each region has characteristic clinical features, although the distinction is blurred in many individual cases where seizures arising from one cortical area spread to another.

Partial seizures arising in the temporal lobe
(Table 1.6)
A number of subclassifications exist, the validity of which is controversial. Categorization into opercular, temporal polar, and basal or limbic types, for instance, seems seldom valid or useful. The distinction into mesial temporal and lateral temporal neocortical types is more widely accepted, and even though symptomatology overlaps and spread from lateral to mesial cortex—and vice versa—is common, this remains a useful distinction.

Epilepsy arising in the mesial temporal lobe (limbic epilepsy). The seizures take the form of simple or complex partial seizures. The complex partial seizure typically has a relatively gradual evolution compared to extratemporal seizures, develops over 1–2 min, has an indistinct onset with partial awareness at the onset, and lasts longer than most extratemporal complex partial seizures (2–10 min). The typical complex partial seizure of temporal lobe origin has three components.

Aura. An aura can occur in isolation as a simple partial seizure or the initial manifestation of a complex partial seizure. It typically comprises visceral, cephalic, gustatory, dysmnestic or affective symptoms. A rising epigastric sensation is the most common. Autonomic symptoms include changes in skin colour, blood pressure, heart rate, pupil size and pilo-erection. Speech usually ceases or is severely reduced if the seizure is in the dominant temporal lobe. In the non-dominant lobe, speech may be retained throughout the seizure or meaningless repetitive vocalizations may occur. Simple auditory phenomena, such as humming, buzzing, hissing and roaring, occur if the discharges occur in the superior temporal gyrus; and olfactory sensations, which are

Table 1.6 Clinical features of partial seizures of temporal lobe origin.

- Past history of febrile convulsions (in those with mesial temporal sclerosis)
- Tripartite seizure pattern (aura, absence, automatism), although only one feature may be present
- Auras are common and include: visceral, cephalic, gustatory, dysmnestic, affective, perceptual or autonomic auras (mesial temporal lobe epilepsy); hallucinations, illusions and complex perceptual changes (lateral temporal lobe epilepsy)
- Partial awareness commonly preserved, especially in early stages
- Prominent motor arrest or absence (the 'motionless stare') especially in mesial temporal lobe epilepsy
- Dystonic posturing of the contralateral upper limb common in the early stages of the seizure (especially mesial temporal lobe epilepsy)
- In seizures arising in the dominant temporal lobe, speech arrest common during the seizures and dysphasia common postictally
- Seizures longer than frontal lobe seizures (typically >2 min), with a slower evolution and more gradual onset/offset
- Postictal confusion and dysphasia are common
- Autonomic changes (e.g. pallor, redness and tachycardia) are common
- Automatisms: less violent than in frontal lobe epilepsy, and usually take the form of oro-alimentary (lip smacking, chewing, swallowing) or gestural (e.g. fumbling, fidgeting, repetitive motor actions, undressing, walking, sexually directed actions, walking, running) and sometimes prolonged. Vocalization also common, and other motor automatisms can occur

usually unpleasant and difficult to define, with seizures in the sylvian region. More complex hallucinatory or illusionary states are produced with seizure discharges in association areas (e.g. structured visual hallucinations, complex visual patterns, and musical sounds and speech). A cephalic aura can also occur in focal temporal lobe seizures, although is more typical of a frontal lobe focus.

Absence. Motor arrest or absence (the 'motionless stare') is prominent, especially in the early stages of seizures arising in mesial temporal structures, and more so than in extratemporal lobe epilepsy. There is frequently dystonic posturing or spasm of the contralateral arm to the seizure discharge, and this is a useful lateralizing sign.

Automatism. The automatisms of mesiobasal temporal lobe epilepsy are typically less violent than in frontal lobe seizures, and are usually oro-alimentary (lip-smacking, chewing, swallowing) or gestural (e.g. fumbling, fidgeting, repetitive motor actions, undressing, sexually directed actions, walking, running) and sometimes prolonged. Upper limb automatisms are usually more prominent ipsilateral to the seizure focus.

Postictal confusion and headache are common after a temporal lobe complex partial seizure and, if dysphasia occurs, this is a useful lateralizing sign indicating seizure origin in the dominant temporal lobe. Amnesia is the rule for the absence and the automatism. Secondarily generalization is much less common than in extratemporal lobe epilepsy. Psychiatric or behavioural disturbances often accompany the epilepsy.

The most common pathology underlying this type of epilepsy is hippocampal sclerosis (synonyms: Ammon's horn sclerosis, mesial temporal sclerosis). This is characteristically associated with a history of febrile convulsions and the subsequent development of complex partial seizures in late childhood or adolescence. Other aetiologies include dysembryoplastic neuroepithelial tumours and other benign tumours, arteriovenous malformations, glioma, neuronal migration defects or gliotic damage as a result of encephalitis.

The EEG in mesial temporal lobe epilepsy often shows anterior or mid-temporal spikes. Superficial or deep sphenoidal electrodes can assist in their detection in some cases. Other changes include intermittent or persisting slow activity over the temporal lobes. The EEG signs can be unilateral or bilateral. Modern magnetic resonance imaging (MRI) will frequently reveal the abnormality underlying the epilepsy.

Epilepsy arising in the lateral temporal neocortex. There is considerable overlap between the clinical and EEG features of mesial and lateral temporal lobe epilepsy. However, differences in degree exist. The typical aura includes hallucinations which are often structured and of visual, auditory, gustatory or olfactory forms, which can be crude or elaborate, or illusions of size (macropsia, micropsia), shape, weight, distance or sound. Affective, visceral or psychic auras are less common than in mesiobasal temporal lobe epilepsy. Consciousness may be preserved for longer than in a typical mesial temporal seizure. The automatisms can be unilateral and have more prominent motor manifestations than in mesial temporal lobe epilepsy. Postictal phenomena, amnesia for the attack and the psychiatric accompaniments are indistinguishable from the mesial temporal form.

There is usually a detectable underlying structural pathology, the most common being a glioma, angioma, hamartoma, dysembryoplastic neuroepithelial tumour or other benign tumour, neuronal migration defect and post-traumatic change. There is no association with a history of febrile convulsions. The age of onset of the epilepsy will depend on the aetiology.

The interictal EEG often shows spikes over the temporal region, maximal over the posterior or lateral temporal rather than inferomesial electrodes. Magnetic resonance imaging will reliably demonstrate the structural lesions responsible for the epilepsy.

Epilepsy arising in the frontal lobe (Table 1.7)
Seizures of frontal lobe origin can take the form of complex partial seizures, simple partial seizures and secondarily generalized attacks.

Table 1.7 Clinical features of complex partial seizures of frontal lobe origin.

Frequent attacks with clustering
Brief stereotyped seizures (< 30 s)
Nocturnal attacks common
Sudden onset and cessation, with rapid evolution and awareness lost at onset
No complex aura
Version of head or eye common
Prominent ictal posturing and tonic spasms
Prominent complex bilateral motor automatisms involving lower limbs; often bizarre and misdiagnosed as pseudoseizures
No postictal confusion
Frequent secondarily generalization
History of status epilepticus

The clinical and EEG features of the complex partial seizures overlap with those of temporal lobe origin, not least because of the rapid spread from seizure foci in the frontal lobe to other cortical areas and to the mesial temporal lobe. There are, however, several core features which are strongly suggestive of a frontal lobe origin. Typically, complex partial seizures of frontal lobe origin are frequent with a marked tendency to cluster. The attacks are brief, with a sudden onset and offset and without the gradual evolution of the temporal lobe seizure. Some types of frontal lobe seizure occur largely during sleep, and in some patients the epilepsy comprises frequent short nocturnal attacks sometimes known misleadingly as paroxysmal nocturnal dystonia. The tripartite pattern of aura/absence/automatism is seldom as well defined in frontal lobe as in mesial temporal lobe complex partial seizures.

A brief non-specific 'cephalic aura' can occur, but not the rich range of auras of temporal lobe epilepsy. The absence (motor arrest) is usually short, and may be obscured by the prominent motor signs of the automatism. There are qualitative differences between frontal and temporal lobe automatisms, although seldom are these specific enough to be reliably of diagnostic value. Frontal lobe automatisms are typically gestural, especially comprising bilateral leg movements (e.g. cycling, stepping, kicking) rather than oro-alimentary. The behaviour in the automatism is often highly excited, violent or bizarre and not infrequently leads to a misdiagnosis of non-epileptic movements (pseudoseizures). In other frontal seizures, posturing or muscle spasms predominate. Urinary incontinence is frequent in frontal lobe complex partial seizures as is vocalization. The automatisms are usually short, with minimal postictal confusion and recovery is usually rapid.

Frontal lobe partial seizures have a more marked tendency to evolve into secondarily generalized than do partial seizures of temporal lobe origin, and the evolution is more rapid. There is also commonly a history of status epilepticus, both of the tonic–clonic and non-convulsive types.

Other partial seizure patterns occur with marked motor manifestations (clonic jerking or posturing) either bilateral or contralateral. Because consciousness can be retained in the presence of bilateral limb jerking, these attacks are commonly misdiagnosed as non-epileptic attacks. Apparently generalized tonic–clonic seizures without lateralizing features are particularly characteristic of seizures arising in the cingulate or dorsolateral cortex, but can occur from other frontal lobe locations. Mesial frontal foci can result in absence seizures which can be almost indistinguishable on clinical or EEG grounds from generalized absence. Seizures arising in the dorsolateral convexity sometimes take the form of a sudden assumption of an abnormal posture (usually bilateral and asymmetrical) with or without loss of consciousness, lasting a second or two only and which cluster, with numerous attacks over a few minutes. Drop attacks are a common feature of frontal partial seizures arising especially medially or anteriorly. Version of the head and eyes is common in many types of frontal lobe and is less frequently seen in temporal lobe epilepsy, and is sometimes the only seizure manifestation (versive seizures). When version occurs in full consciousness at the onset of a seizure, this is useful evidence of a focus in the contralateral frontal dorsolateral convexity, but in other situations the direction of version is of little lateralizing value. Occasionally, seizures with adversion of the head and the body occur, in which the patient circles. Autonomic features are common in frontal lobe epilepsy and may occasionally be an isolated manifestation of an epileptic focus, usually in the orbitofrontal cortex. Dysphasia in frontal seizures is often accompanied by adversive or clonic movements. In epileptic discharges from the perisylvian areas the aphasia is often preceded by numbness in the mouth and throat or salivation, swallowing or laryngeal symptoms.

The scalp EEG in frontal lobe epilepsy is often rather disappointing. This is partly because the large area of frontal cortex is covered by relatively few scalp electrodes. Because much of the frontal cortex is hidden in sulci, the medial or inferior surfaces of the frontal lobe are distant from the dorsolaterally placed electrodes. Many frontal lobe seizures either fail to show a focus, or only demonstrate widespread poorly localized foci. Apparently generalized irregular or bilateral and synchronous spike and wave or polyspike discharges with anterior predominance can occur. Sometimes the interictal and ictal EEGs show non-specific generalized slow activity only.

Epilepsy arising in the central (peri-rolandic) region (Table 1.8)

The primary manifestations are motor or sensory. The motor features can take the form of jerking, dystonic spasm, posturing or occasionally paralysis, often with clear consciousness (i.e. simple partial seizures). The jerking can affect any muscle group, usually unilaterally, the exact site depending on the part of the precentral gyrus involved in the seizure, and the jerks may move (the Jacksonian march) from

Table 1.8 Clinical features of partial seizures of central origin.

Often no loss of consciousness (simple partial seizure)

Contralateral jerking (which may or may not march)

Contralateral tonic spasm or dystonia

Posturing, which is often bilateral

Speech arrest and paralysis of bulbar musculature

Contralateral sensory symptoms

Short, frequently recurring attacks

one part of the body to another as the discharge spreads over the motor cortex. The seizure discharge may remain limited to one small segment for long periods of time, and when it does spread it is typically very slow. The clonic jerks consist of brief tetanic contractions of all the muscles that cooperate in a single movement. The seizures spread through the cortex, producing clonic movements according to the sequence of cortical representation. A seizure which begins in the hand usually passes up the arm and down the leg; if it begins in the foot it passes up the leg and down the arm. A seizure beginning in the face is most apt to originate in the mouth because of the correspondingly large area of cortical representation. In seizures arising anywhere in the central region, head and eye version is common. Arrest of speech (anarthria) can occur if the motor area representing the muscles of articulation is affected (phonatory seizure) and is usually associated with spasm or clonic movements of the jaw. After focal seizure activity there can be localized paralysis in the affected limbs (Todd's paralysis), which is usually short-lived.

If the seizure is initiated in or evolves to affect supplementary motor areas, posturing of the arms may develop, classically with adversive head and eye deviation, abduction and external rotation of the contralateral arm and flexion at the elbows. There may also be posturing of the legs, and speech arrest or stereotyped vocalizations. Consciousness is usually maintained unless secondarily generalization occurs. The classical posture was named by Penfield the fencing posture, resembling as it does the *en garde* position, but other postures also occur. The posturing is often bilateral and asymmetrical. The fencing posture or fragments of it can also occur in seizures originating in various other frontal and temporal brain regions, presumably resulting from spread of the seizure discharge to supplementary motor cortex. In contrast to Jacksonian seizures, supplementary motor area seizures are often very brief,

occur frequently and in clusters, sometimes hundreds each day, and are sometimes also precipitated by startle.

Somatosensory manifestations (simple hallucinations) occur if the seizure discharge originates in, or spreads to, the postcentral region. Typically these take the form of tingling, numbness, an electrical shock-like feeling, a tickling or crawling feeling, burning, pain or a feeling of heat. These symptoms are usually accompanied by jerking, posturing or spasms as the epileptic discharges usually spread anteriorly. The sensory symptoms may remain localized or march in a Jacksonian manner. Ictal pain is occasionally a prominent symptom and can be severe and poorly localized.

Interictal and ictal scalp EEGs in focal epilepsy in central regions are often normal as the focus may be small and buried within the central gyri.

Epilepsy arising in the parietal and occipital lobe
(Table 1.9)

Focal seizures arise from these locations less commonly than from frontal, central or temporal lobe regions. The typical manifestations of the seizures are subjective sensory and visual disturbances. Additional features are common and are the result of spread to adjacent cortical regions.

Parietal lobe seizures typically include sensory manifestations. These may comprise tingling or a feeling of electricity which can be confined or march

Table 1.9 Clinical features of parietal and occipital lobe epilepsy.

Somatosensory symptoms (e.g. tingling, numbness or more complex sensations—may or may not march)

Sensation of inability to move

Sexual sensations

Illusions of change in body size/shape

Vertigo

Gustatory seizures

Elementary visual hallucinations (e.g. flashes, colours, shapes, patterns)

Complex visual hallucinations (e.g. objects, scenes, autoscopia—often moving)

Head turning (usually adversive, with sensation of following or looking at the visual hallucinations)

Visual–spatial distortions: e.g. of size (micropsia, macropsia), shape, position

Loss or dulling of vision (amaurosis)

Eyelid fluttering, blinking, nystagmus

in a Jacksonian manner. Sensations of sinking, choking or nausea can occur. There can be accompanying loss of tone or a sensation of paralysis. Illusions of bodily distortion are characteristic, such as a feeling of swelling or shrinking, or lengthening or shortening particularly affecting the tongue, mouth or extremities. Ictal apraxia, alexia and agnosia have been reported. Sexual feelings can occur, sometimes with erection or ejaculation. Gustatory seizures have their origin in the suprasylvian region (adjacent to the mouth and throat primary sensory region). Ictal vertigo also originates in the suprasylvian region.

Seizures from the occipital, parieto-occipital and temporo-occipital cortex are usually characterized by visual symptoms. Elementary visual hallucinations (sensations of colours, shapes, flashes and patterns) are most common, which can be intermittent, stationary or appear to move. More complex stereotyped hallucinations/illusions can take the form of scenes, animals, people (including self-images), or of topographical or spatial distortion, alterations of size and shape, perseveration or repetition of visual objects, or the break-up of visual objects or movement. Forced head and eye turning are common, with the patient believing that the visual hallucination is being tracked voluntarily. Rapid blinking or eyelid flutter are frequent in some types of occipital seizures, as are headache and nausea which make the distinction from migraine difficult in some cases.

The EEG in occipital or parietal epilepsy can be normal or show appropriate focal discharges, although often the epileptic disturbance is poorly localized without correlation to the ictal symptoms. Occipital spike wave is characteristic of some types of focal occipital seizures, which can be confused with primary generalized epilepsy.

FURTHER READING

Commission on Classification and Terminology of the International League Against Epilepsy (1981) Proposal for revised clinical and electroencephalographic classification of epileptic seizures. *Epilepsia*, **22**, 489–501.

Commission on Classification and Terminology of the International League Against Epilepsy (1989) Proposal for revised classification of epilepsies and epileptic syndrome. *Epilepsia*, **30**, 389–99.

Duncan, J.S., Shorvon, S.D. & Fish, D.R. (1995) *Clinical Epilepsy*. Churchill Livingstone, London.

Engel, J. & Pedley, T.A. (eds) (1997) *Epilepsy: a Comprehensive Textbook*. Lippincott-Raven, Philadelphia.

Hauser, W.A. & Kurland, L.T. (1975) The epidemiology of epilepsy in Rochester, Minnesota, 1935 through 1967. *Epilepsia*, **16**, 1–66.

Hopkins, A., Shorvon, S. & Cascino, G. (1995) *Epilepsy* (2nd edn). Chapman & Hall, London.

Sander, J.W.A.S. & Shorvon, S.D. (1987) Incidence and prevalence studies in epilepsy and their methodological problems: a review. *J Neurol, Neurosurg and Psych*, **50**, 829–39.

Shorvon, S.D., Dreifuss, F., Fish, D. & Thomas, D. (eds) (1996) *The Treatment of Epilepsy*. Blackwell Science, Oxford.

Wallace, H., Shorvon, S.D. & Tallis, R. (1998) Age-specific incidence and prevalence rates of treated epilepsy in an unselected population of 2,052,922 and age-specific fertility rates of women with epilepsy. *Lancet* **352**, 1970–73.

Precipitation, Causes and Differential Diagnosis of Epilepsy

PRECIPITATION OF SEIZURES

Although individuals with epilepsy often have firm views about factors which precipitate seizures, rigorous proof is frequently lacking. The desire to make sense of the world by establishing cause and effect can lead many a patient, and their medical attendants, in a fruitless quest for evidence of seizure precipitation. Nevertheless, there are a number of factors which are often related to worsening of seizure frequency and the most common are listed in Table 2.1.

Emotional stress in particular can be difficult to define or to pin down, and yet is commonly thought to provoke attacks in many individuals. Where measurement has been possible, studies usually show a modest association between worsening seizures and stress, although this can be a complex association in any individual and stress reduction frequently has a disappointing lack of effect on seizure frequency. A wide variety of often spurious psychic explanations have been made in this difficult area.

Sleep deprivation is an undoubted precipitant of seizures in many people, and a few have attacks only in this situation. Young adults with the syndrome of idiopathic generalized epilepsy seem particularly liable to seizure precipitation by sleep deprivation. Electroencephalogram (EEG) abnormalities, and therefore presumably also seizures, are enhanced by sleep deprivation in some people with partial epilepsy. Fatigue is also thought to provoke attacks by many people with epilepsy. While this seems likely to be so, formal studies are lacking.

Acute alcohol intoxication and, even more potently, acute alcohol withdrawal, can precipitate generalized seizures. A 20-fold increase in the incidence of seizures is found in patients consuming large quantities of alcohol, and the avoidance of alcohol is often all that is required to prevent seizures in some of these cases. Antiepileptic drug treatment in alcoholic patients is often fraught with difficulty and should be avoided where possible. Seizures are also common in the 24 h after alcohol withdrawal, taking the form of myoclonus and tonic–clonic convulsions sometimes with photosensitivity. This period can be covered with benzodiazepine or clomethiazole therapy carried out under medical supervision.

Other acute metabolic and toxic disturbances can also result in provoked seizures, and further epileptic attacks are usually avoided by correction of the metabolic derangement. The relation of seizures to the menstrual cycle is outlined on p. 77.

In the syndrome of idiopathic generalized epilepsy, all seizure types (absence, myoclonic and tonic–clonic seizures) are particularly likely to occur within an hour or so of awakening or, less commonly, when drifting off to sleep, or in the first 2 h of sleep—most commonly in non-rapid eye movement (non-REM) sleep. About 60% of children with benign rolandic epilepsy have attacks confined to sleep. In the genetic syndrome of autosomal dominant frontal lobe epilepsy, attacks occur only in sleep and numerous attacks can occur each night without a single event during the day. Some patients with other forms of generalized or partial epilepsy also have attacks only in sleep, and it has long been recognized that focal EEG disturbances can be activated by light sleep. The EEG disturbances in electrical status epilepticus slow wave sleep (ESES) and in the Landau–Kleffner syndrome are also greatly enhanced by sleep.

Seizures occurring in sleep often have less serious social consequences than daytime attacks. Therapy

Table 2.1 Factors which can influence seizure precipitation.

Stress
Sleep deprivation and fatigue
Sleep/wake cycle
Alcohol and alcohol withdrawal
Metabolic disturbances
Toxins and drugs
Menstrual cycle

may not need to be as intensive as in daytime epilepsy, and patients may prefer not to have any drug treatment. In some cases, therapy converts a pattern of regular nocturnal attacks into less frequent daytime seizures with catastrophic social consequences. It should not be forgotten, however, that nocturnal tonic–clonic seizures carry a particular risk of sudden death, especially if the patient sleeps alone and the seizures are unwitnessed. Advice about the choice of treatment should therefore be given on an individual basis.

REFLEX EPILEPSIES

Reflex epilepsies are those in which seizures are precipitated by a specific cause. In some cases the association can be highly specific and in others less so. The term is not usually applied to patients whose seizures are related to internal influences (e.g. menstruation), nor to situations where the precipitating factors are vague or ill-defined (e.g. fatigue, stress). Reflex epilepsies are sometimes divided into simple and complex types: in the simple forms the seizures are precipitated by simple sensory stimuli (e.g. flashes of light, startle) and in the complex forms by more elaborate stimuli (e.g. specific pieces of music). The complex forms are much more heterogeneous and the syndromes are less well-defined than simple reflex epilepsies. In hospital practice, about 5% of patients show some features of reflex epilepsy. The stimuli reported to cause seizures include flashing lights and other visual stimuli, startle, eating, bathing in hot water, music, reading and movement.

Photosensitivity

The most common reflex epilepsies are those induced by visual stimuli. Flashing lights, bright lights, moving patterns, eye closure and viewing specific objects and colours have all been described. 'Photosensitive epilepsy' is a term used to designate these individuals. Photosensitivity is present in a population with a frequency of about 1.1 per 100 000 persons, and 5.7 per 100 000 in the 7–19 years age range. About 3% of persons with epilepsy are photosensitive and have seizures induced by viewing flickering or intermittent light, bright lights, patterns or television. The flicker frequency precipitating photosensitivity varies from patient to patient, but is most commonly in the 15–20 Hz range. The peak age of presentation of photosensitive epilepsy is 12 years, and the male : female ratio is 2 : 3. Most patients with

photosensitive epilepsy have the syndrome of idiopathic generalized epilepsy, although occasionally patients with focal epilepsy, usually arising in the occipital region, will be photosensitive. Other factors facilitate seizures, and photosensitive patients are often more likely to have photic-induced seizures when sleep-deprived. Individual patients may be sensitive to certain frequencies or patterns.

Seizures in some photosensitive patients can be prevented by wearing glasses with tinted or polarized lenses and by avoiding situations known to induce photosensitive responses. Television and, far less often, computer screen or video game screens can produce seizures in some photosensitive people, and the following precautions can reduce the risk of seizures in susceptible individuals.
• Use a small screen or view the screen from a distance.
• View the screen from an angle.
• Use a remote control for changing channels.
• Use a 100-Hz television screen or a non-interlaced computer screen with a high refresh rate or liquid crystal display.
• Close or cover one eye.
• Keep the screen contrast and brightness low.
• Avoid exposure when sleep-deprived.
• Avoid looking at a fixed flickering pattern.
• Use polarizing glasses.
Treatment with valproate usually completely abolishes photosensitivity, even at a dosage which does not provide complete seizure control.

Startle-induced seizures

Startle can be one precipitant of seizures in susceptible persons, and occasionally the only precipitant. Startle-induced seizures usually occur in patients with a frontal lobe focus. The seizures usually take a form similar to a tonic seizure, and the EEG is commonly normal or shows various rather non-specific changes. A susceptibility to startle is more common in late childhood and adolescence and may resolve as the patient gets older. The most common stimulus is a loud noise, but touch, sudden movement or fright can also precipitate attacks. Startle-induced epilepsy must be differentiated from hyperekplexia which is a familial condition with dominant inheritance in which the attacks are of brainstem origin and are not a form of epilepsy. Treatment can be difficult, although carbamazepine and the benzodiazepine drugs have been said at an anecdotal level to be most likely to control the attacks.

Primary reading epilepsy

This is a specific epilepsy syndrome in which clonic jerking of the jaw, which can evolve to a generalized convulsion, is precipitated by prolonged reading. Content, comprehension and context have been shown to be important but different stimuli apply in individual patients. Recorded stimuli include orofacial movement, reading difficult or unfamiliar passages, music, nonsense passages and foreign languages. Reading induces the EEG discharges only after a period of sometimes many minutes of reading and the physiological basis of this curious syndrome is unclear. There is a genetic basis and a positive family history in about 25% of cases. The seizures can usually be aborted if reading is terminated as soon as the clonic jerking develops. Antiepileptic drugs have been used with variable success.

Other forms of reflex epilepsy

Other simple reflex epilepsies include seizures induced by movement, touching or tapping. These should be differentiated from paroxysmal kinesogenic choreoathetosis and stimulus-sensitive myoclonus. Hot-water epilepsy is a remarkable syndrome, common in parts of India but rare elsewhere, in which seizures are induced by pouring hot water over the head or immersion in hot water. The attacks take the form of tonic–clonic or partial seizures.

Other reflex epilepsies with complex forms include seizure precipitated by the act of eating, by hearing certain sounds or even certain pieces of music, by psychic processes including decision-making, mental arithmetic, chess-playing and deep thought. These conditions are heterogeneous in terms of aetiology, EEG and seizure type, the stimulus is only occasionally highly specific and non-reflex seizures also occur. The mechanisms underlying these, and other reflex epilepsies are uncertain and specific 'reflex arcs' have not been identified. Prevention of the precipitating cause is sometimes helpful, as is drug treatment along conventional lines.

CAUSES OF EPILEPSY

The range of aetiology of epilepsy varies in different age-groups and geographical locations. Broadly speaking, congenital and genetic conditions are the most common causes of epilepsy in early childhood. In older children and young adults, inherited predisposition, hippocampal sclerosis, alcohol or drug abuse and trauma are important causes. In the elderly, vascular disease is common. Tumours and sporadic infections occur at all ages, although malignant tumours are more likely over the age of 30 years. In certain areas, endemic infections are common. Epilepsy is often multifactorial and in any acquired condition is more likely to occur if an inherited predisposition is present, as has been shown in epilepsy after head injury or caused by alcohol or alcohol withdrawal. The specific epilepsy syndromes are also very much age-dependent.

A population-based study (National General Practice Study of Epilepsy, NGPSE) reported the frequency of different aetiologies in an unselected series of 784 patients with newly diagnosed epilepsy (Table 2.2). One predominant cause per case was assumed. There are two main limitations of the study, with cases ascertained between 1984 and 1987. First, the study predated the widespread use of magnetic resonance imaging (MRI), and undoubtedly the proportion of idiopathic or cryptogenic epilepsies is higher than would now be the case. This is especially so in regard to hippocampal sclerosis, which was undetectable *in vivo* prior to MRI. Secondly, the idiopathic or cryptogenic category did not differentiate those cases with idiopathic generalized epilepsy and other genetic disorders, from the truly cryptogenic cases.

Category	Percentage	Comment
Cryptogenic/idiopathic	61	83% if aged 0–9 years
		38% if aged >60 years
Symptomatic		
Vascular disease	15	49% if aged >60 years
Alcohol	6	27% if aged 30–39 years
Cerebral tumour	6	1% if aged <30 years
		19% if aged 50–59 years
		11% if aged >60 years
Trauma	3	
Infection	2	
Other	7	

Table 2.2 National General Practice Study of Epilepsy: aetiological diagnosis in cases with newly diagnosed epileptic seizures in a general population, excluding febrile convulsions.

With these provisos however, this study does give useful information about the disposition of causes in an unselected population.

Tables of causes of epilepsy often combine conditions or diseases, syndromes and mechanisms (Table 2.3). A logical classification scheme is difficult to devise. In any individual case, several factors may predispose to epilepsy. The childhood epilepsy syndromes, idiopathic generalized epilepsy and the myoclonic syndromes are described on pp. 53–74.

Inherited genetic disorders

In the following sections, a selection of conditions with known genetic mechanisms will be briefly described.

The epileptogenic potential of different parts of the brain varies, and the development of epilepsy in any focal pathology relates as much to its site as to the nature of the process. Lesions below the tentorium are not epileptogenic. The same generally applies to deep hemisphere lesions. Cortical lesions, on the other hand, are epileptogenic, especially the temporal and frontal lobes, including the hippocampus.

Genetic disorders causing epilepsy alone

Heredity has an important role in epilepsy. While hereditary or genetic factors play a significant part in various idiopathic or primary epilepsy syndromes and probably in some secondary epilepsies, known single-gene disorders underlie the epilepsy in no more than 1–2% of cases. In these conditions, asso-

ciated neurological signs and cognitive impairment are frequently present.

The most common inherited epilepsies are the idiopathic generalized epilepsies. Their mode of inheritance is not clear and these are discussed further on p. 72. The mechanisms of inheritance of the progressive myoclonic epilepsies are being rapidly elucidated, and these conditions are discussed further on p. 60.

A number of linkage studies in idiopathic epilepsies, particularly partial epilepsies, have now been reported. These include benign familial neonatal convulsions (EBN1 (20q), EBN2 (8q), JME (6p, some families), familial frontal-lobe epilepsy (20q, some families), partial epilepsy (10q)).

Inherited conditions with other neurological features

DNA expansion syndromes. A number of dominant-inherited diseases where the phenomenon of anticipation has been observed are caused by a specific kind of mutation, namely an expansion of a trinucleotide repeat sequence. These expansions may be found in a non-coding part of the gene, as in fragile X syndrome, a common hereditary form of learning disability, or in a coding part of the gene, as in Huntington's disease and dentato-rubro-pallido-luysian atrophy. Epilepsy may be a prominent part of the clinical picture in these conditions, particularly in early presentations where a large number of repeats are usually found.

Other inherited conditions with extrapyramidal features. Seizures may also occur in Wilson's disease (6% of cases), Hallervorden–Spatz syndrome and neuroacanthocytosis. Niemann–Pick disease type C is an autosomal recessive inherited disorder, with widespread abnormal deposition of lipid. Progressive neurological deterioration becomes evident in infancy, childhood, adolescence or adulthood. Clinical features include impaired up-gaze and ataxia, followed by dementia, extrapyramidal signs and seizures of different types. There is associated hepatosplenomegaly, more marked in younger age-groups. Diagnosis is based on the finding of lipid-laden histiocytes on bone-marrow biopsy.

Other inborn errors of metabolism. Other inborn errors of metabolism with seizures include pyridoxine dependency, phenylketonuria and other amino acid disorders, organic acid disorders, urea cycle disorders, lactic acidosis (including biotinidase deficiency), dis-

Table 2.3 Aetiology of epilepsy.

Inherited genetic
Epilepsy alone
Epilepsy and other neurological manifestations

Acquired
Trauma
Neurosurgery
Infection
Vascular disease
Hippocampal sclerosis
Tumours
Neurodegenerative disorders
Metabolic disorders
Toxic disorders (including alcohol, drugs)
Miscellaneous: coeliac, Whipple's disease, demyelinating diseases, vasculitis

Congenital (inherited or acquired)
Cortical dysplasia/dysgenesis
Cerebral tumour
Vascular malformations
Prenatal injury

Table 2.4 Some known inherited/genetic conditions.

EPILEPSY ALONE
Benign familial neonatal convulsions (autosomal
    dominant)
    EBN1 (linked to 20q)
    EBN2 (linked to 8q)
Benign familial infantile convulsions (autosomal
    dominant)
Juvenile myoclonic epilepsy (linked to 6p in some
    families)
Familial frontal-lobe epilepsy (autosomal dominant,
    linked to 20q in some families)
Idiopathic generalized epilepsy (see p. 72)

EPILEPSY WITH OTHER MANIFESTATIONS
Chromosomal abnormalities
Down syndrome (trisomy 21)
Trisomy 13, 18, 22
Wolf's syndrome

With myoclonic epilepsy and cerebral degeneration
Unverricht–Lundborg disease
Lafora body disease
Neuronal ceroid-lipofuscinosis
Sialidosis
Biotinase deficiency
Mitochondrial disease
Storage disorders (GM_1 and GM_2 gangliosidosis,
    Gaucher's disease)

With extrapyramidal features
Wilson's disease
Hallervorden–Spatz
Neuroacanthocytosis
Niemann–Pick disease type C
Huntington's disease
Dentato-rubral-pallido-luysian atrophy

EPILEPSY WITH OTHER MANIFESTATIONS
(*continued*)

With muscular dystrophy and mental subnormality
Fukuyama's muscular dystrophy

With mental subnormality
Progressive epilepsy with learning disabilities
Fragile X syndrome

Neurocutaneous syndromes
Tuberous sclerosis
Neurofibromatosis
Others (see text)

With intermittent disturbances
Porphyria

*Other inherited conditions with neurological and
    systemic manifestations*
Phenylketonuria
Progressive neuronal degeneration with liver disease
    (Alpers' disease)
Leucodystrophies (metachromatic, globoid cell,
    adrenoleucodystrophy, Canavan's disease)
Amino acidurias
Urea cycle disorders
Purine and pyramidine metabolic disorders
Organic acidaemias
Menkes' disease

orders of B_{12} metabolism, peroxisomal disorders, poliodystrophies, Menkes' disease (steely-hair syndrome), GM_1 gangliosidosis, Krabbe's disease, Canavan–van Bogaert disease and leucodystrophies (e.g. metachromatic and adrenoleucodystrophy).

Progressive neuronal degeneration with liver disease (Alpers' disease) is a rare, rapidly progressive and fatal autosomal recessive disorder and usually presents in infants and young children. Features include hypotonia in infancy, failure to thrive, psychomotor retardation and, later, intractable seizures and liver failure. In some 25% of cases a more explosive onset, with intractable epilepsy as a first symptom, occurs. A similar presentation, with visual and sensory symptoms and signs and intractable seizures, including myoclonus, has also been reported in young adults with similar pathological changes. Intractable status epilepticus is common.

X-linked adrenoleucodystrophy (ADL), mapped to Xq28, is one of the group 2 peroxisomal disorders, where peroxisomes are normal but there is a single enzyme defect. In group 1 disorders, peroxisomes are reduced or absent. Adrenoleucodystrophy is diagnosed by demonstrating abnormally high levels of very-long-chain fatty acids in plasma. It can present with the childhood cerebral form, with hyperactivity and attention deficit disorders followed by seizures, cognitive decline, ataxia and auditory and visual disturbances. Progression is rapid thereafter, with other neurological signs and finally a vegetative state, leading to death. Other less common presentations include adult-onset adrenomyeloneuropathy (AMN) and adrenal insufficiency alone (>20% of ADL patients). Of heterozygous females 20% develop AMN. Individuals may also be asymptomatic. These variations in presentation, often within the same family, suggest the influence of an autosomal modifier gene. Early diagnosis is important, as treatment is ineffective in advanced disease. The role of dietary treatment before the onset of neurological signs or of bone-marrow transplants when neurological involvement is still mild is uncertain.

Inherited metabolic disorders with intermittent disturbances

Porphyria. Seizures may be part of the clinical presentation in porphyria along with intermittent attacks of abdominal pain, psychiatric disturbances and motor neuropathy. If antiepileptic drugs are required, those that may precipitate attacks must be avoided.

Neurocutaneous syndromes

Tuberous sclerosis (Bourneville's syndrome). This is a relatively common autosomal-dominant condition of variable penetrance and a frequency of one per 10 000 live births. This has been linked to 9q and 16p. Common features include epilepsy (80%), mental subnormality (50%), hypomelanotic patches on ultraviolet-light examination (90%), retinal phakoma/haematoma (50%), periungual fibromas (25%), cardiac rhabdomyomas (40%) and angiolipomas of bone (50%). Tuberous sclerosis is described in more detail on p. 63.

Neurofibromatosis. Types 1 and 2 neurofibromatosis (NF1 and NF2) are both associated with an increased incidence of both epilepsy and neurological tumours. Neurofibromas, neurofibrosarcomas, optic-nerve gliomas and other astrocytomas occur in NF1 and schwannomas, meningiomas and ependymomas in NF2. The epileptogenic potential is partly related to the site of the tumour. However, there is an increased risk of epilepsy independent of the presence of cerebral tumours.

Other neurocutaneous syndromes. Other neurocutaneous syndromes include neurocutaneous melanosis, Chediak–Higashi syndrome, Klippel–Trenaunay–Weber syndrome, midline linear sebaceous naevus syndrome, hypomelanosis of Ito and incontinentia pigmenti.

Acquired or congenital (acquired or genetic) disorders

Included here are a selection of conditions which are acquired or congenital but without a well-understood genetic basis.

Vascular malformations

Sturge–Weber syndrome. This is an uncommon sporadic developmental disorder of uncertain cause. The principal clinical features are a unilateral or bilateral port-wine naevus, epilepsy, hemiparesis, mental impairment and ocular signs. The port-wine naevus is usually but not exclusively in the distribution of the trigeminal nerve. It can cross the midline and spread into the dermatomal distribution of the upper cervical nerve. If it affects the lip or the gum these can be enlarged. In one-third of cases the naevus is bilateral.

The epilepsy can be focal or generalized. It is often the earliest symptom, and most patients with Sturge–Weber syndrome develop seizures within the first year of life and almost all have developed epilepsy before the age of 4 years. Seizures developing in the neonatal period can be very difficult to control and carry a poor prognosis. The hemiplegia and mental impairment can deteriorate following a severe bout of seizures, and in this condition there is little doubt that brain damage can result directly from epileptic attacks. Severe learning disability is less common as a result of better control of the epilepsy. There are a variety of ophthalmological complications, including increased intraocular pressure with glaucoma or buphthalmos; a homonymous field defect is common, particularly when the cerebral lesion is in the occipital region (as is frequent); episcleral haemangioma, choroidal naevi and colobomas of the iris can occur. The underlying brain pathology is a cerebral angiomatosis (often occipital) sometimes with gyral calcification. The affected cerebral hemisphere is often atrophic and gliotic. The lesion is probably caused by abnormal persistence of embryonic primordial vascular plexus and subsequent prenatal growth separates these elements into deep, cerebral and superficial skin elements.

The epilepsy should be aggressively treated to prevent neurological deterioration and, if drug therapy is ineffective, consideration of surgical resection of the affected region or even hemispherectomy is worthwhile, particularly if carried out early in life.

Arteriovenous malformations. Arteriovenous malformations (AVM) cause arteriovenous shunting, with tortuous feeding arteries and draining veins. Pathologically, there is no intervening capillary bed in the tangle of vessels. Intralesional and perilesional gliosis is present, sometimes with associated haemosiderin. The rate of spontaneous haemorrhage is estimated at 2–3% per year. There may be associated aneurysms. Epilepsy is a common manifestation, occurring more frequently in larger lesions and as the presenting symptom in 19%.

Aneurysms. Unruptured aneurysms, particularly if large, can occasionally present as epilepsy. Epilepsy is common if the haemorrhage, after rupture, results in an intracerebral haematoma.

Cavernous angiomas. These epileptogenic lesions are distinct from AVM. Pathologically, they consist of endothelium-lined caverns filled with blood and surrounded by a matrix of collagen and fibroblasts. A typical haemosiderin ring is seen on MRI. The rate of acute haemorrhage is unknown, but is less than in AVM and may be of the order of 1% per year. Multiple lesions occur in up to 20–40% of cases. Inheritance is thought to be autosomal dominant with incomplete penetrance, with some 30% of cases with single lesions occurring in families and 80–90% if multiple. *De novo* cases have also been documented and the cavernomas can develop through life. Epilepsy, which may be intractable, is frequent in supratentorial lesions. With the more widespread use of MRI, more information will become available on the extent, characteristics and natural history.

Hippocampal sclerosis

Hippocampal sclerosis is the most common pathology underlying temporal lobe epilepsy. It is the underlying cause of epilepsy in over one-third of people with refractory focal epilepsy attending hospital clinics in whom there is no other structural lesion. It is less frequent in patients with mild epilepsy.

The pathological changes include shrinkage in the hippocampus with neuronal loss and gliosis, mossy fibre sprouting, dentate gyral dispersion or duplication and a wide range of neurochemical alterations. Structural and pathological changes also occur in the extrahippocampal parts of the temporal lobe and more widely. The cause of hippocampal sclerosis is controversial and may be multifactorial. There is a very clear association with a history of childhood febrile convulsions (see p. 55 and Table 3.24) and one postulation is that the febrile convulsions, especially if prolonged or complex, damage the hippocampus and result in hippocampal sclerosis. Serial MRI studies have demonstrated that status epilepticus can also result in hippocampal sclerosis. Animal models have shown that prolonged partial seizures can cause hippocampal damage, and also

that single short temporal lobe seizures can result in subtle hippocampal changes. There is also evidence that, in some cases, hippocampal sclerosis is a congenital lesion and a form of cortical dysgenesis.

Cortical dysgenesis (cortical dysplasia, malformations of cortical development)

The widespread use of MRI scanning has demonstrated the importance of these conditions, which were previously undetectable and under-recorded, as a cause of epilepsy. The type of abnormality produced depends on the stage at which development was disturbed as well as the site of abnormality. For example, disorders of neural tube formation can result in anencephaly or holoprosencephaly. Defects in gyration can lead to polymicrogyria, defects in lamination to double cortex syndrome, abnormal neuroblast proliferation or migration to heterotopias and hamartomas, and a failure of programmed cell death to agenesis of the corpus callosum or hemimegencephaly. Almost any congenital disturbance of the brain can result in seizures, but the most numerous are disorders of neuronal migration. The classification of these syndromes is controversial, but a pragmatic

Table 2.5 A classification of cortical dysgenesis.

Abnormalities of gyration
  Agyria/macrogyria
  Lissencephaly
  Polymicrogyria
  Schizencephaly
  Minor gyration changes

Megencephaly/hemimegencephaly

Heterotopias
  Subependymal heterotopia
  Subcortical heterotopia
  Subarachnoid heterotopia

Tuberous sclerosis

Focal cortical dysplasia

Cortical dysgenesis with neoplasia
  Dysembroplastic neuroepithelial tumour
  Other developmental tumours

Dysgenesis of the archicortex
  Duplication/dispersion of the dentate granular layer
  Some forms of hippocampal sclerosis

classification based on MRI appearance is widely used (Table 2.5). There are many potential causes of these development anomalies, although in most cases no cause can be uncovered. There is a genetic basis to many cases, but environmental factors which can affect intrauterine development include toxins, viral infections and drugs. The epilepsy in these conditions is extremely variable, although often refractory to treatment.

Certain conditions are usually encountered in the clinical setting of epilepsy. Agenesis of the corpus callosum is associated with a variety of chromosomal disorders and several genetic syndromes, including tuberous sclerosis, Aicardi's syndrome, Menkes' syndrome and Andermann's syndrome. Schizencephaly is characterized by bilateral or unilateral clefts, joining the cortex to the periventricular area. Clinical features vary, although epilepsy and intellectual impairment are common. Hemimegancephaly presents with epilepsy in infancy and developmental delay and contralateral hemiplegia. It may accompany other types of dysgenesis. Subependymal heterotopia is a common form of dysgenesis and epilepsy is often the only clinical feature. It can be associated with other dysgeneses and also with hippocampal sclerosis. Polymicrogyria can be focal or diffuse and refers to an abnormally high number of cerebral convolutions and increased cortical thickness and can be associated with other dysgeneses.

Table 2.6 Broad estimates of seizure risk in some central nervous system infections.

Infection	Percentage
Bacterial meningitis	
Acute seizures	30
Chronic epilepsy in survivors	
If early seizures	10
If no early seizures	3
(Epilepsy is more likely if neurological deficit is present)	
Viral encephalitis including herpes simplex	
Chronic epilepsy in survivors	
If early seizures	25
If no early seizures	10
Bacterial cerebral abscess	72
(Epilepsy is more likely if the abscess is frontal or temporal)	
Cerebral toxoplasmosis in AIDS	25

AIDS, acquired immunodeficiency syndrome.

Clinical manifestations vary and epilepsy is common. Focal cortical dysplasia causes epilepsy and sometimes other features, including intellectual impairment and focal neurological signs. Laminar heterotopia (double cortex syndrome) presents with epilepsy and variable learning disability. The mildest abnormality of neuronal migration is known as microdysgenesis. This condition is detectable on histological examination only, and refers to the alteration of neuronal disposition in cortex and subcortical regions. This has been demonstrated in 38% of brains in people with epilepsy compared with 8% in controls and will frequently accompany other changes, such as hippocampal sclerosis.

Immunization

The National Childhood Encephalography Study suggested that the pertussis vaccine resulted in severe brain damage in one per 310 000 immunizations, a figure that is generally considered now to be methodologically flawed and an overestimate. The result of a population-based case–control study did not show an increased risk of onset of serious acute neurological illness in the 7 days after diphtheria–tetanus–pertussis (DTP) vaccine. However, when the analysis was restricted to children with encephalopathy or complicated seizures and adjusted for factors possibly affecting vaccine administration, the odds ratio for having been vaccinated in the previous week was 3.6 (95% confidence intervals 0.8–15.2), but it fell below 1.0 in subsequent weeks. Thus, overall odds ratios over a 28-day period were not significantly elevated. The data were compatible with induction by fever of an illness to which the child was predisposed. Although benefits associated with protection against pertussis clearly outweigh the potential risk, a causal relationship between serious acute neurological illness and DTP vaccine in occasional children can not be dismissed with absolute certainty. There is a small excess of febrile convulsions after measles vaccination.

Acute and chronic infections and their sequelae

Epilepsy can occur in many infective diseases with cerebral involvement. During the acute phase of bacterial or viral meningoencephalitis, seizures are frequent. The occurrence of early seizures, as in the case of trauma, makes chronic epilepsy more likely (see Table 2.6). Cerebral tuberculosis frequently causes epilepsy. Tuberculomas may be multiple and may enlarge during treatment. They may be missed on computerized tomography (CT) if performed without enhancement. Parasitosis, including schistosomiasis, hydatid disease, cysticercosis, trypanosomiasis (African and rarely American), malaria and toxoplasmosis may all cause epilepsy.

Seizures in human immunodeficiency virus (HIV) infection can be a presenting feature but are much more likely to occur in later stages. In about one-half of cases, there is a demonstrable secondary infection or neoplasm and in the remainder the HIV infection is responsible.

Seizures, including myoclonus, are a feature of subacute sclerosing panencephalitis. Of interest is the possible role of chronic or latent viral infections in the pathogenesis of partial epilepsies. An example of a chronic infection causing epilepsy is the epidemic Russian spring–summer tick-borne encephalitis, where epilepsia partialis continua (EPC), sometimes associated with mono- or hemiplegia, persists for years after a febrile illness, with localized encephalitis shown on biopsy. Although evidence is scant, it is possible that latent viral infections, perhaps of the herpes group, is involved in the pathogenesis of evolving localization-related epilepsy syndromes, including temporal lobe epilepsy, via reactivation or persistent chronic focal infection.

Cerebral tumours

Overall, only 6% of newly diagnosed cases of epilepsy in the NGPSE were caused by cerebral tumours. The peak incidence is in middle age. About 40% of adults presenting with newly developing focal epilepsy have an underlying cerebral tumour, usually of the cerebral cortex (frontal or temporal). Indolent tumours are more likely to be associated with epilepsy, which occurs in 90% of oligodendrogliomas, two-thirds of meningiomas or astrocytomas and one-third of gliomas. The site of a tumour is an important factor in predicting whether epilepsy will be present. Tumours of the cerebral cortex, especially in the frontal or temporal regions, are most likely to result in seizures. Epilepsy is unusual in deep white-matter tumours and rare in subtentorial tumours or in tumours of the pituitary gland. In children, as most tumours are subtentorial, tumour is an unusual cause of epilepsy.

Post-traumatic epilepsy

Civilian head injuries, usually from road traffic accidents, falls or recreational injuries, account for about 2–12% of all cases of epilepsy. It has been estimated that approximately 5% of patients requiring hospitalization for closed head trauma will subsequently develop epilepsy. Seizures occurring after cerebral trauma are commonly divided into early and late categories. Early seizures occur within one week of trauma and are most common in young children and have an incidence of 2–6%. These do not usually lead to subsequent seizures, although if a seizure occurs more than 1 h after the injury, it does convey an increased risk of late seizures.

The severity of the head injury is the predominant factor in determining the risk of late epilepsy. Mild head injury (head injury without skull fracture and with less than 30 min of post-traumatic amnesia) is not associated with any increased risk of epilepsy. Moderate head injury (a head injury complicated by skull fracture or post-traumatic amnesia for more than 30 min) is followed by epilepsy in about 1–2% of cases. About 10% of patients overall will develop epilepsy following a severe head injury (head injury with post-traumatic amnesia of more than 24 h, intracranial haematoma or cerebral contusion). Post-traumatic epilepsy is even more frequent after open head injury, and in particular in penetrating wartime injuries with over 50% of patients suffering subsequent epilepsy.

Overall, the risk of late epilepsy, if early epilepsy is present, is about 25% compared to 3% in patients who did not have early seizures. The risk of late epilepsy in situations where factors coexist has been calculated. For instance, in the absence of a depressed fracture, intracranial haematoma or early seizures, the risk of late epilepsy is less than 2% even if a post-traumatic amnesia exceeds 24 h. If early epilepsy has occurred without haematoma or depressed fracture, the risk of late epilepsy is 19%. The risk of late epilepsy following an intracranial haematoma alone is 35% and after depressed fracture alone is 17%. The risk of epilepsy after open head injury is greatest if the extent of cerebral damage was large and involved the frontal or temporal regions.

About 50–60% of cases have their first (late) seizure within 12 months of the injury, with most cases developing within 4–8 months after the injury, and 85% within 2 years. There is a slightly increased risk of late epilepsy developing after a severe injury over 5–10 years. The seizures can take the form of generalized or partial epilepsy and status epilepticus is common. Post-traumatic epilepsy can be difficult to treat and in one series after open head injury 53% of patients still had active epilepsy 15 years after the injury. The risk of epilepsy is increased in those who have a family history of epilepsy, confirming the often multifactorial nature of epilepsy.

There is controversy about the role of prophylactic antiepileptic drug treatment in patients who have suffered head trauma. Early retrospective reports suggested that such prophylactic treatment reduced the incidence of subsequent epilepsy, although subsequent prospective trials failed to show any effect. Other promising but as yet unproven therapies include the use of antioxidants, antiperoxidants, steroids and chelating agents in an attempt to prevent the changes in the brain following head injury which result in epileptogenesis.

Epilepsy after neurosurgery

Epilepsy can also occur following neurosurgery. It is obviously important to define this risk, as it will often influence the decision about whether or not to undertake neurosurgery, and for counselling preoperatively.

The incidence of seizures varies according to the nature of the underlying disease process, its site and its extent. A large retrospective study found an overall incidence of 17% for postoperative seizures in 877 consecutive patients undergoing supratentorial neurosurgery for non-traumatic conditions. The patients had no prior history of epilepsy and the minimum follow-up was 5 years. The incidence of seizures ranged from 4% in patients undergoing stereotactic procedures and ventricular drainage, to 92% for patients being surgically treated for cerebral abscess. The risk of craniotomy for glioma was 19%, for intracranial haemorrhage 21% and for meningioma removal 22%. All these risks were greatly enhanced if seizures occurred preoperatively. Among patients developing postoperative seizures, 37% did so within the first postoperative week, 77% within the first year and 92% within the first 2 years. If early seizures occurred (i.e. those occurring in the first week), 41% of patients developed late recurrent seizures. Studies after surgery for unruptured aneurysm have also been carried out, with an overall risk of about 14%. The risk of surgery for middle cerebral aneurysms resulting in epilepsy is 19%, for anterior communicating aneurisms and posterior communicating aneurysms about 10%. If the aneurysm has bled, causing an intracranial haematoma, the incidence of epilepsy is much higher, as it is if patients have perioperative complications, including hemiparesis or meningitis, implying parenchymal damage. An overall risk of epilepsy following shunt procedures is about 10%, although this depends on the site of the shunt insertion.

As is the case following cerebral trauma, the risks of epilepsy following neurosurgery are greatest in the first postoperative year although a substantial proportion of cases (perhaps 25%) experience their first seizures in the second postoperative year. Whether or not the prophylactic use of anticonvulsants after neurosurgical procedures is worthwhile is highly controversial. The best studies seem to show no effect, although all investigations in this area have been open to criticism. More definitive investigations are required, but currently it is usual to prescribe prophylactic anticonvulsant drugs for several months after major supratentorial neurosurgery and then gradually to withdraw the medication unless seizures have occurred.

Cerebrovascular disease

Epilepsy can complicate all forms of cerebrovascular disease. The risk of chronic epilepsy caused by intracranial haemorrhage has varied from series to series but is probably in the region of 3–7%. The incidence of early epilepsy (seizures in the first week) is much higher, up to 25% in some series, with status epilepticus in about 10%. The epilepsy risk is greater with large haemorrhages and with haemorrhages which involve the cerebral cortex. The incidence of epilepsy is low in deep haematomas. About 40% of patients with large arterior venous malformations have epilepsy, and epilepsy is the presenting symptom in about 20%. Epilepsy also results, not uncommonly, from smaller low-flow cavernous haemangiomas (cavernomas), which are often demonstrable only by MRI and in which chronic epilepsy is often the only symptom.

The incidence of chronic epilepsy following ischaemic stroke is lower. Seizures typically occur early and when late seizures do happen, they are usually easily controlled by treatment and the overall prognosis for the epilepsy is good. Cortical venous infarcts are particularly epileptogenic, at least in the acute phase, and may underlie a significant proportion of apparently spontaneous epileptic seizures complicating other medical conditions and pregnancy.

Epilepsy can also complicate occult cerebrovascular disease. Patients with late onset epilepsy are significantly more likely to have otherwise asymptomatic ischaemic lesions on CT than age-matched controls and it has been estimated from such CT-based studies that overt or occult cerebrovascular disease underlies about half of the epilepsies developing after the age of 50 years. Late onset epilepsy can be the first manifestation of cerebrovascular disease, and in the absence of other causes should prompt a screen for vascular risk factors. Between 5 and 10% of patients presenting with stroke have a history of prior epileptic seizures in the recent past.

Seizures also occur with cerebrovascular lesions secondary to rheumatic heart disease, endocarditis, mitral valve prolapse, cardiac tumours and cardiac dysrhythmia, or after carotid endarterectomy. Infarction is also an important cause of seizures in neonatal epilepsy. Epilepsy is also common in eclampsia, hypertensive encephalopathy and malignant hypertension, and in the anoxic encephalopathy which follows cardiac arrest or cardiopulmonary surgery.

Antenatal or perinatal injury
Most minor events in the perinatal period (contrary to popular belief) do not predispose to the development of later epilepsy. Antenatal or perinatal intracerebral and intraventricular haemorrhage or infarction, or other serious events on the other hand often result in epilepsy. In these cases, imaging will often demonstrate structural damage, for instance vascular changes or a porencephalic cyst.

Drugs, alcohol, toxins and metabolic disturbances
Alcohol is a relatively common association of seizures, either caused by alcohol withdrawal or by a direct toxic effect. It may also precipitate seizures in established epilepsy. In alcohol withdrawal, seizures occur in about half the cases within 12–24 h after withdrawal and EEG may show photosensitivity. Many drugs—medicinal or recreational—precipitate seizures, either as a toxic effect or during withdrawal. Some antiepileptic drugs may precipitate seizures on withdrawal, even in the absence of epilepsy. Drugs and other agents that can precipitate seizures are listed in Table 2.7.

Acute metabolic disorders frequently cause provoked seizures. These include changes in glucose, calcium, sodium, potassium and magnesium. Seizures are common in severe or late-stage liver and renal disease. In the first month of life, hypoglycaemia and hypocalcaemia are important causes of seizures and pyridoxine deficiency, although rare, is important to detect. In older children and adults, rapid changes in blood electrolytes or glucose concentrations can result in seizures as can hyperam-

Table 2.7 Drugs that may induce seizures.

Antibiotics Penicillin (especially intravenous or intrathecal) Isoniazid (especially in slow acetylators) Cycloserine	Anaesthetics Methohexital Ketamine Halothane Propofol Althesin
Hypoglycaemia drugs Insulin Phenformin and other oral hypoglycaemia drugs	Withdrawal seizures Alcohol Benzodiazepines Barbiturates
Hormonal/metabolic drugs Prednisone Oral contraceptives Oxytocin (causing water retention)	Other antiepileptic drugs Amphetamine Opiates
Cardiac dysrhythmic agents Lidocaine (intravenous) Procainamide (intravenous) Disopyramide	Radiographic contrast media Meglumine derivatives (Conray, Dimer-X) Metrizamide
Antidepressant/antipsychotic drugs Phenothiazines Tricyclic antidepressants (especially amitriptyline and imipramine) Anticholinergic drugs Lithium Clozapine	Antimalaria drugs Mefloquine Chloroquine Proguanil
Stimulants Aminophylline Doxapram Theophylline Amphetamine	Antispastic drug Baclofen

monaemia, changes in blood pH, blood oxygenation, renal disease, hepatic disease and cardiac failure.

Epilepsy can follow the ingestion of a variety of toxins, and the encephalopathy caused by lead poisoning can present with epilepsy, as can ergotism and organophosphate intoxication. Hyperthermia, but not hypothermia, frequently results in seizures.

Degenerative disorders
Epilepsy occurs in about one-third of cases in Alzheimer's disease. It is usually relatively mild and develops only in the later stages of the disease. Seizures are rare in Pick's disease. Five per cent of patients with Huntington's disease have epilepsy, usually in the later stages. Epilepsy is more common in the juvenile form. Six per cent of patients with Wilson's disease have epilepsy and seizures can occur at any stage of the disease and may be the presenting feature. Typically, they develop after the initiation of treatment. The seizures can take any form, respond well to treatment and in three-quarters of cases can be fully controlled. Epilepsy, and indeed status epilepticus, can be the presenting feature of Creutzfeldt–Jakob disease, and generalized tonic–clonic or partial seizures occur in 10% of established cases. Myoclonus occurs in 80% of cases and can be induced by startle or other stimuli. The EEG usually shows the repetitive periodic discharges. In the terminal stages of the condition, the myoclonus and the epilepsy usually cease.

Other diseases
Coeliac disease is associated with epilepsy. This may occur in the absence of prominent gastrointestinal symptoms. Partial or generalized seizures may be associated with calcification on CT scanning. Cortical myoclonus has also been reported.

Whipple's disease, a multisystem chronic and relapsing disease of infective aetiology, can also cause epilepsy. Suggestive clinical features include hypothalamic disturbance, supranuclear and nuclear gaze palsies, ocular involvement, myoclonic ocular, jaw and facial movement disorders, and dementia. The male : female ratio is reported to be 6 : 1. Although rare, because it is treatable, it is important to diagnose.

Multiple sclerosis is associated with an increased risk of true epilepsy, estimated at 1–5%. Seizures are usually easily controlled, although persistent focal seizures may occur in association with acute relapses. In acute attacks, large white-matter plaques may involve adjacent grey matter, with surrounding oedema.

Vasculitides, including systemic lupus erythematosus (SLE), often include seizures as part of the clinical picture. Other features are likely to be present, but epilepsy may be the only symptom of SLE for many years.

DIFFERENTIAL DIAGNOSIS OF EPILEPSY

An assessment of a patient suspected of having epilepsy includes the following.
• A detailed history of the attack(s) from the patient and witnesses, history of antecedent illness or events, family history, history of any coexisting disease and history of previous treatment.
• Clinical examination which, if positive, may relate to the underlying condition or be consequent to epileptic seizures or their treatment.
• Supportive investigations for the diagnosis and classification of the epilepsy, which include: interictal and ictal EEG, imaging, ictal video (from a hand-held home video to video-EEG), psychometry and investigation of any suspected underlying condition.

History
A careful clinical history remains the single most important component in the assessment of a patient with possible epilepsy. It is worth emphasizing that true epileptic attacks, particularly frontal seizures, may take bizarre (although stereotyped) forms, or may be followed by a period of agitation or behavioural change leading to an erroneous diagnosis of non-epileptic attacks, especially where accompanied by non-specific ictal scalp EEG. While it will not always be possible to achieve a definite diagnosis in episodic events, every effort should be made to do so in subjects with continuing symptoms. If attacks are frequent, video or video-EEG recording is invaluable, not only in terms of EEG changes (if present), but also for the opportunity of careful observation of the clinical event.

History of the attack from the patient. This needs to include the situation from which the event arose (body position, circumstances, sleep or wakefulness), trigger factors (fatigue, alcohol, sleep deprivation, flickering light), pattern (diurnal pattern, single events or clusters, relation to menstruation), prodromal symptoms, the onset of the attack including aura or focal motor features, the attack itself (if the person retained consciousness), fall or injury during the attack, duration of loss of consciousness, evidence for automatisms during attack, evidence of incontinence or other autonomic disturbance, and postictal symptoms (headaches, muscle aches, fatigue, sore tongue/lip) and affective symptoms before or after the attack.

History of attack from a witness. This is essential for the assessment of possible epilepsy, as frequently the patient is unable to give an adequate account. Witnesses may also need prompting, for example for the presence or laterality of automatisms or dystonic posturing in complex partial seizures, a consistent focal onset of a generalized attack, or any focal deficit (dysphasia or hemiparesis) during or after an attack. A history of any change in colour or respiration should be ascertained, as well as details of the recovery period, in particular if followed by a period of confusion.

Specific enquiry should be made about other seizure types, which may not be spontaneously mentioned by the patient or witness, for example of auras alone, absences or myoclonic jerks.

Conditions which may be mistaken for epilepsy

Syncope

Syncope is a sudden and brief loss of consciousness caused by generalized cerebral ischaemia. There are various clinical types (Table 2.8).

In vasovagal syncope, there may be characteristic prodromal symptoms. These include a vertiginous sensation, profuse sweating, epigastric discomfort, nausea, vomiting, greying or blackout of vision and an altered quality to sounds. Pallor at onset is noted by observers.

In vasovagal syncope of brief duration, abrupt loss of consciousness with generalized hypotonia associated with a fall occurs, followed by quick recovery of consciousness with no postictal confusion. In more severe attacks, clonic jerks may be seen at onset or on recovery, as well as incontinence and dilated pupils. Clonic movements in syncope are usually irregular and short-lived and do not have the pattern of evolution of a tonic–clonic seizure. Nevertheless, they are frequently misinterpreted as convulsions and lead to a misdiagnosis of epilepsy.

Vasovagal syncope is the most common form of syncope—and it is also far more common than epilepsy. Two mechanisms underlie the occurrence of vasovagal syncope, as implied by the name; the first is vagally mediated bradycardia or cardiac arrest, and

Table 2.8 Classification of syncope by group and cause.

Reflex (vasovagal)
Venesection
Pain
Emotion
Hot surroundings
Upright posture
Micturition
Post-traumatic

Cardiac
Rheumatic heart disease (especially aortic stenosis)
Ischaemic heart disease
Congenital heart disease
Dysrhythmias from any cause
Outflow obstruction
Prolonged QT interval syndromes and other
  conduction defects

Postural
Alcohol and drugs
Old age
Hypovolaemia
Diabetes
Shy–Drager syndrome
Peripheral neuropathy (areflexive syncope)
Other causes of autonomic failure

Vascular
Degenerative (embolism, thrombosis, spasm)
Other (congenital, arteritis, carotid sinus
  stimulation, stretch syncope, migraine)

Respiratory
Coughing
Weight-lifting
Trumpeting
Breath-holding attacks

the second is peripheral vasodilatation. Both or either may be present. It is not generally appreciated that such attacks can occur while lying or sitting, although they are much less likely to do so, and recovery is quicker if the person is supine.

The most important clues in the diagnosis of vasovagal syncope are the circumstances (position, provoking factors) from which it arises. These are numerous and include emotion, pain, gastrointestinal disturbance, upright posture, heat, a particular odour, intercurrent illness, dehydration and drugs.

Cardiac syncope is due to a primary fall in cardiac output and does not have the biphasic features of vasovagal syncope nor the prodromal symptoms, nor the characteristic precipitants. Two conditions that need to be considered, as they may present in otherwise apparently well, young individuals with blackouts, are prolonged QT interval and obstructive cardiomyopathy.

In patients with autonomic failure, there are likely to be other features, which suggest the diagnosis. In such cases, a secondary depletion of intravascular volume exacerbates symptoms. Standing still for any length of time is more likely to result in syncope in the heat or after meals. In postural syncope caused by autonomic failure the skin is warm, the pulse unchanged and sweating absent (areflexic syncope). Alcohol and certain medications enhance the propensity to postural reflex syncope.

Post-traumatic syncope occurs in 5.6% of cranial trauma. It is more likely in adult males, and occurs within hours or weeks of the event in most cases. It is usually a transient phenomenon. Micturition syncope occurs at the beginning, during or immediately after micturition and affects males or females. Cough syncope is thought not to include a vagal component, but to be caused by a reduction in perfusion. Carotid sinus syncope occurs in individuals with hypersensitivity to carotid sinus stimulation.

Breath-holding attacks in young children may lead to syncope if severe. Pallid and cyanotic attacks are described.

Investigations of syncope may be performed in selected cases in controlled settings and include tilt-testing, Valsalva's manoeuvre and ocular compression.

Transient ischaemic attacks

This term is used to imply a focal disturbance of cerebral circulation, rather than the more global impairment seen in syncope. Disturbances affecting one hemisphere are not associated with loss of consciousness. Symptoms are more likely to be negative (loss of function), although positive phenomena can occur, mainly sensory and rarely motor (limb shaking or repetitive involuntary movements). Vertebrobasilar ischaemia is usually associated with other disturbances of brainstem function (bilateral facial or limb sensory or motor symptoms, diplopia, visual disturbance, unsteadiness, vertigo). Transient ischaemic attacks do not evolve over time in the same manner as epileptic seizures and are usually longer lasting. They are at their worst immediately and then gradually resolve.

Transient global amnesia

These episodes typically have an acute onset, last for hours and the amnesia is retrograde and anterograde. Consciousness is preserved. Patients' behaviour can seem superficially normal. Of 114 patients who fulfilled the criteria for transient global amnesia, which excluded patients known to have active epilepsy and episodes of amnesia, only eight (7%) developed epilepsy on follow-up. These patients were more likely to have recurrent or brief attacks lasting less than 1 h.

Migraine

Attacks of migraine with focal neurological symptoms or signs can be difficult to distinguish from partial epilepsy, particularly those with occipital manifestations. Syncope may occur in migraine. Visual prodromes in migraine characteristically last 5–20 min and spread slowly, and the time course is usually sufficient to differentiate migraine from epilepsy. There may be recognized precipitants and a family history. Headache is common in migraine and also postictally in epilepsy. Occasionally, migraine will precipitate and lead on to a genuine epileptic seizure (convulsive migraine).

Cataplexy

This involves sudden loss of tone, which may lead to drop attacks with no associated loss of consciousness. More minor attacks with loss of tone in only neck or facial muscles also occur. The attacks are usually precipitated by laughter or by emotion and are associated with narcolepsy, sleep paralysis and hypnagogic hallucination. There is an association with the human leucocyte antigen DR2 (HLA-DR2).

Acute rise in intracerebral pressure

Tumours of the third ventricle may present with episodes of loss of tone (drop attacks), loss of consciousness, visual disturbance or headache. Although rare, they are potentially life-threatening and should be excluded by urgent neuroimaging. Abnormalities causing brainstem distortion, such as Arnold–Chiari malformations, may rarely present with sudden loss of consciousness or drop attacks.

Parasomnias and normal physiological movements in sleep

Normal physiological movements in sleep include whole-body (hypnic) jerks, fragmentary physiological myoclonus and periodic movements of sleep. The latter are common with increasing age and are particularly associated with restless-leg syndrome.

Parasomnias may be divided into REM and non-REM forms. The latter include sleepwalking and night terrors arising from slow-wave sleep at least

30 min, but not usually more than 4 h, after sleep commenced. Night terrors usually occur in childhood, are infrequent and often occur only at times of stress or when sleeping in a strange bed. The attacks are characterized by sudden awakening, intense fear and autonomic changes, and a sensation of a frightening dream or experience. It may be difficult to arouse the child and there may be some momentary confusion. Vocalization—often a scream—is very common. Brief episodes may mimic complex partial seizures. Sleepwalking can be prolonged and injury can occur. The differentiation for an epileptic fugue though is usually straightforward.

REM parasomnias are most common in the middle-aged or elderly. The sufferer may call out, thrash about or display directed violence in the early hours (later portion of sleep). The normal atonia that occurs in REM sleep is lacking. Attacks last minutes or seconds. If awoken, the patient may recall dream fragments. If left undisturbed, the patient will usually not awaken. There is an association with drugs, alcohol and degenerative central nervous system disorders, although they may also occur in otherwise healthy subjects.

Vestibular disorders

Although vertigo may be a feature of a temporal or parietal epileptic seizure, it is much more commonly caused by peripheral vestibular disease. Associated symptoms, if present, are helpful in distinguishing the two, but where vertigo is the only symptom differentiation may be difficult. Ménière's disease is occasionally mistaken for epilepsy.

Hyperekplexia

This must be differentiated from startle epilepsy. In startle epilepsy, spontaneous seizures and EEG changes are often present. Hyperekplexia is associated with neonatal hypertonia and is an autosomal dominant disorder. Excessive startle to sudden auditory or tactile stimuli occurs. Attacks consist of intense brief generalized hypertonia and collapse which can closely mimic tonic seizures. The attacks are precipitated by startle or by a sudden noise or unexpected touch. The condition, which responds to clonazepam, has been mapped to chromosome 5q.

Tonic seizures in multiple sclerosis

Multiple sclerosis (MS) can cause epilepsy. It can also cause non-epileptic tonic attacks. These usually occur in known MS and are rarely the presenting feature. They can mimic supplementary motor, tonic or focal motor seizures.

Cardiac dysrhythmia

Transient cardiac dysrhythmias can cause episodes of abrupt loss of consciousness (cardiac syncope). Prodromal features sometimes include palpitations, chest pain and shortness of breath, but often the attacks occur without warning. The attacks are usually short and recovery quick. Stokes–Adams attacks are especially commonly confused with epilepsy. Other types of dysrhythmia causing loss of consciousness include ventricular tachycardia or fibrillation. In contrast, supraventricular tachycardias are usually well tolerated unless there is other cardiovascular disease, and can persist for hours or days. Occasionally, cardiac dysrhythmia results in focal neurological disturbance, presumably caused by critical hypoperfusion of specific brain regions. Cardiac valve disease, especially mitral valve prolapse and aortic stenosis, can present with cardiac syncope.

Microsleeps

These are brief daytime naps lasting for a few seconds. They are often consequential upon impaired night sleep resulting from other disorders, the most important being obstructive sleep apnoea. This occurs most commonly in middle age and in obese persons with short necks, reduced oropharyngeal space or other upper respiratory tract problems. The condition is commonly exacerbated by alcohol. There is usually a history of severe snoring. Airflow may cease during sleep many times for 10–30 s causing numerous arousals during sleep and preventing sustained periods of deeper sleep. Narcolepsy can cause brief episodes of sleep which are occasionally misinterpreted as epilepsy.

Hypoglycaemia

Hypoglycaemic attacks causing loss of consciousness are rare, usually occurring iatrogenically in patients with treated diabetes mellitus or due to an insulin secreting tumour, or the malicious injection of insulin. The attacks are usually preceded by a prodromal period of tachycardia, sweating and lightheadedness, a feeling of hunger and faintness, irritability, mood change, bizarre or irrational behaviour, or involuntary movements. This prodromal period can persist for some minutes and, if glucose is taken, the attacks can be aborted.

Involuntary movement disorders and other neurological conditions

Episodic involuntary movement disorders are occasionally confused with epilepsy. The most common is paroxysmal kinesogenic choreoathetosis. These attacks are precipitated by sudden and specific movements, they are of short duration (a few seconds to minutes) and consciousness is fully preserved. The movements are dystonic or clonic, and vary considerably from case to case, although for an individual, are stereotyped. Some cases are due to an inherited channelopathy. Sometimes patients with idiopathic torsion dystonia, Wilson's disease or, rarely, other movement disorders show severe acute exacerbations which mimic convulsions. People with learning difficulty often have stereotyped or repetitive movements, which may include head banging or body rocking, in daytime or in sleep, and these can be difficult to differentiate from epilepsy. Tics can also be mistaken for partial seizures. They are stereotyped movements which are usually restricted to one particular action (e.g. eyeblink) but may be multiple in nature. Consciousness is not lost, and the tics can usually be temporarily voluntarily suppressed at the cost of a rise in psychological tension and anxiety that is then relieved by the patient allowing the tics to recur.

Drop attacks

Sudden falling (drop attack) is unusual in epilepsy without other diagnostic features. The most common non-epileptic form is the so-called idiopathic drop attack, which is characterized by sudden falling without loss of consciousness particularly in elderly or middle-aged females. Characteristically, the patients remember falling and hitting the ground. Recovery is instantaneous but injury may occur. The pathogenesis of such attacks is uncertain. Vertebrobasilar ischaemia probably accounts for very few drop attacks. This condition occurs in the elderly, with evidence of vascular disease and cervical spondylosis, and the attacks can be precipitated by head turning or neck extension. Other brainstem symptoms or signs may be present. Other non-epileptic conditions which manifest as drop attacks include vasovagal syncope, cardiac syncope, hyperekplexia, myoclonus, falls in extrapyramidal disease, cataplexy, midline cerebral structural abnormalities or third ventricular tumours and vestibular disorders.

Psychotic hallucinations and delusions

Hallucinations and delusions are the hallmark of psychotic illnesses, but can be mistaken for epilepsy. Psychotic episodes occur without insight, are usually more long-lasting than isolated epileptic seizures, and have a more complex nature with an evolving or pseudological theme, are commonly auditory, involve ideas of reference, instructions or third-person language, have paranoid content or associated thought disorder. Ruminations and pseudohallucinations can occur in obsessive–compulsive and affective disorders.

Fugue states. Non-epileptic fugue is commonly caused either by alcoholism or by psychogenic causes. The context of the fugue will usually allow a diagnosis to be made, although occasionally differentiation from non-convulsive status epilepticus can be difficult. The episodes can be brief or very prolonged, lasting for days or even weeks. True amnesia is a feature only of non-convulsive status, although amnesia will often be incomplete in this condition. If seen at the time of an episode of psychogenic fugue, inconsistencies are often found on examination of the mental state, and an EEG will be unremarkable. In non-convulsive status, confusion will usually be evident.

Panic attacks, pseudoseizures and hyperventilation

These can all be difficult to differentiate from complex partial seizures. Panic attacks comprise symptoms referable to hyperventilation, autonomic system activation and to anxiety. Features include dissociation, loss of contact, faintness, dizziness, light-headedness, orofacial and/or peripheral paraesthesia, carpopedal spasm, twitching of the peripheries, blurred vision or nausea. Often, but not always, there is a clear precipitant, such as a crowded space, supermarket, lift, public transport, emotional experience or tension. Hyperventilation has similar precipitants and has overlapping features, including a feeling of faintness, dissociation, weakness, fatigue and perioral and orofacial paraesthesia.

Pseudoseizures (non-epileptic attack disorder, NEAD), broadly speaking, fall into two main categories: (i) attacks of motionless collapse; and (ii) attacks with motor phenomena. The former are often prolonged, continuing for minutes or sometimes hours and such a phenomenon is rare in epileptic seizures. It is often possible to demonstrate partial awareness (e.g. the resistance to eye opening). Tone is usually flaccid and attacks are sometimes triggered by external events or stress. The latter attacks also differ from epileptic attacks in important ways. There is often a slow build-up, and periods of motor activity which wax and wane. Movements can include semipurposeful thrashing of all four limbs, prominent pelvic movements and back arching. During attacks, patients may resist eye opening and show signs of volition or semipurposeful movement on examination. Urinary incontinence is uncommon but may occur, as can self injury. The rate of recovery is variable but usually faster than would be expected in an epileptic seizure. The longer the duration of such episodes the less likely they are to be epileptic. Patients with pseudoseizures often have a history of abnormal illness behaviour or previous psychiatric disturbance. This condition is much more common in females than males and usually commences in adolescence or early adulthood. A history of childhood abuse is common. Videotapes of seizures obtained using a handheld camcorder can provide useful diagnostic data. Some patients have both epileptic and non-epileptic attacks, but usually one type clearly predominates.

FURTHER READING

Annegers, J.F., Hauser, W.A., Coan, S.P. & Rocca, W.A. (1998) A population-based study of seizures after traumatic brain injuries. *N Engl J Med*, **338**, 20–4.

Berg, A.T., Shinnar, S., Darefsky, A.S. *et al.* (1997) Predictors of recurrent febrile seizures. A prospective cohort study. *Arch Pediatr Adolesc Med*, **151**, 371–8.

Berkovic, S.F., Anderman, F., Carpenter, S. & Wolfe, L.S. (1989) Progressive myoclonus epilepsies: specific causes and diagnosis. *N Engl J Med*, **315** (5), 296–305.

Bittencourt, P.R.M., Gracia, C.M., & Lorenzana, P. (1988) Epilepsy and parasitosis of the central nervous system. In: *Recent Advances in Epilepsy 4* (eds Pedley, T.A. & Meldrum, B.S.), pp. 123–159. Churchill Livingstone, Edinburgh.

Carpio, A., Escobar, A. & Hauser, W.A. (1998) Cysticercosis and epilepsy: a critical review. *Epilepsia*, **39**, 1025–40.

Cockerell, O.C., Eckle, I., Goodridge, D.M.G., Sander, J.W.A.S. & Shorvon, S.D. (1995) Epilepsy in a population of 6000 re-examined: secular trends in first attendance rates, prevalence and prognosis. *J Neurol Neurosurg Psychiatry*, **58**, 570–6.

Commission on Classification and Terminology of the International League Against Epilepsy (1981) Proposal for revised clinical and electroencephalographic classification of epileptic seizures. *Epilepsia*, **22**, 489–501.

Commission on Classification and Terminology of the International League Against Epilepsy (1989) Proposal for classification of epilepsies and epileptic syndromes. *Epilepsia*, **26** (3), 268–78.

Duncan, J.S. & Panayiotopoulous, C.P. (1995) Juvenile absence epilepsy: an alternative view. In: *Typical Absences and Related Epileptic Syndromes*, pp. 161–7. Churchill Communications Europe, London.

Duncan, J.S. & Panayiotopoulous, C.P. (eds) (1995) *Typical Absences and Related Epileptic Syndromes*. Churchill Communications Europe, London.

Elmslie, F. & Gardiner, M. (1995) Genetics of the epilepsies. *Curr Opin Neurol*, **8**, 126–9.

Engel, J., Pedley, T.A. (1997) *Epilepsy: a comprehensive textbook*, Lippincott Raven, Philadelphia.

European Chromosome 16 Tuberous Sclerosis Consortium: Nellist, M., Janssen, B., Brook-Carter, P.T. *et al.* (1993) Identification and characterization of the tuberous sclerosis gene of chromosome 16. *Cell*, **75**, 1305–15.

Foy, P.M., Chadwick, D.W., Rajgopalan, N., Johnson, A.L. & Shaw, M.D.M. (1992) Do prophylactic anticonvulsant drugs alter the pattern of seizures after craniotomy? *J Neurol Neurosurg Psychiatry*, **55**, 753–7.

Gardiner, M., Sandford, A., Deadman, M. *et al.* (1990) Batten disease (Spielmeyer–Vogt disease, juvenile onset neuronal ceroid-lipofuscinosis) gene (CLN3) maps to human chromosome 16. *Genomics*, **8**, 387–90.

Hopkins, A. (1995) The causes of epilepsy, the risk factors for epilepsy and the precipitation of seizures. In: *Epilepsy*, 2nd edn (eds Hopkins, A., Shorvon, S.D. & Cascino, G.), pp. 59–85. Chapman and Hall, London.

Jennett, W.B. (1982) Post-traumatic epilepsy. In: *A Textbook of Epilepsy*, 2nd edn (eds Laidlaw, J. & Richens, A.), pp. 146–54. Churchill Livingstone, London.

McKusick, V.A. (1994) *Mendelian Inheritance in Man: Catalogs of Autosomal Dominant, Autosomal Recessive and X-linked Phenotypes*, 7th edn. Johns Hopkins Press, Baltimore.

Panayiotopoulos, C.P., Obeid, T. & Waheed, G. (1989) Differentiation of typical absences in epileptic syndromes. A video EEG study of 224 seizures in 20 patients. *Brain*, **112**, 1039–56.

Raymond, A.A., Halpin, S.F.S., Alsanjari, N. *et al.* (1994) Dysembryoplastic neuroepithelial tumours, features in 16 patients. *Brain*, **117**, 461–75.

Roger, J., Bureau, M., Dravet, Ch., Dreifuss, F.E., Perret, A. & Wolf, P. (eds) (1992) *Epileptic Syndromes in Infancy, Childhood and Adolescence*. John Libbey, London.

Sander, J.W.A.S., Hart, Y.M., Johnson, A.L. & Shorvon, S.D. (1990) National General Practice Study of Epilepsy: newly diagnosed epileptic seizures in general population. *Lancet*, **336**, 1267–70.

Shorvon, S.D. (1994) Status occurring in the late childhood and adult life. In: *Status Epilepticus*, pp. 84–98. Cambridge University Press, Cambridge.

Shorvon, S.D. (1995) Epilepsy and driving. *Br Med J*, **310**, 885–6.

Shorvon, S.D., Dreifuss, F., Fish, D. & Thomas, D. (eds) (1996) *The Treatment of Epilepsy*. Blackwell Science, Oxford.

Sung, C.Y. & Chu, N.S. (1990) Epileptic seizures in elderly people: aetiology and seizure type. *Age Ageing*, **19**, 25–30.

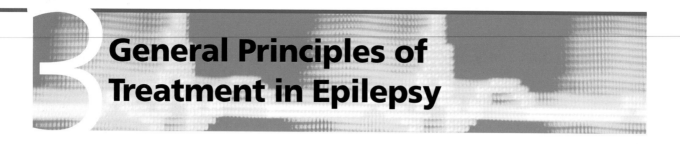

General Principles of Treatment in Epilepsy

PHARMACOKINETIC PRINCIPLES

To use drugs effectively, the prescriber should be aware of certain pharmacokinetic principles. These are enumerated here; to ignore, in routine clinical practice, these elements of simple pharmacology will expose a patient to potential risks and inefficiencies.

Drug absorption

Oral absorption

This process depends both on the physical and pharmacological properties of the drug and biological properties of the person to whom it is administered. Physical properties include the formulation of the tablets, the lipid solubility, the binding and the degree of ionization at the pH levels in the gastrointestinal tract. Solutions are usually rather more quickly absorbed than tablets or capsules. The movement from gastrointestinal tract to plasma for most drugs is a passive process which depends on: (i) the concentration gradient across the gut membrane; (ii) the lipid solubility of the drug. As the non-ionized form of the drug is generally the most lipid-soluble, absorption is quickest of drugs which are not ionized at physiological pH level; and (iii) the absorption area, and time in contact with the absorption surface. Although acidic drugs are less ionized in the stomach than in the small intestine, most orally administered drugs, whether acidic or basic, depend largely on small intestine for absorption because of the very large absorptive area of the small intestine. Several antiepileptics are absorbed by an active transport system (e.g. gabapentin and possibly, phenytoin). The gabapentin absorption mechanism has a limited capacity and higher doses may saturate the system. At saturated levels, further increases in dose do not greatly increase drug uptake. The following measures are important aspects to consider for any drug being administered orally.

pKa. The pH at which there is maximum ionization.

The equation pH = pKa + Log [ionized/total drug] will provide the concentration of drug available for absorption in the gastrointestinal tract environment with its varying pH levels. Some drugs have different structural properties at different pH and may have different pKa values for each structural subtype.

Oral bioavailability. This is the proportion of the oral dose that is absorbed and therefore available for use by the body (Table 3.1). It is important to know to what extent factors such as age, gender or food taken with the drug alter its bioavailability. For drugs requiring an active system for absorption, the bioavailability may be reduced at higher doses as the system becomes saturated (e.g. as for gabapentin). Because of the dependence of absorption on gut motility, drugs with a low bioavailability tend to show high dose-to-dose variability of absorption. Motility is also reduced in some gastrointestinal diseases and in acute illness. Certain drugs interact with antiepileptics to reduce absorption, an example is the interaction of antacids and phenytoin. Several hours should elapse between taking individual drugs which have the potential to interact.

T_{max}. The time taken for peak serum levels to be reached following oral ingestion (Table 3.2). This reflects a balance of absorption, distribution and elimination, and is in effect the beginning of the time when elimination exceeds absorption. For practical purposes, for most drugs the rate of absorption is, however, the major factor. At steady state, T_{max} is earlier than after the initial dose, as a result of higher tissue concentrations and also autoinduction; the importance of the latter is shown with carbamazepine, where initial T_{max} can be 10–24 h and the T_{max} at steady state 1–3 h.

Modified-release formulations. The absorption of the standard preparation of many antiepileptics is relatively fast. Modified release formulations can be used to slow down absorption for more prolonged effect

Table 3.1 Bioavailability of drugs.

Drug	Oral bioavailability
Carbamazepine	75–85%
Clobazam	90%
Clonazepam	>80%
Ethosuximide	<100%
Felbamate	90%
Gabapentin	60%
Lamotrigine	<100%
Levetiracetam	<100%
Oxcarbazepine	<100%
Phenobarbital	80–100%
Phenytoin	95%
Piracetam	<100%
Primidone	<100%
Tiagabine	96%
Topiramate	<100%
Valproate	<100%
Vigabatrin	<100%

or to produce less fluctuation in serum level. The slow (or controlled) release formulations are manufactured by such devices as coating the tablets in an acid-insoluble covering, increasing the size of the drug particles or embedding the drug in a matrix. The bioavailability of such preparations can differ from that of the unmodified parent. The slow release formulation of carbamazepine, for example, is 30% less bioavailable than the standard preparation.

Generic formulations. Generic formulations of a compound are required to have a bioavailability which is approximately similar to the proprietary compound. Rates of absorption, however, do vary

Table 3.2 Time taken for drugs to reach peak levels.

Drug	Time to peak levels
Carbamazepine	4–8 h
Clobazam	1–4 h
Clonazepam	1–4 h
Ethosuximide	<4 h
Felbamate	1–4 h
Gabapentin	2–4 h
Lamotrigine	1–3 h
Levetiracetam	0.6–1.3 h
Oxcarbazepine	4–5 h
Phenobarbital	1–3 h (but variable)
Phenytoin	8–12 h
Piracetam	30–40 min
Primidone	3 h
Tiagabine	1 h
Topiramate	2 h
Valproate	1–8 h (dependent on formulation
Vigabatrin	2 h

somewhat, even if the extent of absorption does not. For all but the occasional patient, generic formulations are perfectly acceptable, and the reader is advised to ignore the commercially driven research which purports to show otherwise. Only in the case of phenytoin, at levels close to saturation, do generics pose any particular problem in epilepsy, and even then serum level monitoring can guide dosage.

Rectal administration

Some drugs are readily absorbed by the rectal mucosa. This is an important mode of administration in emergency practice, as the rate of absorption is often very rapid. Solutions are better absorbed than lipid-based suppositories. The conveniently packaged Stesolid preparation of diazepam is a good example of a valuable liquid formulation which has greatly improved the therapy of febrile seizures; in contrast the wax-based diazepam suppository is absorbed rectally much too slowly.

Parenteral administration

Most antiepileptics cannot be given by intramuscular administration, as the rate of absorption is inadequate. Only phenobarbital or midazolam are usefully given intramuscularly, for emergency therapy. Phenytoin, which crystallizes at tissue pH, can result in muscle necrosis. Intravenous administration is possible for many antiepileptics and special formulations are available to minimize thrombophlebitis and other local complications (e.g. the Diazemuls formulation of diazepam and the fosphenytoin formulation of phenytoin).

Drug distribution

Once in the plasma, drug molecules are available for transfer to other body areas ('compartments'); the resulting drug concentrations at different sites is determined by the process of distribution. Drug distribution is complex, depending on diverse factors, some of which differ over time in the same individual. Distribution to most sites is by concentration-driven passive transfer across lipid membranes. Lipid solubility is an important determinant of this. The more lipid-soluble the drug, the greater its penetration into tissue. The blood–brain barrier has particularly tight intercellular junctions and only lipid-soluble drugs are able to cross to enter the brain. A few antiepileptic drugs, for instance vigabatrin, have an active transport system across the blood–brain barrier. Other lipid tissue (e.g. muscle and fat) compete with the brain for lipid-soluble drugs, and the concentration of a drug in any one compartment will depend on equilibrium with the others. The distribution of less lipid-soluble drugs may depend on blood flow through an organ (e.g. intravenous phenobarbital into the brain during status epilepticus). Mathematical modelling of drug concentrations in the various compartments is possible but, in routine clinical practice, a detailed understanding of drug distribution is necessary only in the emergency situation (e.g. in status epilepticus). The amount of drug available for distribution is the free fraction in the plasma, which is considerably lower than total plasma concentrations for protein-bound drugs (e.g. valproate, phenytoin).

Apparent volume of distribution (V_d)

This is a proportionality constant which provides an estimate of the extent of distribution of the drug in tissues (Table 3.3). It is defined as the volume of fluid which would be required to contain the drug if a single compartment were assumed (i.e. if the body was simply a bag of fluid). The larger the volume of distribution, the greater the distribution in tissues, and the greater the risk of accumulation. Thus, if V_d is approximately 0.05 L/kg (5% of body volume) for a drug confined to the vascular compartment; 0.15 L/kg for a drug confined to the extracellular water; 0.5 L/kg for a drug distributed throughout the total body water. Higher values indicate that the drug is concentrated in tissue. V_d can also be used to estimate peak plasma level after the initial dose (very approximately equal to dose/V_d).

Protein binding (Table 3.4)

The protein binding of a drug is defined as the pro-

Table 3.3 Volume of distribution of drugs.

Drug	Volume of distribution (L/kg)
Carbamazepine	0.8–1.2
Clobazam	–
Clonazepam	2.0
Ethosuximide	0.65
Felbamate	0.75
Gabapentin	0.9
Lamotrigine	0.9–1.3
Levetiracetam	0.5–0.7
Oxcarbazepine	0.3–0.8
Phenobarbital	0.42–0.75
Phenytoin	0.5–0.8
Piracetam	0.6
Primidone	0.6–1.0 (derived phenobarbital)
Tiagabine	1.0
Topiramate	0.6–1.0
Valproate	0.1–0.4
Vigabatrin	0.8

Table 3.4 Proportion of total plasma concentration bound to plasma proteins.

Drug	Protein binding (%)
Carbamazepine	75
Clobazam	83
Clonazepam	86
Ethosuximide	Nil
Felbamate	20–25
Gabapentin	Nil
Lamotrigine	55
Levetiracetam	Nil
Oxcarbazepine	38 (MHD)
Phenobarbital	45–60
Phenytoin	70–95
Piracetam	Nil
Primidone	25 primidone; 45–60 derived phenobarbital
Tiagabine	96
Topiramate	15
Valproate	85–95
Vigabatrin	Nil

portion of the total plasma concentration which is bound chemically to plasma proteins. The bound portion is not available for distribution. Plasma protein binding alters in disease states (e.g. hepatic or renal disease), and tends to fall with age. There can be competition for binding sites between drugs, and this is an important mechanism for drug interaction.

Total and free antiepileptic serum level

The total serum level refers to the total plasma concentration of a drug (i.e. both its bound and unbound fractions). The free serum level is the amount of unbound drug (i.e. that available for distribution).

Drug elimination

A drug is cleared (eliminated) from the body by the processes of metabolism and excretion.

Drug metabolism (biotransformation)

Most antiepileptics are metabolized in the liver, by hepatocyte microsomal enzymes (Table 3.5). Metabolism is frequently in two phases. Phase I is usually a process of oxidation, reduction or hydroxylation. The metabolites are usually less biologically active—although this is not always the case (e.g. phenobarbital from primidone, desmethylclobazam from clobazam). Most oxidation processes are carried out by the cytochrome microsomal P450 enzyme system. Valproate oxidation is via a non-microsomal branched-chain fatty acid system enzyme involving monoamine oxidase. In phase II, the resulting me-

Table 3.5 Biotransformation and excretion of antiepileptic drugs.

Drug	Metabolism and excretion
Carbamazepine	Hepatic epoxidation and then conjugation
Clobazam	Hepatic oxidation and then conjugation
Clonazepam	Hepatic reduction and then acetylation
Ethosuximide	Hepatic oxidation and then conjugation
Felbamate	Hepatic hydroxylation and then conjugation (60%); renal excretion as unchanged drug (40%)
Gabapentin	Renal excretion without metabolism
Lamotrigine	Hepatic glucuronidation (without phase I reaction)
Levetiracetam	Partially hydrolysed in the blood to inactive compound
Oxcarbazepine	Hepatic hydroxylation then conjugation
Phenobarbital	Hepatic oxidation, glucosidation and hydroxylation, then conjugation
Phenytoin	Hepatic oxidation, glucosidation and hydroxylation, then conjugation
Piracetam	Renal excretion without metabolism
Primidone	Metabolized to phenobarbital and phenylmethylmelanamide
Tiagabine	Hepatic oxidation then conjugation
Topiramate	Mainly renal excretion without metabolism (majority of the drug dose)
Valproate	Hepatic oxidation and then conjugation
Vigabatrin	Renal excretion without metabolism

tabolite is conjugated, usually by glucuronidization. The resulting conjugate is usually biologically inert and more polar, and therefore more easily excreted, than the parent drug. Biotransformation rather than renal excretion of unchanged drug is the main route of elimination for most antiepileptics. Pharmacokinetic drug interactions are very commonly the result of either induction of enzyme activity (including autoinduction, for instance in the case of carbamazepine) or competitive inhibition of metabolism.

Kinetics of biotransformation. Metabolism is an enzyme-catalysed process which is potentially saturable, described by the Michaelis–Menten equation:

$$V = V_{max} \, C/(Km + C)$$

where V is the velocity of the process, V_{max} is the maximum velocity possible, Km is the Michaelis–Menten constant, and C is the drug concentration. For most drugs, the required serum concentrations are well below their Km values, and in these circumstances V is virtually equal to V_{max} (i.e. metabolism is not saturated). These drugs have a linear relationship between drug dose and serum level in the ranges which are clinically useful; so-called 'first-order kinetics'. A few antiepileptic drugs, however, have levels close to saturation (e.g. phenytoin, thiopental and ethotoin). When concentrations reach levels which overwhelm the capacity of the system (i.e. where V is close to V_{max}), the velocity of metabolism cannot be increased. In this situation, such parameters as clearance and half-lives become dose-dependent, and small increases in dose may result in large and unpredictable rises in blood level.

Steady-state values. Steady-state values are those that are achieved when, for any particular drug dose, the pharmacokinetic processes reach equilibrium. In long-term treatment, steady-state values (e.g. for serum levels, clearance, V_d, half-life, T_{max}) are generally of greater use to clinicians than values for initial dosing.

Time to steady state (Tss). This is defined as the time it takes to reach steady state. It is dependent on many factors, but as a rule of thumb is equal to five times the drug's elimination half-life.

Drug excretion

Most drugs after being metabolized, are excreted via the kidney. Nearly all the various processes of renal excretion are mediated by concentration-dependent passive transfer, although acidic molecules, including the glucuronide conjugates, are also actively pumped into the proximal renal tubules. The more polar the molecule the less resorption occurs in the distal tubule. Severe renal disease affects this process and can result in impaired excretion and greater drug accumulation in the body. Mild disease rarely has any important effect on antiepileptic drug handling. Some antiepileptics are excreted without prior metabolism (e.g. gabapentin and piracetam) but most are excreted as a conjugated metabolite after hepatic biotransformation.

Drugs can also be excreted by exhalation and in tears and maternal milk. With the exception of the pulmonary excretion of gaseous anaesthetics used in status epilepticus, these routes of excretion are of no importance in regard to the antiepileptic drugs. Drug concentrations in maternal milk though do have implications for prescribing in breast-feeding women (see p. 84).

Elimination half-life (Table 3.6). This is the period of time after absorption, in which half of the drug is eliminated from the body. This depends primarily on metabolism. There can be marked interindividual variation as well as intraindividual changes over time. Drug interactions can also have marked effects on elimination half-life. About three-quarters of a drug is eliminated in two half-lives, and 15/16 of a drug in four half-lives. Once steady state has been reached, at a very rough approximation, dosing a drug at intervals equivalent to one half-life will keep trough levels within 50% of peak concentrations.

Fraction (of dose) excreted unchanged in urine ($Fu_{(x)}$). After a drug is given intravenously and the patient's urine is collected for seven half-lives, the proportion of the drug present in an unchanged form ($Fu_{(x)}$) measures the contribution of renal excretion to total drug elimination (the rest being eliminated by metabolism). If this fraction ($Fu_{(x)}$) is high, renal impairment may require drug dosage to be lowered; if it is low,

renal impairment is unlikely to seriously affect drug kinetics. Similarly, high values of $Fu_{(x)}$ imply that modification of drug dosage will be unnecessary in hepatic disease, and low $Fu_{(x)}$ values that such modification may be necessary. In the elderly, because renal excretory capacity falls, it is wise to consider lower than average doses of drugs with high $Fu_{(x)}$ values.

Clearance (Table 3.7). This is defined as the amount of drug excreted over a unit time. Plasma clearance is a measure of the amount of drug removed from the plasma. Renal clearance is a measure of the amount of drug removed by the kidneys. As a general rule, if $Fu_{(x)}$ is low, then clearance is largely dependent on hepatic metabolism; conversely, if $Fu_{(x)}$ is high, clearance is largely dependent on renal excretion. When drugs are avidly taken up by the liver, clearance values can be as high as 1.4 L/kg/h (i.e. the rate of hepatic blood flow).

Serum level measurements

When steady state has been reached, there is a fairly consistent relationship between plasma concentration and the concentration in brain, or other tissues. It should therefore be possible to define those plasma levels that are associated with optimal clinical effects (i.e. an optimal balance between effectiveness and side-effects). Because of biological variation, such levels may well vary from individual to individual, but nevertheless a range can be developed which is based on statistical or population parameters. This is the 'therapeutic range' (also known as the 'target range' or the 'optimal range').

Table 3.6 Elimination half-lives of antiepileptic drugs.

Drug	Elimination half-life (h)
Carbamazepine	5–26 (but variable)
Clobazam	10–50 (clobazam); 50 (N-desmethylclobazam)
Clonazepam	20–80
Ethosuximide	30–60
Felbamate	20 (13–30; lowest in patients comedicated with enzyme inducers)
Gabapentin	5–9
Lamotrigine	30 (monotherapy approx.); 15 (enzyme-inducing comedication); 60 (valproate comedication)
Levetiracetam	6–8
Oxcarbazepine	8–10 (MHD)
Phenobarbital	75–120
Phenytoin	7–42 (mean, 20: dependent on plasma level)
Piracetam	5–6
Primidone	5–18 primidone; 75–120 derived phenobarbital
Tiagabine	3.8–4.9
Topiramate	18–23 (varies with comedication)
Valproate	4–12
Vigabatrin	4–7

MHD, 10-monohydroxy metabolite.

Table 3.7 Plasma clearance rates of antiepileptic drugs.

Drug	Plasma clearance
Carbamazepine	0.133 L/kg/h (but very variable)
Clonazepam	0.09 L/kg/h
Ethosuximide	0.010–0.015 L/kg/h
Felbamate	0.027–0.032 L/kg/h (but variable)
Gabapentin	0.120–0.130 L/kg/h
Lamotrigine	0.044–0.084 L/kg/h
Levetiracetam	0.6 mL/min/kg
Phenobarbital	0.006–0.009 L/kg/h
Phenytoin	0.003–0.02 L/kg/h (dependent on plasma level)
Primidone	0.006–0.009 L/kg/h (derived phenobarbital)
Tiagabine	12.8 L/h
Topiramate	0.022–0.036 L/kg/h
Valproate	0.010–0.115 L/kg/h
Vigabatrin	0.102–0.114 L/kg/h

In practice, skill is needed to interpret serum drug concentrations wisely. The clinician should know when to ignore as well as heed blood level measurements. The following guidelines should be followed (Tables 3.8–3.12 and Fig. 3.1).

Timing of blood samples. Generally, blood samples should be taken at steady state (i.e. at a period greater than five times the drug's elimination half-life after any dosage change). Steady-state serum levels of

Table 3.8 The clinical utility of serum level monitoring of antiepileptic drugs.

Drug	Serum level monitoring
Carbamazepine	Useful
Clobazam	Not useful
Clonazepam	Not useful
Ethosuximide	Useful
Felbamate	Value not established
Gabapentin	Not useful
Lamotrigine	Value not established
Levetiracetam	Value not established
Oxcarbazepine	Value not established
Phenobarbital	Useful
Phenytoin	Useful
Piracetam	Not useful
Primidone	Primidone, not generally useful. Derived phenobarbital, useful
Tiagabine	Not useful
Topiramate	Not generally useful
Valproate	Not generally useful
Vigabatrin	Not useful

Table 3.9 Target range for antiepileptic drugs.

Drug	Target range (μmol/L)
Carbamazepine	20–50
Clobazam	–
Clonazepam	–
Ethosuximide	300–700
Felbamate	200–460
Gabapentin	–
Lamotrigine	4–60
Levetiracetam	–
Oxcarbazepine	50–125
Phenobarbital	40–170
Phenytoin	40–80
Piracetam	–
Primidone	<60 primidone; 40–170 derived phenobarbital
Tiagabine	–
Topiramate	6–74
Valproate	300–600
Vigabatrin	–

Table 3.10 Factors influencing antiepileptic drug levels.

Drug factors
Chemical constitution
Drug formulation
Drug interactions
Timing of blood sampling/dosage schedules

Patient factors
Genetic/constitutional factors (influenced by such factors as age, sex)
Absorption (influenced by such factors as food, gastrointestinal disease)
Metabolism (influenced by such factors as metabolic enzyme status, hepatic disease)
Distribution (influenced by serum proteins, nutritional status, body weight, pregnancy)
Excretion (influenced by such factors as renal disease)

drugs with short half-lives fluctuate through the day in patients on oral medication. Blood sampling should be taken at a similar time (the trough level—that taken before the morning dosing—is a conven-

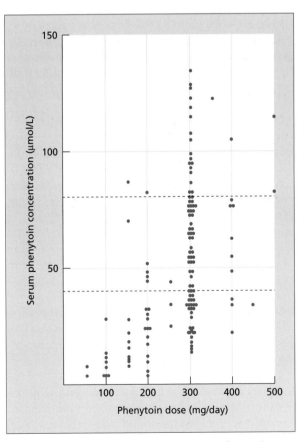

Fig. 3.1 Distribution of steady-state serum phenytoin concentrations in 131 adult epileptic patients on admission to a residential centre. Note the large variability observed in patients receiving the same dosage.

tional preference) to assess blood level changes. For drugs with a long half-life (e.g. phenobarbital) there is little diurnal fluctuation and timing is unimportant.

Rapid assay. Technology exists for rapid assay of the commonly used drugs. It can be extremely helpful to have blood level data available before a consultation, and in large clinics it is cost-effective to offer an immediate assay service (equivalent to having the blood sugar results during a diabetic clinic).

Individual drugs. The value of monitoring drug concentrations varies. A fair moment-to-moment relationship exists between response (particularly side-effects) and serum level for some drugs (notably phenytoin, carbamazepine, ethosuximide and phenobarbital). For these drugs, therefore, a serum level measurement will allow the clinician to tailor drug dosage on the basis of levels. Where such a relationship does not exist (e.g. for vigabatrin, topiramate and gabapentin) blood level monitoring has less value. Finally, monitoring is useful for drugs with non-linear kinetics in view of the sharp rises in serum levels which may occur with small dosage increases when the enzyme systems are saturated. Phenytoin is the classic example, and adjusting therapy with phenytoin almost always requires blood level surveillance.

Therapeutic range. The therapeutic range is based on population statistics. There are many individuals whose epilepsy is well controlled with 'suboptimal' levels (at least one-third of patients treated with phenytoin, for example). There are also others whose seizures are only controlled, without side-effects, at 'supra-optimal' levels. Furthermore, those with frequent seizures or those with partial epilepsy often require higher 'therapeutic ranges' than those with less severe forms of epilepsy.

Tolerance. Pharmacodynamic tolerance is common on benzodiazepine and barbiturate drugs and this will modify the serum concentration–response relationship.

Total vs. free serum drug concentrations. Routine analytical methods measure the total drug concentration (i.e. the protein-bound and unbound (free) fractions). The free fraction is available for biological action. Measurement of the total level is satisfactory as there is usually a consistent relationship between the free and the total levels. However, in

certain states this relationship can be altered (e.g. hypoalbuminaemic states, severe renal disease, severe hepatic disease, pregnancy, old age, neonatal period). In these situations the free levels may be higher than would be predicted from the total concentration, and the low total concentration may mislead clinicians. Some advocate the direct measurement of free levels in these situations, but assay techniques are difficult and in practice free-level estimations are rarely required.

Active metabolites. Some drugs are converted into active metabolites (Table 3.11), and interpretation of parent drug level measurements without accounting for the potential contribution of the active metabolite may lead to therapeutic errors. Carbamazepine is metabolized to a 10,11-epoxide which can cause side-effects similar to those of the parent drug. Measurement of the parent drug only can be misleading, especially as the proportion of carbamazepine converted to carbamazepine 10,11-epoxide can markedly vary (for instance in the presence of enzyme-inducing comedication).

Salivary vs. serum concentrations. The salivary concentration of certain drugs (e.g. ethosuximide, carbamazepine, phenytoin) correlates well with the unbound (free) serum concentration. Salivary measurements avoid the need for venepuncture and so are particularly acceptable in children. However, measurement is more difficult and more prone to error than serum measurements, and can be compli-

Table 3.11 Active metabolites of antiepileptic drugs.

Drug	Active metabolites
Carbamazepine	Carbamazepine epoxide
Clobazam	*N*-desmethylclobazam
Clonazepam	Nil
Ethosuximide	Nil
Felbamate	Nil
Gabapentin	Nil
Lamotrigine	Nil
Levetiracetam	Nil
Oxcarbazepine	10-Monohydroxy metabolite (MHD)
Phenobarbital	Nil
Phenytoin	Nil
Piracetam	Nil
Primidone	Phenobarbital
Tiagabine	Nil
Topiramate	Nil
Valproate	Nil
Vigabatrin	Nil

cated by gingivitis and dose residues in the mouth. Salivary measurements have therefore not been widely adopted. Also, with other drugs, for various pharmacological reasons, there is no consistent relationship between serum and salivary levels (e.g. phenobarbital, valproate).

In Table 3.12 the indications for blood level monitoring are given. In practice, drug level monitoring is extensively abused. Zealous adherence to the concept is inappropriate. Drug concentrations are often measured unnecessarily, or interpreted incorrectly. The latter is usually an over-interpretation of the role of the 'therapeutic range'. Common errors include:

1 increasing drug dosage in patients fully controlled simply because the serum level is below the therapeutic range;

2 lowering drug dosage in patients without side-effects because the serum level is above the therapeutic range; and

3 ignoring adverse effects because the levels are within the therapeutic range.

The importance of the maxim 'treat the patient, not the serum level' cannot be overstated (Table 3.12).

NEWLY DIAGNOSED PATIENTS

Few decisions are more critical in the course of epilepsy than the decision to initiate drug therapy. In addition to its biological effects, therapy confers illness status, confirms the state of 'being epileptic', and can affect self-esteem, social relationships, education and employment. The decision to treat depends essentially on a balance of benefit vs.

drawbacks of therapy, and should be tailored to the requirements of the individual patient; there are no inviolate rules (Table 3.13).

The balance is difficult to define. The benefits of therapy include the lower risk of recurrence of seizures, and thus of potential injury and even death, and the psychological and social benefits of more security from seizures. The drawbacks of therapy include the potential drug side-effects, the psychological and social effects, the cost, stigmatization and inconvenience. Chronic, long-term or subtle side-effects are not easily detected, and weigh heavily on the decision to treat. One example is the potential adverse effect on learning in children, and partly because of this paediatricians initiate therapy less early than adult neurologists.

Practice varies in different countries. In the USA, for instance, a higher proportion of patients are treated after a single seizure than in the UK and more often too by emergency loading therapy. Practice is also divided in Europe. The lack of consensus reflects more the differing social rather than medical contexts of therapy.

One proposition recently researched is that early effective therapy will improve long-term outcome; and thus that early antiepileptic drug therapy will prevent the establishment of chronic epilepsy. There is a striking lack of clear evidence to support this canard, and there seems no reason currently to modify the traditional approach.

Factors influencing the decision to treat

Diagnosis
It is essential to establish a firm diagnosis of epilep-

Table 3.12 Indications for serum level monitoring.

Poor response in spite of adequate dose: to identify unusual pharmacokinetic patterns or poor compliance
Physiological or pathological conditions known to be associated with altered or changing pharmacokinetics (hepatic disease, kidney disease, pregnancy, etc.)
Establishing drug toxicity
Minimizing the problems caused by non-linear kinetics with phenytoin
Minimizing the problems caused by drug interactions (e.g. to identify which drug is causing adverse reactions)
To assess changes in bioavailability caused by changes in drug formulation

Table 3.13 Criteria for starting antiepileptic drug therapy.

Diagnosis of epilepsy must be firm
Risk of recurrence of seizures must be sufficient
Seizures must be sufficiently troublesome
Type of seizures
Frequency of seizures
Severity of seizures
Timing of seizures
Precipitation of seizures
Good compliance must be likely
Patient has been fully counselled
Patient's wishes have been fully accounted for

sy before therapy is started. This is not always easy, particularly in the early stages of epilepsy. Rarely should treatment be started before a definitive diagnosis is made. There is equally almost no place at all for a 'trial of treatment' to clarify the diagnosis; it seldom does.

A good first-hand witnessed account is essential, as diagnostic tests are often non-confirmatory. Electroencephalogram, magnetic resonance imaging (MRI) scan and biochemical and haematological tests can be useful, but the differential diagnosis is wide. In practice, the misdiagnosis rate is quite high. About 20% of all patients referred to a tertiary level epilepsy service, for instance, have psychogenic attacks. The diagnosis is also often delayed. In one study, a firm diagnosis could be made within 24 months after the onset of seizures, in less than two thirds of seizures.

Risk of recurrence of seizures after a first attack

This is obviously a key factor in the decision to start therapy. Investigations have produced conflicting findings with figures varying from 27 to 84%; the differences being largely a result of methodological issues. Most would now accept that about 50–80% of all patients who have a first non-febrile seizure will have further attacks, the greatest risk being in the first 6 months after the first seizure. In a national UK study, the risk of a recurrence after the first seizure was 60% in the initial 6 months, a further 9% in the next 6 months and 8% in the following 12 months. The risk varied with aetiology and with elapsed time since first seizure (Figs 3.2 and 3.3).

The risk of recurrence is influenced by the following factors.

Aetiology. This is probably the most important factor. The risk is greater in those with structural cerebral disease, and least in acute symptomatic epilepsy. The risk of recurrence of 'idiopathic' or 'cryptogenic' seizures is approximately 50%. In those with pre-existing learning disability or cerebral damage, the risk approaches 100%.

Electroencephalogram. Informed opinion concerning the prognostic value of EEG is remarkably conflicting. While there is consensus that the risk of recurrence is high, if the first EEG shows spike and wave discharges, the predictive value of a normal EEG or an EEG with other types of abnormality is much less clear.

Age. The risk of recurrence is somewhat greater in those under the age of 16 or over the age of 60 years, probably because of the confounding effect of aetiology, especially so because acute symptomatic seizures with their good prognosis are more common in young adult life.

Seizure type. Partial seizures are more likely to recur than generalized seizures, again because of the confounding effect of aetiology.

The risk of recurrence after a second attack has not been extensively studied, although is almost certainly higher than after a first attack.

Type, timing and frequency of seizures

Some types of epileptic seizure have a minimal impact on the quality of life; for example, simple par-

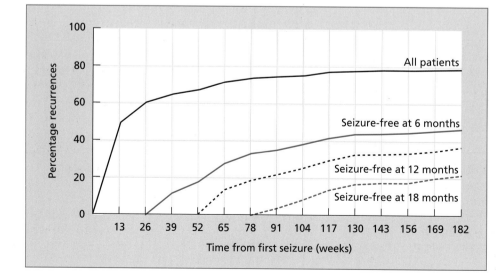

Fig. 3.2 National General Practice Study of Epilepsy (NGPSE): actuarial percentage of recurrence after first seizure. A study of 564 patients followed prospectively from the time of diagnosis. Within 3 years of the first seizure, 78% of patients had a recurrence of their attacks. If attacks had not recurred within 6, 12 or 18 months, the chance of recurrence was substantially reduced, falling to 44, 32 and 17%, respectively.

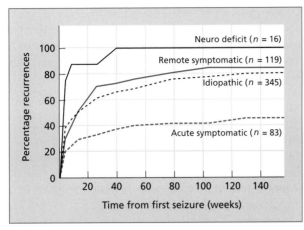

Fig. 3.3 Actuarial percentage recurrences after first seizure by aetiological category.

tial seizures, absence or sleep attacks. The benefits of treating such seizures, even if happening frequently, can be outweighed by the disadvantages.

If the baseline seizure frequency is very low, the disadvantages of treatment can be unacceptably high. It would certainly be unusual to treat a person having less than one seizure a year, especially if this was confined to sleep and a minor or partial seizure.

Type of epilepsy
Some benign epilepsy syndromes have an excellent prognosis without therapy (e.g. benign rolandic epilepsy) and do not require long-term therapy.

Compliance
Antiepileptic drugs need to be taken reliably and regularly to be effective and to avoid adverse events or withdrawal seizures. The decision to treat should be reconsidered in all circumstances in which compliance is likely to be poor.

Reflex seizures and acute symptomatic seizures
Occasionally, seizures occur only in specific circumstances or with certain precipitants (e.g. photosensitivity, fatigue, alcohol). Avoiding these circumstances may obviate the need for drug treatment.

Patient's wishes
Individuals differ greatly in their views about epilepsy and its treatment. The role of the physician is to explain the relative advantages and disadvantages of therapy; the final decision must be left to the patient.

Protocol for initial treatment
It will be clear that there can be no absolute rules about when to start therapy and when not to do so. In general terms, if there is a risk of recurrence of convulsive seizures or seizures with risk of injury or death, treatment will be indicated. In all other circumstances, however, the requirement to initiate therapy can be quite individual. Where seizures are infrequent and minor, where non-convulsive seizures occur exclusively at night, or in the benign syndromes of childhood epilepsy, treatment is often not indicated at all even in established cases. In all situations, the patient should be given advice based on available data and allowed to make the final decision.

A protocol for the initial treatment in newly diagnosed patients is shown in Table 3.14. This scheme will take a number of months to complete, the time depending largely on the seizure frequency. It will require patience and tenacity. The procedure should be explained in advance to the patient to maintain confidence and compliance. It will require the expenditure of time and effort by the doctor, who should be available throughout for guidance and reassurance. Perseverance brings rewards, though, and most people will, following this protocol, become established on effective long-term therapy.

Outcome of therapy
The outcome of therapy in newly diagnosed cases is generally good. In about 70–80% of those developing epilepsy, seizures will cease, usually within the first few years of treatment. If seizures stop, the risk of subsequent recurrence is low (approximately 10% after a 5-year period without attack), and most patients will eventually be able to discontinue medication. About two-thirds of patients started on therapy will enter a 1-year remission within a year of initiating treatment and three-quarters will be in 3-year remission 5 years after starting therapy.

The prognosis is worse if any of the following factors apply: structural cerebral disease; partial seizures; severe epilepsy syndromes; a family history of epilepsy; a high frequency of tonic–clonic seizures before therapy; or neurological or psychiatric handicaps. Of these, the aetiology of the epilepsy is probably the most important influence on outcome. Certain structural cerebral conditions are almost invariably associated with poor prognosis and then are predictable outcomes from other aetiologically well-defined syndromes. Electroencephalogram findings (positive or negative), conversely, have generally been shown to be a poor indicator of prognosis.

Table 3.14 Protocol for treatment of newly diagnosed patients.

---

1 Establish diagnosis

2 Identify precipitating factors—and counsel about avoiding these

3 Decide upon the need for antiepileptic drug treatment

4 Counsel about reasons for starting therapy:
- Goals for therapy
- Likely outcome of therapy
- Logistics of therapy
- Risks of therapy

5 Start monotherapy with the chosen first-line antiepileptic drug (Tables 3.17, 3.22), initially at low doses titrating up to a low maintenance dose. Emergency drug loading is seldom necessary in newly diagnosed epilepsy, except where status epilepticus threatens

6 If seizures continue, titrate the dose upwards to higher maintenance dose levels (guided by serum level monitoring where this is appropriate)

In about 60–70% of patients, these simple steps for initial treatment will result in good seizure control. If seizures are not controlled despite optimal doses of a first drug:

7 Alternative monotherapy should be tried with other appropriate first-line antiepileptic drugs. The second drug should be introduced incrementally at suitable dose intervals (Table 3.22) and the first drug then withdrawn in decremental steps. The second drug should be titrated first to a low maintenance dose, and then if seizures continue, the dose should be increased to maximal doses (guided by serum level monitoring where appropriate)

8 If seizures continue or recur after initial control:
- Diagnosis should be reassessed as in this situation it is not uncommon to find that the attacks do not have an epileptic basis
- Investigations should be considered to exclude the possibility of a progressive structural lesion
- Possibility of poor compliance should be explored

9 If seizures continue, other first-line drugs should be tried in monotherapy (procedures as above)

10 If seizures are controlled after steps 5, 6, 7 or 9 the drug should be continued, with serum level monitoring where appropriate, at the lowest dose which controls seizures and is without unacceptable side-effects

---

PATIENTS WITH CHRONIC AND ACTIVE EPILEPSY

Drug treatment

The goal of therapy should, generally speaking, be complete seizure control without side-effects. This is achieved with initial first-line therapy in most cases. In others it may take time to find the right medication, and seizure control may be possible only at the expense of side-effects. In some the goal cannot be realized.

Monotherapy vs. combination therapy

Single-drug therapy will provide optimal seizure control in about 80% of all patients with epilepsy, and should be chosen whenever possible. The advantages of monotherapy are:
- better tolerability and fewer side-effects;
- simpler and less intrusive regimen;
- no potential for pharmacokinetic or pharmacodynamic interactions with other antiepileptic drugs; and
- less risk of teratogenicity.

Combination therapy is needed in about 20% of all those developing epilepsy, and in a much higher proportion of those with epilepsy which has remained uncontrolled despite initial monotherapy (chronic active epilepsy). The prognosis for seizure control in these patients, even on combination therapy, is far less good. Nevertheless, skilful combination therapy can make a substantial difference by optimizing control of the epilepsy and minimizing the side-effects of treatment. The choice of drugs in combination has not been satisfactorily studied, and is rather arbitrary. There is little convincing evidence to support the recent and heavily trailed proposition that mixing drugs with differing modes of action has a synergistic effect. Patients need to be advised carefully about the implications of polytherapy in terms of drug interactions, teratogenesis and potential pharmacodynamic effects.

Treatment protocol for chronic epilepsy

When first seeing a patient with chronic uncontrolled epilepsy, the following steps should be followed (Table 3.15).

Assessment

Review the diagnosis of epilepsy. An eye-witness account of the attacks should be obtained, and the previous medical records inspected. A series of normal EEG results should alert one to the possibility that the attacks are non-epileptic, although this is not an infallible rule.

Establish aetiology. It is important at this stage to ascertain the cause of the epileptic attacks, and especially to exclude progressive pathology.

Table 3.15 Treatment of chronic active epilepsy.

Review diagnosis and aetiology
    History
    EEG
    Neuroimaging
    Other investigations

Classify epilepsy (seizure type and syndrome)

Review compliance

Review drug history
    Which AEDs were useful in the past?
    Which AEDs were not useful in the past?
    Which AEDs have not been used in the past?
    Drug and blood levels of previous therapy

Review non-pharmacological factors

Set a treatment plan
    Sequence of drug changes
    Background medication
    Sequence of addition of drugs
    Sequence of withdrawal of drugs
    Duration of treatment trials
    Serum level monitoring

Consider surgical therapy

Recognize limitations of therapy

AEDs, antiepileptic drugs.

Classify seizure type. This has some value in guiding the choice of first- and second-line drugs.

Review previous treatment history. This is an absolutely essential step, often omitted. The response to a drug is, generally speaking, relatively consistent over time. Find out which drugs have been previously tried, what was the response (effectiveness/side-effects), what was the maximum dose, why was the drug withdrawn?

Table 3.16 Methods of improving compliance.

Information to patients about drug treatment
    Role
    Limitations
    Efficacy/side-effects
Drug therapy
    Monotherapy
    Simplify drug regimens
    Drug wallet
Regular clinic follow-up
Use of cues and *aides-mémoire*

Review compliance. This may have been a reason for poor seizure control. A drug wallet, filled up for the whole week, can be a great assistance for patients who often forget to take the medication. Other methods for improving compliance are listed in Table 3.16.

Treatment

Form a treatment plan. Do this on the basis of the assessment. The plan should take the form of a series of drug combinations, to be tried in turn (treatment trials). The emphasis of this stepwise treatment plan is to try each available antiepileptic in a reasonable dose singly or as two-drug therapy or, more rarely, three-drug combinations (Table 3.17). This will involve deciding which drugs to introduce, which drugs to withdraw and which drugs to retain. Decisions will also be needed about the duration of each treatment trial. There is often a nihilistic inertia in the treatment of chronic epilepsy which should be resisted. An active and logical approach to therapy can prove very successful.

(a) Choice of drug to introduce or retain. Generally these should be drugs which are appropriate for the

Table 3.17 Antiepileptic drugs for different seizure types.

Seizure type	First line drugs	Second line drugs
Simple and complex partial seizures, primary and secondarily generalized tonic–clonic seizures	Carbamazepine, valproate and phenytoin	Acetazolamide, clobazam, clonazepam, ethosuximide, felbamate, gabapentin, lamotrigine, levetiracetam, oxcarbazepine, phenobarbital, primidone, tiagabine, topiramate, vigabatrin
Generalized absence seizures	Valproate, ethosuximide	Acetazolamide, clobazam, clonazepam, lamotrigine, phenobarbital, primidone
Atypical absence, tonic and clonic seizures	Valproate	Acetazolamide, carbamazepine, clobazam, clonazepam, ethosuximide, felbamate, lamotrigine, oxcarbazepine, phenobarbital, phenytoin, primidone, topiramate
Myoclonic seizures	Valproate	Clobazam, clonazepam, ethosuximide, lamotrigine, phenobarbital, piracetam, primidone

This is a list based upon the author's current practice. There is a dearth of good comparative data; this list is therefore, to an extent, empirical and subjective. Similar seizure types in different syndromes may, furthermore, respond in a different manner.

seizure type and which have either not been previously used in optimal doses or which have been used and did prove helpful. Rational choices depend on a well-documented history of previous drug therapy. Attention needs to be paid to drug interaction, see Table 3.18.

(b) Choice of drug to withdraw. These should be drugs which have been given an adequate trial at optimal doses and which were either ineffective or caused acceptable side-effects. There is obviously little point in continuing a drug which has had little effect, yet remarkably this is frequently done.

(c) Duration of treatment trial. This will depend on baseline seizure rates. The trial should be long enough to have differentiated the effect of therapy from that of chance fluctuations in seizures.

(d) It is usual to maintain therapy with either one or two suitable antiepileptic drugs. If drugs are being withdrawn, it is wise to maintain one drug at a good dose as an 'anchor' to cover the withdrawal period.

Drug withdrawal. Drug withdrawal needs care. The withdrawal or sudden reduction in dose of antiepileptics can result in a severe worsening of seizures or in status epilepticus—even if the withdrawn drug was apparently not contributing much to seizure control. Why this happens is not clear. Experience from telemetry units suggest that most withdrawal seizures have physiological features similar to the patient's habitual seizures. It is therefore customary, and wise, to withdraw medication slowly. This caution applies particularly to barbiturate drugs (phenobarbital, primidone), benzodiazepine drugs (clobazam, clonazepam, diazepam) and to carbamazepine. Table 3.19 lists the fastest decremental rates that are recommended in normal clinical practice. In many situations even slower rates of withdrawal are safer. The only advantage to fast withdrawal is better compliance and the faster establishment of new drug regimens. Only one drug should be withdrawn at a time. If the withdrawal period is likely to be difficult, the dangers can be reduced by covering the withdrawal with a benzodiazepine drug (usually clobazam 10 mg per day), given during the phase of active withdrawal. A benzodiazepine can also be given in clustering of seizures following withdrawal. It is sometimes difficult to know whether seizures during withdrawal are caused by the withdrawal or simply the background epilepsy. Whenever possible a long-term view should be taken and over-reaction in the short-term to seizures avoided. Sometimes the withdrawal of a drug will result in improved seizure control simply by improving well being, assuring better compliance and reducing interactions.

Drug addition. New drugs added to a regimen should also be introduced slowly, at least in the routine clinical situation. This results in better tolerability, and is particularly important when adding lamotrigine, topiramate, carbamazepine, primidone or benzodiazepines. Too fast an introduction of these drugs will almost invariably result in side-effects. It is usual to aim initially for a low-maintenance dose. In severe epilepsy, however, it is sometimes advisable to build up to high doses immediately.

Concomitant medication. Changing the dose of one antiepileptic, either incrementally or decrementally, can influence the levels of other drugs, and the changing levels of concomitant medication will often contribute to changing side-effects or indeed effectiveness. The serum levels or doses of concomitant antiepileptics may need to be monitored in this situation.

Limits on therapy. Drug therapy will fail in about 10–20% of patients. In this situation, the epilepsy can be categorized as 'intractable' and the goal of therapy changes to defining the best compromise between inadequate seizure control and drug-induced side-effects. Individual patients will take very different views about where to strike this balance.

Intractability is inevitably an arbitrary decision. There are over 10 widely used antiepileptic drugs, and far more combinations (with 10 first-line antiepileptic drugs there are 45 different two-drug and 36 different three-drug combinations). All combinations cannot therefore be tried. The chances of a new drug controlling seizures after five appropriate agents have failed to do so is small (less than 5%). At a pragmatic level, therefore, one can categorize an epilepsy as intractable when at least five of the major antiepileptics have proved ineffective in adequate doses. A recent excellent suggestion is to define intractability by the number of ineffective drugs tried; thus second-level intractability is defined as the failure of two drugs, third-level intractability by the failure of three drugs, and so on.

PATIENTS WITH EPILEPSY IN REMISSION

Most people developing epilepsy will find the seizures rapidly controlled by appropriate drug therapy. Epilepsy can be said to be in remission when

Table 3.18 The commonly encountered and significant interactions between antiepileptic drugs. (This table shows the common significant interactions in routine practice. There is however considerable interindividual variation, and in occasional cases other interactions occur. Furthermore, for some of the newer drugs, information is sparse.)

Drugs causing interaction	Drug affected by interaction																
	CBZ	CLB	CLN	ESM	FBM	GBP	LTG	LEV	OXC	PB	PHT	PIR	PRM	TGB	TOP	VPA	VIG
Carbamazepine	AI	NE	↓CLN	↓ESM	↓FBM	NE	↓LTG	NE	NE	↑PB	↑↓PHT	NE	↓PRM	↓TGB	↓TOP	↓VPA	NE
Clobazam	NE		NE	NE	NE	NE	NE	NE	NE	NE	NE	NE	NE	NE	NE	↑VPA	NE
Clonazepam	↓CBZ	NE		NE	NE	NE	NE	NE	NE	NE	↑↓PHT	NE	NE	NE	NE	NE	NE
Ethosuximide	NE	NE	NE		NE	NE	NE	NE	NE	NE	↑PHT	NE	NE	NE	NE	NE	NE
Felbamate	↓CBZ ↑CBZ-E	NE	NE	NE		NE	NE	NE	NE	↑PB	↑PHT	NE	↑PRM	NE	NE	↓VPA	NE
Gabapentin	NE	NE	NE	NE	NE		NE	NE	NE	NE	NE	NE	NE	NE	NE	NE	NE
Lamotrigine	↑CBZ-E	NE	NE	NE	NE	NE		NE	NE	NE	NE	NE	NE	NE	NE	NE	NE
Levetiracetam	NE	NE	NE	NE	NE	NE	NE		NE	NE	NE	NE	NE	NE	NE	NE	NE
Oxcarbazepine	NE	NE	NE	NE	NE	NE	NE	NE		NE	NE	NE	NE	NE	NE	NE	NE
Phenobarbital	↓CBZ	NE	↓CLN	↓ESM	↓FBM	NE	↓LTG	NE	NE		↑↓PHT	NE	NE	↓TGB	↓TOP	↓VPA	NE
Phenytoin	↓CBZ	NE	NE	↓ESM	↓FBM	NE	↓LTG	NE	NE	↓↑PB		NE	↑PRM	↓TGB	↓TOP	↓VPA	NE
Piracetam	NE	NE	NE	NE	NE	NE	NE	NE	NE	NE	NE		NE	NE	NE	NE	NE
Primidone	↓CBZ	NE	↓CLN	↓ESM	↓FBM	NE	↓LTG	NE	NE	NE	↑↓PHT	NE		↓TGB	↓TOP	↓VPA	NE
Tiagabine	NE	NE	NE	NE	NE	NE	NE	NE	NE	NE	NE	NE	NE		NE	NE	NE
Topiramate	NE	NE	NE	NE	NE	NE	NE	NE	NE	NE	↑↓PHT	NE	NE	NE		NE	NE
Valproate	↑CBZ-E	NE	NE	↑ESM	↑FBM	NE	↑LTG	NE	NE	↑PB	↑↓PHT	NE	↑PRM	NE	NE		NE
Vigabatrin	NE	NE	NE	NE	NE	NE	NE	NE	NE	NE	↓PHT	NE	NE	NE	NE	NE	

Antiepileptic drugs (with grateful acknowledgements to Dr P.N. Patsalos) Key: ↓, decreased level; ↑, increased level; NE, no interaction expected (in most cases); CBZ, carbamazepine; CBZ-E, carbamazepine epoxide; CLB, clobazam; CLN, clonazepam; ESM, ethosuximide; FBM, felbamate; GBP, gabapentin; LEV, leviteracetam; LTG, lamotrigine; OXC, oxcarbazepine; PB, phenobarbital; PHT, phenytoin; PIR, piracetam; PRM, primidone; TGB, tiagabine; TOP, topiramate; VPA, valproate; VIG, vigabatrin.

Table 3.19 Fastest recommended decremental rates of drug withdrawal in seizure-free patients.

Drug	Dose decrement every 4 weeks (mg/day)
Carbamazepine	200
Clobazam	10
Clonazepam	1
Ethosuximide	250
Felbamate	300
Gabapentin	400
Lamotrigine	100
Levetiracetam	500
Oxcarbazepine	300
Phenobarbital	30
Phenytoin	50
Piracetam	1600
Primidone	125
Tiagabine	10
Topiramate	100
Valproate	200
Vigabatrin	500

seizures have not occurred for long time periods (conventionally 2 years or 5 years). The drug treatment of such patients is the subject of this section.

Regular monitoring of patients in remission

On-going therapy is usually straightforward. Drug doses should be minimized, and it is usually possible to avoid major adverse effects. In most cases, little medical input is required with appropriate care provided at primary care level. The seizure type, epilepsy syndrome, aetiology, investigations and previous treatment should be recorded. Routine haematological or biochemical monitoring is usually not necessary in an asymptomatic individual. At some point, though, the calm of this ideal situation is likely to be disturbed by the question of discontinuation of therapy.

Discontinuation of drug treatment

It is often difficult to decide when, if ever, to discontinue drug treatment. The decision should be made by a specialist who is able to provide an estimate of the risk of reactivation of the epilepsy. This risk is influenced by the factors listed below, but it must be stressed that withdrawal is never entirely risk-free. The decision whether or not to withdraw ther-

apy will depend on the level of risk the individual patient is prepared to accept.

Probability of remaining seizure-free after drug withdrawal

The best information comes from the Medical Research Council (MRC) antiepileptic drug withdrawal study, which included 1013 patients who had been seizure-free for 2 years or more. Within 2 years of starting drug withdrawal 59% remained seizure free, compared to 79% of those who opted to stay on therapy. Other studies have had essentially similar findings. Certain factors influence the risk of recurrence (Fig. 3.4 and Table 3.20).

Period of seizure freedom. The longer the patient is seizure-free, the less is the chance of relapse. A 5-year period of seizure freedom will reduce the risk of relapse on drug withdrawal to less than 10%.

Duration of active epilepsy. This is probably an understudied factor. One has a strong impression that the shorter the history of active seizures (i.e. the

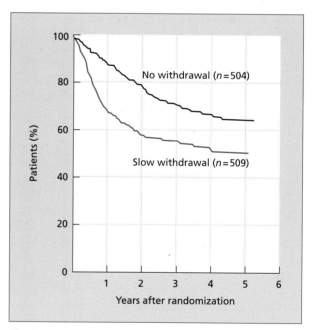

Fig. 3.4 Actuarial percentage of patients seizure-free amongst those randomized to continuing or to slow withdrawal of antiepileptic drugs. A study of 1013 patients seizure-free for at least 2 years, randomized to either slow withdrawal of their antiepileptic drug therapy or to continuing drug therapy. Two years after randomization 78% of those who continued treatment and 59% of those who had treatment withdrawn were seizure-free, but thereafter the differences in recurrence rate between the two groups diminished.

Table 3.20 Factors predictive of seizure recurrence following withdrawal of therapy, in patients free of seizures for two years or more (MRC antiepileptic drug withdrawal study).

Age over 16

Taking more than one antiepileptic drug

Seizures after starting antiepileptic treatment

History of secondarily generalized tonic–clonic seizures

History of myoclonic seizures

Electroencephalogram with spike and wave discharges

Short period of freedom from seizures

duration of time from the onset of epilepsy to the onset of remission), the less is the risk of relapse.

Type and severity of epilepsy. The type of epilepsy and its aetiology are important influences on prognosis. The presence of symptomatic epilepsy, secondarily generalized and myoclonic seizures, neurological deficit or mental retardation greatly lessen the chance of remission, and also increase the chances of recurrence should remission occur. The higher the number of seizures prior to remission, the greater the number of drugs being taken to control the seizures and the presence of two or more seizure types (a surrogate for severity of epilepsy) all increase the risk of relapse.

Electroencephalography. The value of EEG in predicting outcome is controversial, as it is in almost all other areas of prognostication. The persistence of spike wave in those with primary generalized epilepsy is probably the most useful EEG feature, indicating a higher chance of relapse. Other EEG abnormalities have no great utility in this regard and are at best of marginal benefit.

Age. There is no clear overall relationship between age and the risk of relapse, although there are age-specific syndromes which have specific prognostic patterns. There is a low chance of relapse in the benign epilepsies of childhood or in generalized absence epilepsy. These data simply emphasis the obvious point that the overriding determinant of prognosis is the type of epilepsy.

These risk factors are additive, and if two or more adverse factors are present, the risk of recurrence is over 70%. On the other hand, if positive factors exist,

such as a long duration of remission, a short history of epilepsy, mild epilepsy prior to remission, idiopathic epilepsy with a normal EEG, the risks are considerably lower than the 40% found in the MRC study. A predictive model has been developed on the basis of the study, which takes into account some of these features and provides useful estimates of relapse rate.

When a decision to withdraw therapy is made, the drugs should be discontinued one at a time, slowly. Half of patients who are going to experience seizure recurrence on withdrawal do so during the reduction phase, and a further 25% in the first 6 months after withdrawal; this should be explained carefully to the patient, and driving restrictions should be applied during the withdrawal period and the subsequent 6 months. The fastest recommended rates of out-patient withdrawal are given in Table 3.19, although in many instances there is no need to proceed so rapidly. In general terms, the slower the withdrawal, the less likely are seizures to recur. If seizures do recur, the drug should be immediately restarted at the dosage which controlled the attacks.

DRUGS IN PARTIAL AND SECONDARILY GENERALIZED SEIZURES

A central question, which in numerical terms dwarfs all others about drug choice in epilepsy, is which antiepileptic drugs are best used for those with partial onset seizures? These seizures form the bulk of uncontrolled seizures; partial seizures, and their feared partner the secondarily generalized attack, account for at least two-thirds of all epilepsy cases. This is also the pharmaceutical industry's battle ground. It is here that the gloves are off, for these epilepsies are the material of the registrational clinical trials. These are the seizures most commonly refractory to current medical treatment and these are the seizures which sometimes justify the extreme remedy of neurosurgery.

Newly diagnosed partial onset seizures

The principles of treatment are discussed on pp. 41–44. Therapy should be started with a single drug, and the previous fashion for combination therapy has been thoroughly discredited, although on somewhat diaphanous grounds. The older antiepileptic drugs were introduced at a time when the distinction between 'monotherapy' and 'polytherapy' licences was not made. The newer antiepileptics though have fallen foul of the regulations requiring proof of efficacy and safety in single-drug therapy as well as in combination with other drugs. There are few if any examples of an antiepileptic drug effective in combination but not in single-drug therapy, and the main purpose of this rule is perhaps to erect a bureaucratic hurdle to prevent the widespread and costly use of the newer drugs as first-line treatment. Of the newer drugs, oxcarbazepine, lamotrigine, felbamate, gabapentin and topiramate have to date undergone sufficient single-drug trials to have satisfied the licensing authorities that monotherapy is appropriate.

In spite of this emphasis on the need for clinical trials, comparative data are very scarce, because the trials usually compare the drug to placebo added to existing therapy. The landmark study of the traditional drugs was the double-blind multicentre comparison of phenytoin, carbamazepine, phenobarbital and primidone carried out in the American Veterans Association hospitals. Six hundred and twenty-two patients were randomized to treatment to one of the four drugs and followed for 12 months or until toxicity or lack of seizure control required a treatment switch. The patients were adults, and a mixture of newly diagnosed drug-naïve cases and also those with recent-onset epilepsy who had failed to respond to previous initial therapy. Retention rates were best for phenytoin, carbamazepine and phenobarbital, but the proportion of patients rendered seizure-free on the four drugs was similar (between 48 and 63%). This confirmed the widely held view that, in terms of antiepileptic efficacy, there was nothing to choose between the four drugs. Furthermore, there were no significant differences in the side-effect profile of the drugs. A follow-on study comparing carbamazepine and valproate in 480 adult patients showed no differences in control of secondarily generalized seizures, although carbamazepine was more effective in complex partial seizures. Another study of phenytoin, carbamazepine and valproate conversely found carbamazepine and valproate similarly effective in secondarily generalized seizures but both less effective than phenytoin. Other smaller monotherapy studies involving variously carbamazepine, valproate, phenytoin, primidone and clonazepam have generally failed to clarify the situation. The general consensus is that there is little evidence to favour any of these mainline drugs in terms either of efficacy or toxicity. Choice therefore becomes a matter of largely personal preference.

Of the newer drugs, again no controlled study has shown any of the drugs licensed for monotherapy to be any strikingly better than the traditional therapy, either in terms of effectiveness or even in most aspects of tolerability, or in terms of serious side-effects. There is intensive marketing to promote the newer drugs and the relative reputation of the drugs in practice reflects more these marketing pressures than any scientific study.

Cost is one issue which clearly differentiates the newer and older drugs. In Table 3.21 are shown the 1996 unit costs of one year's treatment with high and low doses of the antiepileptic drugs. Although these costs are only indicative (different purchasers paying different prices), there is clearly a huge variation with an over 1000-fold difference between the highest and the lowest cost. Cost is of only limited interest unless related to outcome. The only published study to have looked at the total medical costs of prescribing carbamazepine, phenytoin, lamotrigine or valproate used a cost-minimization model and found that, for the same outcome, the overall costs of prescribing lamotrigine in newly diagnosed epilepsy were about four times those of the other three drugs. Other health economic studies of different drugs in different setting have reached similar conclusions.

Because of this cost differential, it seems reasonable to recommend one of the traditional, and cheaper, medications as first-line therapy, at least until a clear-cut difference can be demonstrated in outcome in terms of either seizure control, tolerability or serious side-effects. The usual choice is between carbamazepine, phenytoin or valproate.

Partial onset seizures unresponsive to initial therapy

The definitive randomized placebo-controlled clinical trials of almost all the antiepileptic drugs have been carried out in populations of patients with partial seizures refractory to their previous medication. One might therefore have anticipated that clear guidelines for clinical practice would exist; sadly this is far from the case and this is a reflection of the inadequacies of the clinical trial process.

Clinical antiepileptic drug trials

The root of the problem lies in the fact that clinical trials are designed for regulatory not clinical purposes. It is vital to recognize this to avoid unjustified extrapolation. The regulatory requirement is for the trial to demonstrate antiepileptic efficacy. To do this, the drug is invariably compared to placebo, in a double-blind fashion, over a short period of time in a highly selected group of patients in a highly artificial clinical context. Perhaps it is not surprising that only limited clinical information can be derived from these studies. While they will provide evidence of

Table 3.21 Relative costs of antiepileptic drugs.

	Dosage (low/high, mg per day)		Yearly cost	
			Cost (US $, to nearest $*)	Relative to phenobarbital therapy at 60 mg per day (times greater)
Carbamazepine	Low	600	85	29
	High	1800	255	87
Gabapentin	Low	1200	1007	345
	High	3600	3022	1035
Lamotrigine	Low	200	973	333
	High	400	1947	667
Phenobarbital	Low	60	3	1
	High	180	9	3
Phenytoin	Low	200	30	10
	High	400	61	21
Topiramate	Low	300	1739	596
	High	600	3445	1180
Valproate	Low	600	105	36
	High	2000	486	166
Vigabatrin	Low	1500	737	252
	High	4000	1964	674

*Based on cheapest proprietary bulk price quoted in the *UK Prescribing Manual* in 1996.

an antiepileptic effect, they absolutely do not provide evidence of relative clinical value.

Efficacy measures. The primary efficacy variable is usually a 50% or more reduction in the number of seizures in the trial period compared to a prospectively controlled baseline figure, or the number of 'responders'—defined as the number of patients whose seizure frequency falls by 50% or more in the trial compared to baseline period. The two end-points are not necessarily equivalent, as some patients will experience more seizures than others and thereby potentially influence the primary end-point more than those with fewer attacks. For most patients with severe epilepsy, a 50% reduction in seizure frequency is an unsatisfactory end-point. More impressive would be the complete cessation of seizures, but this is seldom reported in studies. Secondary end-points have included quality of life scores, but these are highly artificial in the context of a few weeks of clinical trial (what aspect of quality of life change can be measured meaningfully over such a short time?).

Short-term. Almost all of the regulatory trials are very brief with treatment periods typically of 8–16 weeks. This is a short time in the life of a patient with epilepsy, particularly as seizures fluctuate as a result of environmental and emotional factors.

Selected population. Almost all the studies are of adult patients with refractory partial epilepsy. Many are 'professional' trialists having participated in previous studies. Such patients are highly unrepresentative of the generality of epilepsy patients. Furthermore, the trials almost all exclude key groups, such as women of child-bearing age, the elderly, those with learning difficulty, children, pregnant women, patients with unquantifiable or unclassifiable seizures and those with concurrent illness. These patients make up the majority of patients with epilepsy. Drug response in the trial can be a very poor guide to that in the wider epilepsy population.

Seizure type. The trials in refractory partial epilepsy usually exclude other types of seizure or epilepsy. There are many examples of drugs that have greater effects in generalized rather than partial epilepsy, for instance lamotrigine or valproate, yet these effects are often not noticed nor subjected to formal evaluation for many years after the studies in partial epilepsy. A wider set of inclusion criteria would improve this unsatisfactory situation.

Fixed dosage. In the clinical trials, the dose of drugs is usually fixed. Quite often, the dose chosen in the trials turns out not to be the dose most often used in clinical practice. Too high a dose was used in most of the trials of topiramate and vigabatrin, and too low a dose in those of felbamate, gabapentin, lamotrigine and valproate. Trials therefore give scant guidance to dosage in individual patients and indeed can be thoroughly misleading.

Artificial outside clinical context. The inclusion and exclusion criteria, the titration regimens and escape criteria, and the logistics of follow-up result in a highly artificial clinical setting. Alternative 'pragmatic' trial designs would be possible, in which these aspects are not so rigidly controlled, but these have not found favour within the regulatory framework. Pragmatic trials in the post-licensing phase, though, are urgently needed as only they can provide information for routine prescribing.

Side-effects. The side-effects are usually recorded by predetermined checklists (dictionaries). These are interpreted differently by different investigators and are difficult to evaluate—the widely used dictionary term 'abnormal thinking' for instance covers a variety of cognitive effects. Furthermore, rarer side-effects will be missed altogether. Felbamate, for instance, was grossly over marketed as a safe drug until drug-induced aplastic anaemia and hepatic failure resulted in its withdrawal from use.

The first randomized clinical trial in medicine was carried out in 1948, but trials only recently have become the cornerstone of 'evidence-based medicine'. In epilepsy, trials were not widely used until the 1980s. Their value in demonstrating a drug's antiepileptic properties is undisputed, but too rigid a reliance on their findings misleads and obfuscates clinical practice. The situation is greatly exacerbated by the intense marketing of drugs, in the immediate post-trial period, in which trial results are often extrapolated without due thought. A period of post-licensing assessment, in more open clinical settings, is needed to place a drug in its appropriate context, but the marketing onslaught has, in recent years, made this impossible. The result is therefore that we do not have good data on which to base drug choice in routine clinical practice, and have to a large extent to rely on subjective guidelines and anecdote.

Meta-analysis of randomized placebo trials

There has been one attempt to provide a compre-

hensive analysis (meta-analysis) of antiepileptic drug efficacy by combining the results of all randomized clinical trials. This is a landmark study. Twenty trials were include in which gabapentin, lamotrigine, tiagabine, topiramate, vigabatrin and zonisamide were compared with placebo as add-on treatments in patients with drug-resistant partial epilepsy. The review generated overall estimates of the efficacy and tolerability of each drug compared with placebo and allowed broad comparisons of the potency of the new drugs against partial epilepsy.

Of the placebo-treated patients in these studies 0–18% showed a 50% reduction in the frequency of seizures, which probably represents a 'regression to the mean' phenomenon. The estimates of odds ratios for a 50% response showed gabapentin and lamotrigine to be only mildly effective drugs, with odds ratios for 50% response two to three times that of placebo. Tiagabine seems to have a relatively well-defined dose responsiveness, ranging from a mild effect (like that of gabapentin and lamotrigine) at 16 mg a day up to more substantial effects at 56 mg a day. This responsiveness seems to be mimicked by vigabatrin. Topiramate had the best documented dose–response curve, with a clear plateau that helps to define the maximal therapeutic dose at about 600 mg a day (with the odds ratio of response up to six times that of placebo).

However, when the summary estimates of odds ratios for 50% responders with each drug were compared, the 95% confidence intervals overlapped. Therefore, this study provided no conclusive evidence to support apparent differences in efficacy. A reanalysis of the data calculating the 'number needed to treat' to achieve a 50% response was subsequently carried out and this did show that vigabatrin and topiramate were both significantly more efficacious than the other drugs. The study has been criticized on various counts, and there seems little doubt that different results would be obtained if the drug doses were varied. Furthermore, group comparisons, not individual within-patient data were used. Nevertheless, this study is the best systematic comparison that we have of drug trial results. The weaknesses of drug trials cannot be overcome by simply combining the studies, and this meta-analysis does not replace the urgent need for large-scale pragmatic trials, although it does provide a good basis for such a study.

Severe side-effects of antiepileptic drugs

The side-effect profile of drugs which is produced in most clinical trials is of the common dose-related side-effects, which are transient and reversible. In some senses, these are of less importance than the much rarer but much more severe side-effects. How the risk of these is accounted for in choosing a drug can be a difficult decision for the physician and patient. The particular side-effects of individual drugs are listed in Chapter 4.

The anticonvulsant hypersensitivity syndrome is a particular problem. It has been recorded, particularly with phenytoin, phenobarbital, carbamazepine, felbamate and lamotrigine. The triad of fever, rash and organ damage can be fatal. The risk overall is between 1 in 1000 and 1 in 10 000 exposures for phenytoin, carbamazepine or phenobarbital. The risk for lamotrigine may be greater, although definitive figures are not available. Hepatic failure caused by felbamate occurs in about 1 in 10 000 persons and aplastic anaemia at approximately twice this rate. Hypersensitivity usually develops within 12 weeks of first contact with the drug, and fever, lymphadenopathy, rash and pharyngitis are common initial symptoms. The rash can be life-threatening if it is allowed to evolve. The most prominent organ manifestations are hepatitis, eosinophilia, blood dyscrasia and nephritis. Other symptoms include facial angioedema, tonsillitis, oral and genital ulceration, myopathy, late hypothyroidism and disseminated intravascular coagulopathy. The patient should be hospitalized and the offending drug should be stopped immediately in spite of the risk of withdrawal seizures. Cover with other antiepileptics can be given, and benzodiazepines or barbiturates are most useful. Status epilepticus should be managed in the usual way. Meticulous skin care and the prevention of infection are vital in severe skin reactions, and transfer to a burns unit is sometimes needed. Acute respiratory disease, organ failure and ocular disorders may require specific therapy. High-dose corticosteroid therapy is sometimes required, although evidence for its effectiveness is equivocal. Occasionally, cyclophosphamide or intravenous immunoglobulins are given. The pathogenesis of this reaction is unclear, but may involve toxic metabolites caused by genetically determined deficiencies in the patient's metabolic pathways, or a graft vs. host reaction, or a circulating antibody-mediated response.

Seizure-inducing effects of antiepileptic drugs

Not often mentioned in the published results of drug trials is the occurrence of a paradoxical increase in seizures caused by an antiepileptic drug; this phenomenon is sometimes hidden in the 'not improved' category. Sometimes this is an idiosyncratic effect, sometimes the use of an incorrect drug for the particular seizure type and sometimes the result of anticonvulsant intoxication or encephalopathy. Gabapentin has been shown to increase complex partial seizures in a substantial minority of patients. The precipitation of tonic–clonic seizures by ethosuximide, gabapentin, lamotrigine, carbamazepine and diazepam has been reported. Absence seizures can be precipitated by phenobarbital, carbamazepine, and vigabatrin. Carbamazepine can precipitate focal, tonic, myoclonic and absence seizures especially in the Lennox–Gastaut syndrome and benzodiazepines can precipitate tonic status in the same syndrome. Myoclonic seizures can be induced by lamotrigine and vigabatrin. Phenytoin intoxication can markedly increase seizures and valproate can induce an encephalopathy, in some instances caused by drug-induced hyperammonaemia.

Choice of antiepileptic drug

In the absence of definitive preferences from existing drug trials and the lack of large-scale pragmatic studies, drug choice for partial or secondarily generalized seizures is to an extent arbitrary. On cost grounds alone, carbamazepine, valproate and phenytoin should be used initially. Their efficacy is as good as any of the newer agents, and the side-effect profile in most patients no worse. If these are ineffective, the author's preference is for any of the following: clobazam, gabapentin, lamotrigine, levetiracetam, oxcarbazepine or topiramate. The appropriate choice of drug in an individual patient is a balance of efficacy, tolerability and cost. Acetazolamide, clonazepam, ethosuximide, felbamate, phenobarbital (or primidone), tiagabine or vigabatrin are further possible alternatives. The order in which these are started depends on individual circumstance. Where efficacy is the paramount consideration topiramate is preferred, or gabapentin when lack of side-effects but only mild efficacy is required. Clobazam is useful as an adjunctive therapy with few side-effects and excellent efficacy in some patients, and can be given a short trial without the need for long periods of titration or tapering. The initial and maintenance doses are shown in Table 3.22.

CHILDHOOD EPILEPSY SYNDROMES

Neonatal seizures

The clinical and EEG features, the cause and the pathophysiology of seizures in the neonatal period differ from those in later life. Clinical signs are necessarily confined to motor features and are usually

Table 3.22 Commonly used starting and maintenance doses of antiepileptic drugs for adults in routine, non-emergency therapy.

Antiepileptic drug	Starting dose (mg)	Suggested incremental dose (mg per day)	Suggested incremental interval (weeks)	Average maintenance dose (total mg per day)	Doses per day
Carbamazepine	100	100–200	2	400–1600	2–3
Clobazam	10	10	2	10–30	1–2
Clonazepam	0.5	0.5	2	0.5–4	1–2
Ethosuximide	250	250	2	750–2000	2–3
Felbamate	1200	600–1200	2	1200–3600*	3–4
Gabapentin	300	300–900	1	900–3600	2–3
Lamotrigine	25*	50–100	2	100–400*	2
Levetiracetam	1000	500	1	1000–3000	2
Oxcarbazepine	600	300	2	900–2400	2
Phenobarbital	30	30–60	2	30–180	1–2
Phenytoin	100–200	50–100	2	100–300	1–2
Piracetam	7200	24 000	1	Up to 24 000	2–3
Primidone	125	250	2	500–1500	1–2
Tiagabine	20	5	2	30–45	3
Topiramate	25–50	50–100	2	200–600	2
Valproate	400–500	500	2	500–2500	2–3
Vigabatrin	1000	500	2	1000–3000	2

*Dependent on comedication (see text).

focal or multifocal, reflecting the immature synaptic connections in the neonatal brain. The EEG changes are variable and non-specific. Seizures can take the form of tonic attacks, clonic seizures, unilateral focal seizures, electrographic seizures without overt clinical changes and so-called subtle seizures. The seizures can have mild or atypical features, such as grimacing, staring, eye movements, posturing or pedalling movements. Neonatal seizures occur in about 1% of all infants with a higher frequency (up to 23%) in premature babies. While there is no doubt that most neonatal seizures are 'epileptic', some subtle and some tonic seizures are not associated with any EEG changes and may be subcortical in origin resulting from abnormal brainstem release mechanisms. There are a large variety of potential causes, the most common being hypoxic–ischaemic encephalopathy, intracranial haemorrhage, neonatal infection and metabolic disorders (especially hypocalcaemia, hypomagnesaemia, hypoglycaemia) (Table 3.23). The development of neonatal seizures is an ominous sign not only because they often indicate cerebral disease but also because the seizures themselves possibly damage the developing brain. The prognosis depends largely on the underlying cause. Overall, the immediate mortality rate is about 15%, 37% develop neurological deficits and only 48% develop normally. Prognosis is worse in premature infants, especially those with a gestational age under 31 weeks.

If the seizures are considered non-epileptic, antiepileptic drug treatment may not indicated. Indeed, medication may worsen the phenomena by decreasing the level of cortical inhibition over subcortical structures. Whether genuine (cortical) but slight (subtle) epileptic seizures require treatment is uncertain, especially in infants who are not paralysed for artificial ventilation. Not uncommonly such seizure manifestations remit spontaneously after days or weeks and the usefulness of treatment in this situation is difficult to assess. Opinions vary about the need to treat infants with EEG evidence of seizure activity without overt clinical signs. There is also disagreement about the duration of therapy, although most would aim for as short a period as possible. Many neonatal seizures are self-limiting and over-long treatment carries its own risks.

For all other neonatal seizures treatment is urgent. Management demands meticulous specialized paediatric care, usually on an intensive care unit. Electroencephalogram monitoring is desirable and artificial ventilation often required. There is no place for treating these critically ill infants in non-specialist settings. The treatment should be directed primarily at the causal disorder where this is possible, and immediate investigation is required to ascertain the cause. Hypoglycaemia requires immediate correction with 2–4 mL/kg of a 20–30% solution of glucose intravenously. Hypocalcaemia requires the slow intravenous injection of 2–5% calcium gluconate with ECG monitoring. Hypomagnesaemia requires 2–8 mL of 2–3% solution of magnesium sulphate intravenously or 0.2 mL/kg of a 50% solution intramuscularly. Pyridoxine deficiency, although rare, responds dramatically to 50–200 mg of pyridoxine. Infections, other metabolic disorders (e.g. hyperammonaemia, organic aciduria) and mass lesions require specific therapy. Emergency antiepileptic drugs are indicated for all but isolated seizures. Traditional practice is to load the infant with either phenobarbital or phenytoin. Phenobarbital is given to obtain a blood level of 20 mg/mL, which requires a loading dose of 20 mg/kg followed by a maintenance dose of 3–4 mg/kg per day intravenously or intramuscularly. Phenytoin is a second-line drug, with a loading dose of 15–20 mg/kg administered intravenously at a rate not exceeding 1–2 mg/kg/min, and with a maintenance dose of 3–4 mg/kg per day to obtain a plasma level of between 15 and 20 mg/mL. It is mandatory to monitor blood levels because of abrupt changes in half-lives of the drugs in the first 2–3 weeks of life. Others tend to postpone the use of these long-acting antiepileptics until the diagnosis is clarified and/or after shorter-acting agents, such as diazepam, lorazepam or clonazepam have failed. The shorter acting drugs are given for 24–48 h and then withdrawn.

Febrile seizures

Febrile seizures are epileptic events that occur in the context of an acute rise in body temperature. They are common. About 3–5% of children will have at least one attack. The first febrile seizure happens in the second year of life in 50% and in the first 3 years in 90%. Four per cent occur before 6 months and 6% after 6 years. In over 85%, the seizures are generalized and are usually brief. Febrile seizures are more common in males and in those with a family history. The important risk factors seem to be an acute temperature rise and the attainment of a high fever. Viral infection is the underlying cause of the fever in 80%. Eight per cent of first febrile seizures are caused by viral or bacterial meningitis. About 30–50% of susceptible children will have a second attack and 10% three or more. Although most are benign, specialist attention is required especially

Table 3.23 Causes of neonatal seizures.

Hypoxic–ischaemic encephalopathy
Acute cerebrovascular event
Subarachnoid haemorrhage
Intraventricular haemorrhage
Intracerebral haemorrhage
Subdural haemorrhage
Cerebral infarction

Intracranial infection
Meningitis (e.g. group B streptococci, *Escherichia coli*)
Encephalitis (e.g. herpes simplex, toxoplasmosis, coxsackie B, rubella, cytomegalovirus)
Abscess

Cerebral malformations
Neuronal migrational and other developmental defects (e.g. agyria, pachygyria, polymicrogyria, corpus callosal
  agenesis, anencephaly, holoprosencephaly, lissencephaly)
Neurocutaneous disorders (e.g. Sturge–Weber, neurofibromatosis, tuberous sclerosis)
Chromosomal anomalies (e.g. Down syndrome, trisomy 13 and 18)

Metabolic causes
Hypocalcaemia (primary, perinatal asphyxia, small for gestational age, diet, diabetic mother, septicaemia,
  hypomagnesaemia, malabsorption)
Hypoglycaemia (premature, small for gestational age, perinatal asphyxia, meningitis, transfusion, galactosaemia,
  fructosaemia, leucine sensitivity, pituitary hypoplasia, pancreatic tumour, glycogen storage disease)
Hyponatraemia (e.g. inappropriate therapy, inappropriate antidiuretic hormone)
Inborn errors of metabolism, e.g. aminoaciduria, urea cycle defects, organic acidurias, pyridoxine deficiency)
Bilirubin encephalopathy
Hypomagnesaemia

Benign and familial syndromes
Benign familial neonatal convulsions
Benign neonatal seizures
Benign neonatal myoclonus

Toxic or withdrawal convulsions
Toxins (e.g. mercury, hexochlorophene)
Drugs (e.g. penicillin, anaesthetics)
Drug withdrawal (e.g. maternal barbiturate, alcohol, narcotics)

Specific epileptic encephalopathies
Ohtahara's syndrome
Neonatal myoclonic encephalopathy
Early infantile epileptic encephalopathy

after the first attack. The aetiology should be established. Febrile seizures occurring before 6 months of age particularly raise the possibility of bacterial meningitis and urgent lumbar puncture is indicated. In older children, investigation depends on the clinical circumstances, but may include lumbar puncture or brain scanning (Table 3.24).

Prolonged febrile seizures can result in cerebral damage with consequential focal neurological deficit, epilepsy or intellectual effects; the hemiplegia, hemiatrophy, epilepsy (HHE) syndrome typically develops after febrile status. The longer the duration of the attack, the more likely is cerebral damage, and for this reason febrile seizures require emergency therapy if they continue for 15 min or more.

Between 6 and 18% of children with febrile seizures show subsequent learning difficulties. This is usually not a causal association, with both the seizures and the learning difficulty reflecting existing cerebral dysfunction. The occurrence of febrile seizures is also associated with the much later devel-

Table 3.24 Febrile convulsions.

Age range	3 months to 5 years, peak 2–4 years

Forms	Simple
	Complex
	   >30 min
	   and/or focal or lateralizing features
	   and/or recurs within 24 h

Seizure types	Tonic–clonic (80–85%) Tonic (15%) Atonic (2–5%)
Precipitants	Rapid rise in fever High temperature >80% viral infections Small excess after measles vaccination
Sequelae Immediate	Todd's paresis if prolonged Rarely (developed world) Hemiplegia- Hemiatrophy-epilepsy syndrome in febrile status

Late	Recurrence (30–50%)
	   <10% have three or more
	   More likely with
	   early age of onset and
	   positive family history
	Later epilepsy
	   Overall 2–10%
	   No prior neurological disease 2.4%
	Risk factors for later epilepsy
	   <13 months
	   Prior neurological abnormality
	   Complex convulsions

Association *with mental* *handicap*	6–18% of those admitted with febrile convulsions

opment of subsequent epilepsy. Typically, the epilepsy develops years later, between the ages of 6–12 years. The risk of epilepsy is small; less than 10% in children with a history of febrile seizures. The risk is said, albeit on rather poor evidence, to be somewhat higher after complex febrile seizures (defined as an event lasting more than 30 min and/or with focal manifestations and/or recurring within 24 h). Whether this is a causal relationship—febrile seizures resulting in temporal lobe damage which becomes the substrate for subsequent epilepsy—or not is unclear. However, because of the risk of immediate damage and the possible risk of late epilepsy, febrile seizures should be treated as a medical emergency. There are three aspects to this treatment.

Emergency antiepileptic treatment. Standard treatment is the administration of diazepam 0.5 mg/kg intravenously or rectally (the latter using the Stesolid or similar formulation), given if the seizure has continued for 15 min or more, or earlier if there is a history of prior prolonged seizures. The child should also be cooled by any means possible.

Emergency prophylactic treatment. In susceptible children, prophylactic diazepam can be given rectally or orally as soon as a fever develops. Suitable twice daily doses, during the episode of fever, are 0.3–0.5 mg/kg rectally or 5 mg orally for children less than 3 years and 7.5 mg orally for those over 3 years of age. Measures to lower temperature should also be taken to prevent a seizure, including tepid sponging, removing clothing and the administration of paracetamol. Unfortunately, the seizure occurs before the fever is apparent in one-third of cases and such prophylaxis is not feasible.

Long-term prophylaxis. The need for long-term prophylaxis is contentious. In the past, antiepileptics were commonly given. However, because of potential side-effects, and concern about the risks to learning and to development, long-term therapy is increasingly reserved for those who are at particularly high risk of frequent or complex febrile seizures. Typically, treatment is now given only to infants under the age of 1 year who have had episodes lasting 30 min or more, or who have had multiple seizures. The antiepileptic drugs used are either phenobarbital 15 mg/kg per day or valproate 20–40 mg/kg per day in two divided doses.

West syndrome

West syndrome is a severe epileptic encephalopathy. The prognosis is primarily dependent upon the underlying aetiology. Having said this, in about 30% of

Table 3.25 Infantile spasms (West syndrome).

(1 case per 4000 live births)
Age-specific epileptic encephalopathy
Variety of causes
Onset 4–8 months
Salaam attacks
Hypsarrhythmia on EEG
Response to corticosteroids or vigabatrin
Spasms remit on therapy or spontaneously
Prognosis poor: learning difficulty and continuing epilepsy are common sequelae

Table 3.26 Cause of infantile spasm (West syndrome).

Disorders of cerebral development
Neuronal migrational and other developmental defects (e.g. heterotopia, agyria–pachygyria, corpus callosal agenesis, dysplasia, hemimegalencephaly, holoprosencephaly, microcephaly, macrocephaly, porencephaly schizencephaly)

Neurocutaneous syndromes (e.g. tuberous sclerosis, Sturge–Weber syndrome, neurofibromatosis, incontinentia pigmenti and linear naevus syndrome)

Metabolic and degenerative disorders
Metabolic disorders (e.g. phenylketonuria, non-ketotic hyperglycinaemia, pyridoxine deficiency, Leigh's disease, histidinaemia, hyperornithinaemia, hyperammonaemia, homocitrullinaemia, maple-syrup urine disease, leucine-sensitive hypoglycaemia)

Degenerative disorders of uncertain aetiology (e.g. leucodystrophies, Alpers' disease, Sandhoff disease, Tay–Sachs disease)

Perinatal or postnatal chronic acquired cerebral lesions
Hypoxic–ischaemic encephalopathy and cerebral infarction

Cerebral trauma

Cerebral tumour

Maternal toxaemia

Metabolic and endocrine disorders

Infantile spasms evolving from neonatal seizure syndrome (e.g. Ohtahara's syndrome or neonatal myoclonic encephalopathy)

In approximately 40% of cases, no cause is found (of whom 10–15% show some preceding developmental disturbance). The condition is best viewed as an age-specific epileptic response to cerebral injury, and it can thus be caused by many conditions that affect the brain.

cases, no cause can be identified, and the prognosis of these idiopathic cases is generally better. The incidence of West syndrome is 0.25–0.42 per 1000 live births, with a family history it is 7–17%. The condition is defined by the occurrence of infantile spasms. These epileptic seizures may be very frequent with hundreds of attacks a day, and with a strong tendency to occur in repetitive clusters. The spasms rarely develop before the age of 3 months, and 90% develop in the first year of life. The peak incidence is 4–6 months. There is often evidence of developmental retardation before the onset of the spasms. The EEG shows the characteristic pattern of hypsarrhythmia in its fully developed form. Modified EEG forms frequently occur (Tables 3.25 and 3.26).

Urgent treatment of the underlying cause is required where this is possible. The value of antiepileptic therapy in West syndrome is difficult to assess. Hormonal therapy with adrenocorticotropic hormone (ACTH) or corticosteroids have been used since 1958, and is probably more effective in controlling the infantile spasms than most conventional antiepileptics. No controlled study of steroids has, however, been carried out, and there is debate about the relative advantages of ACTH or corticosteroid and also the doses which should be employed. Experienced paediatricians often use low-dose regimens and then higher doses (up to 60–80 IU ACTH) if lower doses fail. Uncontrolled studies of sodium valproate have suggested effectiveness, and uncontrolled studies have also shown benefit from pyridoxine and immunoglobulins. Perhaps the most persuasive evidence of benefit comes from the use of vigabatrin which has been compared in controlled and uncontrolled studies to ACTH. Effectiveness is similar, but vigabatrin has far fewer adverse effects. High-dose corticosteroid (or ACTH) in infants has a number of severe side-effects and the introduction of vigabatrin as an alternative therapy has been widely welcomed.

In the few cases of infantile spasms in which positron emission tomography (PET) scanning shows clear-cut focal abnormalities, surgical resection can be performed with complete abolition of the spasm. The longer-term effects on neurological function of large surgical resection have, however, not been fully established. Equally, it is not clear to what extent cognitive development is affected by such radical treatment.

About 5% of children die in the acute phase of spasms. The death rate was much higher before the introduction of ACTH therapy. On treatment, the spasms remit in almost all cases with few cases having attacks after the age of 3 years. However, both the development of the child and the ultimate neurological status are usually impaired. Of the survivors 70–96% have learning difficulty (severe in over 50%) and in 35–60% chronic epilepsy develops. In a proportion of idiopathic cases (under 5% in all) subsequent development can be normal, and it has been proposed that this subgroup represents a form of benign epilepsy of childhood.

Lennox–Gastaut syndrome
This term is used to describe an ill-defined epileptic encephalopathy with a wide range of causes. The epilepsy takes the form of frequent atypical absence, tonic, myoclonic, tonic and tonic–clonic seizures. There is almost always a mixture of seizure types

Table 3.27 Features of the Lennox–Gastaut syndrome.

Onset age 1–14 years

Severe epileptic disorder with multiple seizure types, including myoclonic, atypical absence, tonic and tonic–clonic seizures

Seizure precipitated by drowsiness or understimulation, not by hyperventilation or photic stimulation

Learning disability

Status epilepticus common, especially non-convulsive forms

EEG shows 1–2.5 Hz spike and wave complexes with various other abnormalities and abnormal background rhythms, without photosensitivity

Many causes, although about 25% are cryptogenic in origin

Poor response to antiepileptic drug treatment

Prognosis for seizure control and mental development poor

and, particularly in long-standing cases, complex partial and other seizure types develop (Table 3.27). The patients fall frequently and are prone to injury. Episodes of convulsive and more typically non-convulsive status occur.

The EEG shows a characteristic pattern. The signature of the condition is the presence of long bursts of diffuse slow (1–2.5 Hz) spike-and-wave activity, widespread in both hemispheres, roughly bilaterally synchronous but often asymmetrical. The spike wave is not induced by hyperventilation and there is no photosensitivity. The background activity is abnormal with an excess of slow activity and diminished arousal or sleep potentials. The ictal and interictal EEG are often similar, especially during periods of non-convulsive status. Associated with the epilepsy is a slowly progressive learning difficulty. In 15–25% of cases, the syndrome develops in children who have already suffered infantile spasms. Subcategories of the syndrome have been proposed although these do not influence treatment strategies. The onset of the condition is usually between 1 and 7 years of age. The prognosis for control of seizures and for intellectual development is generally poor. However, in some series, up to 15% of cases showed long remissions from seizures or intellectual improvement, although case definitions have not been uniform. Seizures do improve in adult life, and rarely is the epilepsy either as frequent or as ferocious as in early childhood. Motor slowness and learning disability (often severe) though are almost invariable, and

many patients require institutional care in childhood or adult life.

The underlying cause should be treated where possible (often it is not). Antiepileptic drug treatment is frequently ineffective. One clinical point deserves special emphasis. This is the importance of resisting the tendency—in the face of severe epilepsy—to escalate treatment. Such an escalation is seldom effective, and high-dose polypharmacy may cause drowsiness which is a potent activator of the atypical absence and tonic seizures and non-convulsive status epilepticus. Phenobarbital and other drugs also can exacerbate the overactivity and aggressive behaviour disorder which commonly accompany the epilepsy.

Sodium valproate or benzodiazepine drugs are currently the least unsatisfactory of the conventional drugs. Valproate is particularly effective against atypical absences, myoclonic or atonic seizures. Clobazam and clonazepam are the most commonly used benzodiazepines, the latter having more side-effects and is generally less well tolerated. ACTH and corticosteroids have been used and are perhaps best used in short-term courses to tide a patient over a bad patch. Prolonged administration can have profound side-effects.

Several of the newer antiepileptic drugs have shown promise in the Lennox–Gastaut syndrome. Clinical trials of lamotrigine, felbamate and topiramate have all shown significant reductions in atypical absence, myoclonic, atonic seizures and drop attacks. Few patients in any study though have become seizure-free. These drugs also have been shown to improve awareness and responsiveness.

Table 3.28 Benign rolandic epilepsy.

15% of all childhood epilepsy

Age of onset 5–10 years

Simple partial seizures with frequent secondarily generalization

Partial seizures involve the face, oropharynx and upper limb

Seizures are typically during sleep and infrequent

No other neurological features: normal intelligence

Family history

EEG shows typical centrotemporal spikes

Excellent response to antiepileptic drugs

Excellent prognosis with remission by mid-teenage years

Other treatments include the use of the ketogenic diet which can have a dramatic effect, especially in young children. Surgical therapy has included unilateral cortical resection, and corpus callosectomy which can reduce drop attacks and tonic seizures (see p. 216).

Benign partial epilepsy syndromes of childhood

There are a variety of 'syndromes' of partial epilepsy at various stages of childhood which have an excellent prognosis (Table 3.28).

Benign epilepsy with centrotemporal spikes (rolandic epilepsy)

This is the most common of these benign syndromes. Seizures develop between the age of 3–12 years and the children are otherwise normal from the developmental and neurological point of view. Three-quarters of the seizures are brief simple partial attacks involving preferentially the facial and oropharyngeal musculature, and occur during sleep. Tonic–clonic seizures also occur in sleep. The EEG shows a characteristic pattern of high voltage spikes in the rolandic region with a normal background tracing.

Treatment is not necessary in all cases. If attacks are infrequent or mild, regular therapy seems inappropriate, especially as some children have only a few attacks before the epilepsy remits. Tonic–clonic seizures carry greater risks than the partial attacks and tip the balance towards therapy. The partial seizures too can warrant treatment, even if infrequent when frightening and distressing. If treatment is decided upon, overmedication and polypharmacy should be avoided. Both carbamazepine and valproate are highly effective, often at low doses. Withdrawal of medication should be considered after 1–2 years free of attacks even if the EEG has not normalized.

Benign occipital epilepsies

The benign occipital epilepsies can take several subforms, although to what extent these justify categorization as separate syndromes is a matter of argument. The principles of therapy are similar in all. The clinical phenomenology of all forms reflect occipital cortical activation. Typical symptoms are visual phenomena, eye and head deviation, blinking and alteration of consciousness. The visual phenomena may be elementary or complex, and can be negative (i.e. hemianopia, temporary blindness) as well as positive. The seizures can be alarmingly prolonged. Tonic–clonic seizures can occur, particularly as a culmination of prolonged partial seizure

Table 3.29 Acquired epileptic aphasia (Landau–Kleffner syndrome).

Uncommon condition with male preponderance

70% of cases onset before age of 6 years

Dysphasia, fluctuating, often severe

EEG shows epileptiform patterns, often amounting to electrographic status

70% of cases have seizures, often not severe

Other intellectual disturbances are often present

Prognosis is variable

activity. Visual symptoms, vomiting and headache are common in childhood migraine, and the differentiation between the two conditions can be difficult in some cases. Rarely, occipital seizures are caused by mitochondrial disease, Lafora body disease, coeliac disease or metabolic disorders. In most cases, however, the prognosis is good and the epilepsy remits in about 80% of cases. In a few cases, seizures persist or evolve into a more usual form.

The principles of treatment are similar to those for benign epilepsy with centrotemporal spikes. Where seizures are infrequent, treatment may not be necessary. Valproate is probably the drug of choice before carbamazepine, and there is a strong clinical impression that the drug is particularly effective in seizures with occipital foci. Clobazam can be used in seizure clusters.

Landau–Kleffner syndrome

This is a disorder of childhood in which persisting aphasia develops in association with severe EEG abnormalities and epilepsy (Table 3.29). It is an uncommon condition with a male predominance and usually without a family history. The aetiology and pathogenesis of the syndrome, if indeed these are unitary, are unknown. The condition develops in children who were previously developmentally normal. Usually a progressive aphasia occurs, gradually over months or subacutely over weeks. Verbal comprehension and expressive speech both become severely affected. The children can become almost mute. Rather fruitless and inconclusive discussion has revolved around whether or not this is a true aphasia or an auditory agnosia. The aphasia fluctuates and indeed, during the course of the condition, speech can become quite normal only to relapse again later. Other inconsistent features include behavioural disorder, personality disturbance and intellectual decline. Overt epileptic seizures occur in about 70% of cases and are usually mild, and 15% of cases have episodes of overt status epilepticus. The epilepsy, but not the EEG disturbance, is usually controlled by simple antiepileptic therapy. The EEG shows repetitive high voltage spikes or spike–wave discharges in a generalized, focal or multifocal distribution. The EEG abnormality is activated by slow wave sleep, and can become continuous. If focal, the EEG disturbance commonly, but not always, involves the dominant temporal lobe. The pathophysiology of the speech disturbance is unclear. It is tempting to see this as a manifestation of continuous focal epileptic activity disrupting language, and there is a general correlation between the course of the speech disturbance and of the EEG changes, although this is not always very close. There is an overlap between this syndrome and that of electrical status epilepticus during slow wave sleep (ESES). The long-term prognosis is variable. Some children make a complete recovery after years of aphasia, and others are left with permanent, sometimes severe, speech disturbance and mental impairment. The EEG changes usually recover, although ESES may persist.

Treatment of the Landau–Kleffner syndrome is difficult. Although seizure control is often possible with rather modest antiepileptic treatment, the EEG abnormalities may not disappear and the aphasia may not be improved. If one accepts that the speech disturbance is caused by the EEG disturbance, then aggressive antiepileptic therapy to suppress the EEG disturbance is a logical approach even in the absence of overt seizures. All antiepileptic drugs have been tried in the syndrome. Vigabatrin and carbamazepine may worsen the EEG abnormalities and are therefore sometimes avoided. Adrenocorticotropic hormone or high-dose corticosteroid are also commonly given for periods of several months. The relative benefits of these approaches is unclear, and there are no controlled trials. Assessment of any therapy is made difficult by the fluctuating course of this curious condition. A fashion for surgical treatment using the technique of multiple subpial transection has also arisen, although results are very variable and even if there is improvement, it may be months or years after the operation. It seems quite unclear, to this author at least, whether the operation ever improves the long-term prognosis. All this is unsatisfactory but, until a better understanding of the underlying pathophysiology and of the prognostic determinants is gained, therapy can only be empirical.

Electrical status epilepticus during slow wave sleep

This term refers to the presence of generalized spike–wave discharges occupying 85% or more of the EEG of non-REM sleep (Table 3.30). Of children with epilepsy, 0.5% show this EEG pattern. The pathophysiology of this condition is not clear. About 30% of children showing this pattern have identifiable brain pathology, such as previous meningitis or brain anoxia. There are no specific clinical signs during sleep, but the EEG pattern usually occurs in children with severe epilepsy and learning difficulty. The seizures can be focal or generalized and episodes of status are common. The pattern is frequent in children with the Landau–Kleffner and Lennox–Gastaut syndromes, and whether it is a specific epileptic syndrome or simply a reflection of severe epilepsy is uncertain. The syndrome is largely a childhood phenomenon, and the pattern usually disappears by the age of 16 years. The epilepsy can also remit, as can the mental impairment, although the prognosis will depend on the underlying pathology.

The EEG pattern does not generally require specific treatment. Indeed, it is often not possible to abolish the spike–wave by oral antiepileptic therapy. If treatment is decided upon, ethosuximide, benzodiazepine drugs, ACTH and corticosteroids as well as other conventional antiepileptic drugs have been used.

Table 3.30 Electrical status epilepticus during slow wave sleep.

Age of onset 1–14 years
0.5% of children with epilepsy
EEG evidence of epileptic activity for >85% of non-REM sleep
Seizures occur in most cases
Learning disability and other associated handicaps
Identifiable cause for the epilepsy in 25% of cases
Associated with Lennox–Gastaut syndrome and acquired epileptic aphasia

EPILEPSY IN CHILDREN AND ADULTS WITH ADDITIONAL HANDICAPS

If one defines 'handicap' as the impossibility of living independently (autonomously), then epilepsy is indeed a frequent cause. Overall, amongst individuals requiring long-term institutional care, between 30 and 50% have epilepsy. Epilepsy has been found to occur in 50% of those with IQ levels less than 20, and 35% of those with IQ levels in the 35–50 range. Seizures are particularly common in those with post-

Table 3.31 Specific problems of diagnosis and treatment of epilepsy in handicapped patients.

Problems of diagnosis Communication
Observation and interpretation of symptoms
Distinguishing between epileptic and non-epileptic behaviours
Neuroleptic and other drug-induced seizures
Electroencephalogram interpretation
Problems of treatment Communication
Insidious side-effects, especially sedation and behavioural changes
Sensitivity to medication and unusual side-effects
Brittle epilepsy and tendency to status epilepticus
Unusual seizure manifestations, which often are poorly responsive to therapy
Attitude of family or carers
Drug formulation

Table 3.32 Points to note in the treatment of seizures in handicapped persons.

Tailor treatment regimens (often unusual)
Avoid overmedication
Special vigilance for side-effects
Written procedures for emergency care
Respect issues of consent

natal cerebral damage. High frequencies of epilepsy also occur in specific prenatal conditions: for instance, in over 70% of cases of Rett's syndrome, 25–50% of fragile X syndrome, 70% of tuberous sclerosis, 80% with Sturge–Weber syndrome and all cases of Aicardi syndrome. The frequency of epilepsy is low in children, but not adults, with Down syndrome, which is the most common chromosomal disorder causing mental handicap. The frequency of handicap amongst those with epilepsy is difficult to ascertain. In 1983, in Finland, in a study of 223 adults with epilepsy, 30% had an IQ of less than 50, 20% were institutionalized and 15% were completely dependent. A more recent study, also from Finland, found handicap in 20% of children with epilepsy compared with 1% of controls.

The principles of epilepsy management in handicapped persons are largely similar to those in other persons. There are, however, several diagnostic and treatment points which need special consideration (Table 3.31).

Diagnosis
There are two common problems. First, there are difficulties in communication. The history, the central plank of epilepsy diagnosis, may therefore not be clear-cut. Interpretation of symptoms can be problematic, and especially those of a psychic nature. Secondly, individuals with learning disability can exhibit strange, often repetitive and stereotyped mo-

tor behaviours, pseudo-automatisms, episodes of self-abuse, apnoea, hyperpnoea and other behavioural disturbances. These are seldom epileptic and should not be treated as such. The EEG can show artefacts that complicate interpretation, and it is not uncommon for the erroneous diagnosis of epilepsy to be made and futile therapy initiated (Table 3.32).

Treatment
Epilepsy in the context of learning difficulty is often severe and resistant to drug therapy. Nevertheless, the usual principles of antiepileptic drug therapy apply. Single-drug therapy should be used where possible and, if seizures continue, alternative drug options should be given as treatment trials. Some points need specific emphasis.
• Vigilance for side-effects is particularly important. In the presence of cerebral damage, drug side-effects tend to be more frequent, to occur at lower serum levels and to take unusual forms. Examples are: confusion; neurological side-effects; behavioural change and mental deterioration and encephalopathy; weight gain which may be attributed to neuroleptics or inactivity; hypotonic children are hypersensitive to the muscle-relaxing effects of benzodiazepines; and dystonia and ataxia in patients with pre-existent motor deficits. The individual with learning difficulty may not be able to clearly communicate the adverse consequences of drug therapy. It is an essential duty of the prescribing physician to maintain extreme vigilance for side-effects, to prevent distress or harm.
• Serial seizures, clusters and episodes of status are common in patients with severe epilepsy and learning difficulty. These can be precipitated by seemingly minor problems, such as intercurrent infections or trivial environmental changes. Emergency therapy is often needed earlier and more frequently than in a non-handicapped population. Drug doses may need to be modified as handicapped individuals often show special sensitivities to the usual drugs. Tailored regimens for emergency intervention need to be defined for each individual, based on previous, often unfortunate experiences. It is helpful to docu-

ment these in writing, and to have these available to all carers and emergency medical services.
• The appearance of epileptic seizures can have consequences for the care of the other handicaps, with the attitude of carers varying from neglect to extreme overprotection. Guidance and counselling from the lead clinician can be valuable.
• Overmedication in the face of intractable epilepsy is a particular problem in handicapped persons. The reasons are complex and include the severity of the epilepsy, the need for a third party to decide upon treatment on behalf of the individual, the difficulty in communicating side-effects, and the carer's tendency to overprotection. It is vital to resist this propensity. Great benefits, without loss of seizure control, are often gained by reducing the overall antiepileptic drug load.
• Surgical therapy can benefit a small number of individuals with epilepsy. The presence of handicap is not *per se* a bar to considering this. However, assessment should be carried out in experienced centres, and other issues such as quality of life gain and informed consent are often problematic.
• The formulation of drugs may need to be in sprinkle or in liquid forms; and it can be difficult to ensure consistent dosing.

Epilepsy in specific syndromes

Down syndrome. The prevalence of epilepsy is about 2% in children with Down syndrome, and is much more common in adults. There are various underlying pathologies ranging from ischaemic–hypoxic brain damage to the changes of premature Alzheimer's disease. All seizure types occur, although tonic–clonic seizures are said to be the most common. Infantile spasms are frequent and seem to have a relatively mild prognosis. Reflex seizures and startle epilepsy are common. Late-onset epilepsy may take the form of myoclonus. Treatment should be chosen according to seizure type.

Fragile X syndrome. After Down syndrome this is the most common chromosomal disorder causing learning difficulty. Hyperkinetic behaviour, hypotonia, macro-orchidism and a specific facies are other features of the condition. Epilepsy occurs in between 10 and 25% of cases. It usually develops early and remits spontaneously during the second decade of life. Tonic–clonic seizures are the most common form. Atypical absence, staring spells, complex partial seizures and akinetic seizures can also occur. The epilepsy can usually be completely controlled with conventional therapy. Single seizures or rare isolated seizures do not require antiepileptic therapy.

Angelman syndrome. The features of this syndrome include learning difficulty, lack of speech, microcephaly, hyperactive behaviour, a characteristic facies and puppet-like motor pattern. Early problems include failure to thrive and feeding problems. Epilepsy develops in 90% and is intractable in about 50% especially in children. By adult life, however, seizures are no longer a major feature of the condition. All seizure types occur, including myoclonus and atypical absence. Convulsive and non-convulsive status are common. A subcontinuous rhythmic limb jerking caused by cortical myoclonus is characteristic and can be mistaken for tremor. Treatment is usually started with valproate, ethosuximide and/ or benzodiazepine drugs.

Rett's syndrome. This X-linked syndrome causes learning difficulty, acquired microcephaly, loss of purposeful hand skills, severe impairment of expressive and receptive language, gait apraxia, growth retardation and other features, such as breathing dysfunction, scoliosis and spasticity. Seizures occur in 70–80% of patients, usually starting between the ages of 3–5 years. The most frequent seizure types are complex partial seizures, atypical absences and generalized tonic–clonic, atonic or myoclonic seizures. Other behavioural abnormalities can be mistaken for seizures including tremor, bruxism, hyperpnoea/apnoea and episodic cyanosis. The epilepsy can become severe and intractable by school age but lessens in severity in adult life. Clinical trials of carbamazepine, clonazepam and valproic acid have been reported, without obvious superiority of any specific antiepileptic drug.

Tuberous sclerosis. This is the most common of the simple Mendelian inherited diseases causing epilepsy, and is inherited in an autosomal dominant fashion. The gene locus has been identified, but not the gene product. It occurs with a frequency of about 1 in 10 000 live births. Epilepsy occurs in about 80% of cases, and the types of seizure are strongly age-related. Neonatal seizures can occur, and tuberous sclerosis is the most common cause of the syndrome of early infantile epileptic encephalopathy, West and Lennox–Gastaut syndromes with seizure manifestations varying with age of onset. The other features of the condition are listed in Table 3.33. Mental deficiency occurs in about 50% of identified cases, and is more likely in those who develop seizures below

Table 3.33 The diagnostic features of tuberous sclerosis.

Primary features (a definite diagnosis can usually be made if only one of these is present)

Classic shagreen patch

Periungual fibroma

Retinal hamartoma

Facial angiofibromas

Subependymal glial nodule (on CT or MRI brain scan)

Renal angiomyolipoma (bilateral and multiple)

Secondary features (two or more features are required to make a diagnosis)

Atypical shagreen patch

Hypomelanotic macule

Gingival fibroma

Bilateral polycystic kidneys

Isolated renal angiomyolipoma

Cardiac rhabdomyoma

Cortical tuber (histological)

'Honeycomb lungs'

Infantile spasms

Myoclonic, atonic or tonic seizures

First-degree relative with tuberous sclerosis

Forehead fibrous plaque

Giant cell astrocytoma

the age of 2 years. In the brain, the characteristic pathological findings are cortical and subependymal nodules, and other features of cortical dysgenesis may be present. The subependymal nodules can undergo malignant transformation in adult life. Affected individuals can show widely varying manifestations, and very occasionally no clinical features at all. At one extreme, the sufferer can be entirely normal and at the other be severely disabled physically, mentally and with severe epilepsy. The diagnosis is made by clinical examination, family history, brain imaging, renal ultrasound, electrocardiogram (ECG), ophthalmic examination, and scrutiny of the skin under Wood's (ultraviolet) light. The patients should be counselled that there is a 50% chance of passing the condition to offspring. The epilepsy is treated on conventional lines, and the prognosis for seizure control and for other aspects of the condition is extremely variable. The infantile spasms respond well to vigabatrin, but there are no other known specific responses to particular antiepileptic drugs.

Cortical dysgenesis (cortical dysplasia and malformations of cortical development). Epilepsy is a common accompaniment of these disorders. The extent of the dysgenesis varies greatly, and so does the epilepsy. Infants with agyria are hypotonic, show poor development and seizures from the first days of birth. The epilepsy is severe, infantile spasms are frequent which can evolve into diffuse multifocal epilepsy. Medical treatment is generally ineffective. The clinical picture of pachygyria varies according to the severity of the malformation. In its severe form, patients can be severely retarded and have early onset multifocal epilepsy. At the other extreme, mild cases can present in adult life with mild focal epilepsy. Some cases conform to the pattern of the Lennox–Gastaut syndrome and treatment follows conventional lines. A similar range of clinical manifestations occur in band heterotopia. The bilateral perisylvian syndrome causes epilepsy, mental retardation and pseudobulbar palsy. Seizures are resistant to medical therapy in half the cases and callosotomy can be beneficial in reducing disabling seizures and drop attacks. Hemimegalencephaly presents with a severe encephalopathy, congenital hemiplegia, developmental delay and intractable seizures. The seizures are usually focal and hemispherectomy can be curative. The phenotype of both schizencephaly and polymicrogyria is extremely variable, with developmental delay and seizures the most common presenting features. Treatment is usually along conventional medical lines, and outcome is variable. Cortical resection of epileptogenic areas can be successful if the lesions are well localized. However, subtle abnormalities often extend beyond lesions detected on routine MRI. The presurgical assessment of these cases is difficult, and should be carried out only in experienced units. There have been no published investigations of the relative benefits of specific antiepileptic drugs in the cortical dysgeneses, and to date there is no known response-specificity.

Institutional care

The needs of individuals with multiple handicaps are often complex, and care is difficult to organize. In patients with severe epilepsy, the seizures usually pose major problems but in others the problems of epilepsy are less pressing than those of other handicaps. Epilepsy adds a dimension which care-providers often find difficult to deal with. The responsibility of dealing with potentially life-threatening seizures is felt to be too great by many otherwise competent persons. It is therefore often difficult to find suitable residential, daytime or vocational placements for handicapped people with epilepsy. A few specialized institutions provide expert epilepsy care and, although these provide a secure environment from the epilepsy point of view, they may be geographically distant, risking family estrangement. All institutions dealing with epilepsy require specialist medical input, and a failure to monitor the epilepsy is a dereliction of care. Teamwork is needed, with facilities for outpatient and inpatient treatment and good communication between the different professional groups and also the family. Care can be shared between an institution and the family, and in both settings a balance has to be set between overprotection and neglect. This balance can be very difficult to define or achieve. Individuals deserve an individually tailored solution, and the issues involved and the risks taken should be explicitly agreed with the individual, the family and the professional carers.

EPILEPSY IN THE ELDERLY

The incidence of epilepsy is highest in the young and the old. About 30% of new cases now occur in people over 65 years. The prevalence rises steeply in the elderly, and indeed the prevalence rate of treated epilepsy in those over 70 years is now almost double that in children. As the number of elderly people in the population is rising, the numbers of elderly people requiring treatment for epilepsy is also greatly increasing. The chief cause of epilepsy in those over 65 years is cerebrovascular disease. The frequency of vascular disease has greatly increased in the past 50 years. Currently, about 0.7% of the elderly population are treated for epilepsy, and epilepsy in the elderly is now the third most common neuro-

Table 3.34 Specific problems of treatment of epilepsy in elderly patients.

Distinctive range of causes of epilepsy
Distinctive differential diagnosis (especially syncope, cerebrovascular disease, cardiac disease, dementia and confusion)
Frequency of concurrent pathologies, unrelated to epilepsy
Pharmacokinetic differences (e.g. effective drug dose, dosage regimens, interactions, complications of polytherapy)
Pharmacodynamic differences (sensitivity to side-effects, dosage, specific drugs)
Distinctive psychological or social effects
Danger of precipitating functional failure

logical condition after dementia and stroke. The medical services must catch up to make adequate provision (Table 3.34).

Seizures in the elderly have a serious impact. Their unpleasantness is self-apparent. Postictal states can be prolonged. The confusional state of over 24 h was found to occur in the wake of 14% of seizures in the elderly, and in some cases confusion lasted over a week. Todd's paresis is also more common, and seizures are commonly misdiagnosed as stroke. Fractures and head injury are a potential risk. The falling in a seizure can mark a watershed in the older person's life, after which there is a sharp decline in functional independence. The loss of confidence and fear of further falls can render the person electively housebound. This loss of confidence can be compounded by other factors including the stigmatization of epilepsy, the assumption of impending death, the reaction of family and friends, the exclusion from activities, marginalization, loss of a driving licence, disempowerment and a shrinkage of life space.

Diagnosis
There are three elements worth special mention.
The differential diagnosis of the epileptic seizure. There is an abundance of causes of 'funny turns' in the elderly. Syncope, hypoglycaemia, transient ischaemic attacks, transient global amnesia, vertigo and non-specific dizziness afflict up to 10% of the older population. Syncope can have cardiac causes, be caused by blood pressure changes or simply impairment of the vascular reflexes linked to posture. Acute confusional states or fluctuating mental impairment can be ictal, postictal or caused by non-convulsive status, but are frequently misdiagnosed as manifestations of functional psychiatric illness, dementia or vascular disease. The discrimination of these events from epilepsy can pose a challenge. The history may be less well defined, the differentiating features less clear-cut than in the younger patient and pathologies may coexist.
The identification of cause. Cerebrovascular disease accounts for between 30 and 50% of cases. This can be occult and the first manifestation of hitherto silent cerebrovascular disease. Evidence of cerebrovascular disease can be found in about 15% of those presenting with apparently idiopathic late-onset epilepsy. In this sense, the seizures can be the harbinger of future stroke. Seizures also follow stroke, with a frequency of about 5% in the acute phase after stroke and 10% in the first 5 years after ischaemic stroke. The frequency after haemorrhagic stroke is somewhat greater than after ischaemic stroke. Large haemorrhag-

es or those affecting cerebral cortex are especially likely to result in seizures. Seizures can also result from cerebrovascular lesions secondary to rheumatic heart disease, endocarditis, mitral valve prolapse, carotid endarterectomy, cardiac dysrhythmias and, rarely, cardiac tumours. Subdural haematoma are another underdiagnosed cause of epilepsy in the elderly, and seizures also uncommonly occur in cerebral aneurysm, ruptured or unruptured. Cerebral tumours account for between 5 and 15% of all late onset epilepsies. The tumours are most commonly metastatic or gliomas. A few are meningiomas which are potentially operable. Ten per cent of the late onset epilepsies are caused by metabolic causes, such as alcohol, pyrexia, dehydration, infections, renal or hepatic dysfunction. Many drugs can cause seizures and drug-induced epilepsy is likely to be common in the elderly both because drugs are given more frequently and also because of the propensity of the elderly to pharmacokinetic vicissitude.

EEG changes. In the elderly, there are a variety of EEG changes which complicate diagnosis, and which are easily mistaken for epileptogenic patterns. Brief runs of temporal slow activity, especially on the left, becomes increasingly evident after the age of 50 years and should be considered a normal variant. Small sharp spikes during sleep and drowsiness also increase in frequency with age. Runs of tempero-parietal activity can occur in individuals over the age of 50 years. This pattern is known as the subclinical rhythmic electrographic discharge in adults (SREDA) pattern, and is not associated with epilepsy. Cerebrovascular disease produces focal and bilateral temporal changes which are also commonly mistaken for epilepsy, and are not predictive of overt epileptic seizures.

General aspects of management

Reassurance is of overriding importance that seizures: do not usually indicate cerebral tumours; do not imply psychiatric disorder or dementia; and can be controlled on safe medication.

Management often involves other professionals. Confidence needs to be rebuilt, mobility restored and the home circumstances reviewed. Advice and input from social services, remedial and occupational therapists are often needed. A home visit to identify sources of potential danger is helpful. A personal alarm can very useful, as can counselling and written advice for friends and relatives.

Factors known to precipitate seizures should be avoided, such as inadequate sleep, excess alcohol or hypoglycaemia.

Drug treatment

The general principles of treatment in the elderly are similar to those in other adults. However, there are potential differences which deserve special mention.

• Pharmacokinetics. There are important pharmacokinetic differences which affect drug handling, and the relationship between dose and serum level can be very different from that in younger adults. For many drugs, age is an important variable in a wide range of pharmacokinetic parameters. Furthermore, the range of variability in the elderly is greater than in young adults, and is often unpredictable. Protein binding can be reduced as albumin concentrations are lower in the elderly. The volume of distribution for lipid-soluble drugs can be increased and clearance lowered as a result of renal or hepatic disease. The half-life of many drugs is thereby increased. The interaction of the many medicaments taken by the elderly also can complicate the handling of drugs, by competition for absorption, protein binding, hepatic metabolism and renal clearance. The prescriber should be aware also that the published pharmacokinetic values are often expressed as mean values which do not necessarily take into account the wide range in the older population. Most drugs have not been subjected to rigorous trials in the elderly, but for all the above reasons this is an omission which should in the future be rectified.

• Compliance with medication can be poor as a result of memory lapses, failing intellect or confusion. In these situations, drug administration should be supervised. The provision of a weekly drug wallet can also be worthwhile.

• The adverse effects of drugs in the elderly may take unfamiliar forms. Confusion, general ill health, affective change or uncharacteristic motor or behavioural disturbances can occur with many of the antiepileptic drugs. Other side-effects in the elderly include the dangers of loss of bone mass from enzyme-inducing drugs, such as phenytoin, carbamazepine or phenobarbital. This is a particular risk in postmenopausal women. Phenytoin and carbamazepine also pose potential risks to cardiac function, and have the potential to promote hypotension and dysrhythmias. They should be used continuously in the elderly. Carbamazepine has an anticholinergic effect which may cause urinary retention and this effect is exacerbated in those with autonomic dysfunction, for instance in diabetes. Drug toxicity occurs generally at lower levels than in young adults.

• The therapeutic ranges defined in younger age groups do not necessarily apply to all elderly patients, who are generally susceptible to drug side-effects at lower serum levels than in younger patients.

• Polypharmacy. In the USA, persons over the age of 65 years comprise 13% of the population yet receive 32% of prescribed medications, and in one study of epilepsy patients aged 75 years, a mean of three medications per patient was taken in addition to the prescribed antiepileptic drugs.

Antiepileptic drugs

Phenytoin

Phenytoin is commonly prescribed to the elderly, in spite of its complex pharmacokinetics. As it is metabolized by saturable processes, age-related declines in hepatic function might be expected to be of real significance. However, published studies are inadequate and results have been conflicting. Some reports suggested that free phenytoin concentrations do indeed increase with age, although others have shown increased clearance in the elderly, partly attributable to the decreased albumin concentrations and others have shown no age-related difference in elimination parameters. The picture is confusing and advice is difficult to give. However, it would be wise to initiate therapy with phenytoin cautiously, at a relatively low dose (initial maintenance of 200 mg per day) followed by small dose increments (50 mg per day) as clinically indicated. The measurement of free phenytoin concentrations can be worthwhile in special circumstances, for example in ill or debilitated elderly patients whose serum albumin concentrations are low, or in those at risk from interactions.

Carbamazepine

There is little information about age-related changes in the pharmacokinetics of carbamazepine; surprisingly, in view of its widespread usage. One study of a small number of patients showed a 40% reduction in clearance in the elderly compared with young adults, whereas a study in healthy volunteers showed no specific age changes either in the area under the concentration–time curve, nor the elimination rate constants, nor in the carbamazepine 10,11-epoxide concentrations. Again, general advice is to initiate carbamazepine therapy slowly in individuals over 65 years, and also only cautiously to increment the dose. A reasonable regimen is to start therapy on 100 mg per day, and to increase the dose by 100 mg increments every fortnight, to a initial maintenance dose of 400 mg per day. This can be then be increased as clinically indicated.

Phenobarbital

Phenobarbital is partly eliminated by the kidneys and, as renal excretion declines with age, one might expect concentrations of phenobarbital to be higher per mg/kg dosage. Studies have shown significant changes in women but not in men. There have been surprisingly few comprehensive studies of metabolism or of absorption, metabolic or elimination parameters, and no studies of interactions in elderly subjects. This is a notable omission as phenobarbital has been widely used in the elderly for many years, and there are intensive pharmacokinetic studies in other age-groups. General advice would be to start phenobarbital dosage at between one-third to one-half less than those used in younger adults. Because of anxieties about the increased sensitivity of the older person to the cerebral side-effects of phenobarbital, dosage increments should be cautious and carefully monitored.

Sodium valproate

The half-life, volume of distribution and total clearance of valproate are little changed in the elderly. However, free valproate concentrations do increase and clearance decreases. One study has shown a 65% decrease in valproate clearance and a 67% increase in free valproate concentrations in old age. Valproate generally has few interactions at the hepatic level, and this is an advantage over other conventional antiepileptic drugs in older patients who are often taking a cocktail of other drugs for various conditions. There is also an impression that encephalopathic side-effects of valproate are more common in the elderly and these should be carefully monitored. It seems sensible therefore to initiate valproate therapy at 200 mg per day and increment the dose in 200 mg increments to an initial maintenance dose of 600 mg.

Gabapentin

Gabapentin is absorbed by a saturable transport mechanism, and it is not known if this is affected by age. As it is not metabolized, and there is minimal protein binding, age-related changes in distribution or metabolism should not be expected. The renal clearance of gabapentin does decrease with age, although the effect is small. For all these reasons, age does not influence gabapentin dosage, and in this respect it is a safe drug in the elderly.

Lamotrigine

The distribution and pharmacokinetics of lamotrigine in the elderly have not been studied. It is about 55% bound to plasma proteins and undergoes extensive hepatic metabolism, and also interacts with other antiepileptic drugs. For these reasons, age-related irregularities might be expected. Advice about dosage in the elderly therefore must be empirical, but again it would probably be wise to aim at low initial maintenance doses: 100 mg in monotherapy, 50–100 mg when comedicated with valproate alone, or 200 mg in patients comedicated with other enzyme-inducing antiepileptic drugs. Further studies though are clearly needed.

Generally, the absence of pharmacokinetic data for the elderly is a disgrace. Elderly patients are usually excluded from clinical trials, and there is therefore a worrying lack of information when a drug is newly licensed. After licensing, there seems little interest in defining pharmacokinetic parameters. Great care is therefore required when treating patients over 75 years. Because of the dearth of research data in this group, guidelines should be taken as generalities only. As concentrations per given dose are generally higher in the elderly than in young adults, it is wise to initiate therapy with low doses, and to aim for low maintenance doses, and to monitor drug concentrations more frequently than in the young adult population. Drug combinations should be avoided where possible. The potential therefore for interactions between the drugs due to hepatic mechanisms particularly, but also protein binding and renal mechanisms should be carefully monitored. Vigilance for unusual side-effects should be maintained—both encephalopathic and also metabolic.

EPILEPSY WITH MYOCLONIA

Myoclonus is defined as a sudden brief involuntary muscle contraction arising from the central nervous system. It can be non-epileptic in origin, arising from subcortical, brainstem or even spinal cord structures—these conditions are not considered further.

It can also occur as a form of epilepsy in a variety of settings.

Myoclonus in idiopathic generalized epilepsy
Myoclonus is most commonly encountered in idiopathic generalized epilepsy. These syndromes are outlined on p. 73.

Benign myoclonic epilepsy in infancy
This is a rare form of idiopathic generalized epilepsy, associated electrographically with spike–wave discharges. The myoclonus develops in infants or children before the age of 3 years, and can sometimes be exclusively startle-induced, or both startle-induced and spontaneous. The children are usually normal neurodevelopmentally, although delaying therapy has been said to carry the risk of slowing developmental progress. The prognosis is generally good and valproate will control the myoclonus in most cases.

Progressive myoclonic epilepsies (PME)
This generic term is applied to a group of rare conditions described in more detail below.

Focal myoclonus
Albeit rarely, focal forms of myoclonus are encountered in focal cortical epilepsy, typically of occipital, parietal or central origin. There is usually underlying structural cerebral disease.

Epilepsia partialis continua
This term is used to refer to continuous focal myoclonus and is a form of focal motor status epilepticus. It can be caused by various underlying disorders of the cerebral cortex, including tumour, stroke, arteriovascular malformations, trauma and infection. Rasmussen's chronic encephalitis is a common cause, especially in children. Epilepsia partialis continua is discussed further on p. 187.

Myoclonus in patients with diffuse cerebral dysfunction
Myoclonus also occurs in those with mental handicap and multifocal epilepsy. The myoclonus often takes several forms, even in the same patient, and frequently results in falls. It can be impossible clinically to differentiate from atonic or even tonic seizures. It is common in the Lennox–Gastaut syndrome, in Angelman syndrome, and in the various forms of childhood myoclonic encephalopathy.

Myoclonic astatic epilepsy (Doose syndrome)
This is a characteristic form of idiopathic myoclonic epilepsy. It develops in previously normal children usually between the ages of 2–5 years. In about one-third of cases there is a family history. Seizures take the form of massive myoclonic, myoclonic–astatic, atonic, atypical absence and tonic–clonic attacks. The seizures tend to cluster and episodes of convulsive and non-convulsive status epilepticus are not uncommon. The non-convulsive status episodes typically result in a stuporous state with apathy, se-

rial head-nodding, irregular twitching of the limbs and face which can persist for hours or days. The prognosis is variable. Some patients improve rapidly. In others, the seizures persist, tonic seizures at night develop as does learning disability. The clinical and EEG features of a severe case are indistinguishable from those of the Lennox–Gastaut syndrome and some authorities consider this condition to be part of a spectrum of the Lennox–Gastaut syndrome.

Progressive myoclonic epilepsy

This term refers to a group of rare conditions which are characterized by relentlessly progressive myoclonus, other seizure types, dementia and other neurological signs. In most parts of the world, there are six common underlying conditions: Lafora body disease; neuronal ceroid lipofuscinosis; mitochondrial disorders; dentato-rubro-pallido-luysian atrophy (DRPLA); sialidosis and Unverricht–Lundborg disease. Less common causes are listed in Table 3.35. The term progressive myoclonic epilepsy should be confined to those cases where the predominant clinical symptom is myoclonus, and differentiated from other progressive encephalopathies with myoclonus and from the so-called progressive myoclonic ataxias.

Differential diagnosis from idiopathic generalized epilepsy—especially juvenile myoclonic epilepsy—can be difficult in the early stages when myoclonus may be the only manifestation, but the diagnosis is usually resolved by evidence of progression, the development of other signs and the lack of response to treatment.

The myoclonus is erratic, generalized, multifocal or asymmetric and affects limbs, the trunk and the face. The myoclonus can become continuous for long periods of time. It can be exacerbated by action or startle, and sometimes there is a massive increase in the frequency and amplitude of the jerks produced by movement. The jerks can reach devastating proportions, rendering the patient bedbound and severely disabled. Focal or restricted myoclonus is a much less common manifestation. Tonic–clonic and other seizures also occur at different frequencies in different aetiologies, but are not generally a serious clinical problem. The underlying cause also determines the degree of cognitive and neurological disturbance and its progression. A causal diagnosis can sometimes be made on the basis of the family history, the age of onset, the rate of progression, the occurrence of associated neurological symptoms and diagnostic tests.

Neurophysiology and neuroimaging. The EEG exhibits generalized spike or polyspike and slow wave discharges, sometimes with photosensitivity. Somatosensory evoked potentials (SEPs) are also abnormal, showing giant cortical responses. The background activity of the EEG is slow, and this differentiates the conditions from idiopathic generalized epilepsy, but does not help in establishing the underlying cause. In neuronal ceroid lipofuscinosis, the electroretinogram is undetectable and the visual evoked response abnormal. EMG may demonstrate a peripheral neuropathy in sialidosis and mitochondrial disease. Neuroimaging can show atrophy, but there are no specific radiological features.

Urine testing. Dolichols may be increased in the urine of patients with neuronal ceroid lipofuscinosis. Oligosaccharides are increased in patients with sialidosis. Organic acids are found in the urine in patients with biotin-responsive encephalopathy.

Blood. Assay of the white cell enzymes can help diagnose sialidosis (alpha-N-acetylneurominidase, beta- galactosidase and Gaucher's disease (beta-glucocerebrosidase). Analysis of mitochondrial DNA may reveal the underlying mitochondrial mutations. Genetic tests are now also available for Unverricht–Lundborg disease, dentato-rubro-pallido-luysian atrophy and Lafora body disease.

Table 3.35 Causes of progressive myoclonic epilepsy.

Unverricht–Lundborg disease (Baltic myoclonus)
Lafora body disease
Mitochondrial disease (MERRF)
Ceroid lipofuscinosis
Dentato-rubro-pallido-luysian atrophy (DRPLA)
Sialidosis
GM$_1$ and GM$_2$ gangliosidosis
Gaucher's disease
Huntington's disease
Juvenile neuraxonal dystrophy
Alpers' disease
Biotin-responsive progressive myoclonus
Phenylketonuria
Menkes' disease

In a significant proportion of patients no cause can be identified.

Biopsy. Examination of the ecrine sweat gland in skin biopsy, looking for polysaccharide-containing inclusion bodies, is the diagnostic test for Lafora body disease. The inclusion bodies can also be identified on liver biopsy. Electron microscopy of the ecrine secretory cells and other tissues demonstrates what are known as fingerprint profiles and curvilinear bodies in neuronal ceroid lipofuscinosis. Mitochondrial cytopathy can be diagnosed by muscle biopsy, and Gaucher's disease by finding the characteristic foam cells on bone marrow examination. Brain biopsy is not generally indicated, but is occasionally needed where there is the question of remediable pathology or where the need for diagnosis is paramount. Neuro-axonal dystrophy and atypical inclusion bodies can be diagnosed *in vivo* only by this method.

Lafora body disease

The age of onset is between 6 and 19 years. The disease presents with progressive myoclonic and associated tonic–clonic and partial seizures, the latter often with visual symptomatology and severe dementia. Ataxia and dysarthria also occur. The condition is progressive and death occurs within 10 years. The EEG may show focal occipital spike discharges although this is not a reliable diagnostic finding. The underlying enzymic defects have not yet been characterized. The condition is inherited by an autosomal-recessive defect. The genetic basis has recently been established.

Unverricht–Lundborg disease (Baltic myoclonus)

The onset is between the ages of 6–15 years. There is marked geographical variation, with the condition being especially frequent in Scandinavia and the Baltic regions. The genetic defect has recently been identified. The condition presents with myoclonus, initially easy to control, but which slowly worsens. Other seizures are infrequent and usually easily controlled. Ataxia and tremor develop and may become the major clinical features. There is a very slow intellectual decline, but this can be mild. Death usually occurs in the third or fourth decade of life.

Mitochondrial disease

Mitochondrial cytopathy presents with myoclonus. The classical phenotype is with myoclonic epilepsy and ragged red fibres (MERFF). The onset of symptoms can be in childhood or adult life and the progression and clinical severity are extremely variable. The myoclonus is usually associated with ataxia and less consistently with tonic–clonic seizures and dementia. Other associated features include, in some cases, short stature, deafness, optic atrophy, endocrine dysfunction, pes cavus and other congenital abnormalities, peripheral neuropathy and myopathy. The conclusive diagnostic test is the demonstration of a mitochondrial DNA mutation and the finding of characteristic ragged red fibres on muscle biopsy.

Neuronal ceroid lipofuscinosis

This is an autosomal-recessive disorder characterized by liposomal inclusions. These have a characteristic appearance on electron microscopy. Diagnosis is made by a demonstration of liposomal inclusions in white blood cells or in biopsy material. There are various clinical phenotypes. The infantile form (Santavuori's disease) has its onset before 2 years and is rapidly progressive with death by the age of 10 years. It is characterized by myoclonus, developmental regression, ataxia, hypotonia and blindness. The late infantile form (Bielschowsky–Janski disease) develops between the age of 2–4 years, presents with myoclonus and progressive ataxia, dementia and spasticity and again death occurs before the age of 10 years. The juvenile form (Batten's disease) is the most common. The onset is between the age of 4–15 years and presents with visual failure and then progressive massive myoclonus and other seizure types. Dementia is usually relatively mild. Pyramidal, extrapyramidal and cerebellar signs develop and death usually occurs by the age of 20 years. Adult onset neuronal ceroid lipofuscinosis (Kufs' disease) presents with progressive myoclonus and prominent dementia. Motor signs develop, including cerebellar, pyramidal and extrapyramidal signs. Visual failure, in contrast to the younger forms, is not a prominent feature. The progression is rapid and death occurs usually within 10 years of onset.

Dentato-rubro-pallido-luysian atrophy

Dentato-rubro-pallido-luysian atrophy is an autosomal-dominant condition with varying frequency around the world. It is most common in Japan and not uncommon in Europe. The condition develops in childhood or adult life and is only slowly progressive. Fifty per cent of cases present a progressive myoclonic epilepsy, and the others with dementia or with cerebellar ataxia. Pyramidal and extrapyramidal signs and psychiatric disturbance develop in the course of the illness. The genetic basis, a trinucleotide repeat, has now been identified, and the diagnosis can be made by genetic analysis.

Treatment of myoclonic epilepsy

As will be obvious from the previous section, myoclonus occurs in a wide range of clinical contexts. The gravity of the seizure disorder, the response to therapy and the outcome will vary accordingly. The principles of therapy, though, are similar for all the myoclonic epilepsies. The myoclonus in idiopathic generalized epilepsies is generally well controlled on single-drug therapy with valproate. The myoclonus in the symptomatic generalized, progressive myoclonic or the focal epilepsies is more difficult to treat, and drug combinations are said by some to confer greater benefit.

Choice of drug for myoclonus

The drug of first choice in all the generalized myoclonic epilepsies is valproate. This should be used initially alone. Second-line therapy includes the following drugs, used either alone or in combination with valproate.

Benzodiazepine drugs. The traditional choice is clonazepam. However, this has a strong tendency to cause drowsiness, and its use has been to a large extent superseded—in some countries at least—by clobazam which has much less sedative action. A major disadvantage of the benzodiazepine drugs generically is the tendency for tolerance to develop and for their effectiveness to be lost. This applies in myoclonus as well as in other seizure types, and to all compounds in this class.

Phenobarbital (and other barbiturates). Phenobarbital has strong antimyoclonic action. Its tendency to cause sedation and behavioural effects in children has limited its use in contemporary practice, but it is still useful as second-line therapy for intractable myoclonus.

Piracetam. This extraordinary compound is the only drug uniquely effective in myoclonus and which has no effect in other types of epilepsy. The mode of action is unknown, but it is a useful addition to the armamentarium of second-line drugs for myoclonus. The dosage required for myoclonus is extremely high, but the drug is very well tolerated. It is primarily effective in cortical myoclonus, but

may also have some value in other myoclonic syndromes (Fig. 3.5).

Lamotrigine. This drug has an unpredictable effect in myoclonus. Some patients respond well but in other cases the drug is ineffective. The effect is unpredictable and the reason for the variable response unknown. Lamotrigine is not currently licensed for use in myoclonus and there have been no controlled trials of the drug in myoclonus.

Topiramate, felbamate and levetiracetam. These are newer drugs in which there is anecdotal evidence of good antimyoclonic action, at least in some patients. Levetiracetam has a close chemical relationship to piracetam and their similar structure may explain the antimyoclonic effects. It is however, not currently licensed for use in myoclonus, and no controlled studies in myoclonus have been carried out.

Steroids can be used as a last resort in many of the refractory myoclonic epilepsies, especially in childhood. Their effectiveness has not been rigorously tested and there is no agreement as to dosage or formulation.

Focal myoclonus can be treated with any drug used for focal epilepsy. There are no controlled, or even open studies but anecdotal experience would favour valproate as first choice.

Drugs which aggravate myoclonus

The antiepileptic drugs vigabatrin and gabapentin frequently aggravate myoclonus and can indeed precipitate myoclonus for the first time in susceptible patients with other seizure types. Phenytoin has been reported to worsen the myoclonus in the progressive myoclonic epilepsies, although the evidence is not conclusive. Both carbamazepine and phenytoin can aggravate myoclonus in juvenile myoclonic epilepsy.

Therapies for specific myoclonic syndromes

Specific therapy has been attempted in a number of the progressive myoclonic epilepsies, although none has an uncontested place in treatment regimens. Anti-oxidant treatments have been used for some years in the treatment of the neuronal ceroid lipofuscinoses. *N*-acetylcysteine has some advocates in Unverricht–Lundborg disease. Although often prescribed, it is doubtful whether these compounds have any major beneficial effect. Alcohol has a beneficial effect on the myoclonus in Unverricht–Lundborg

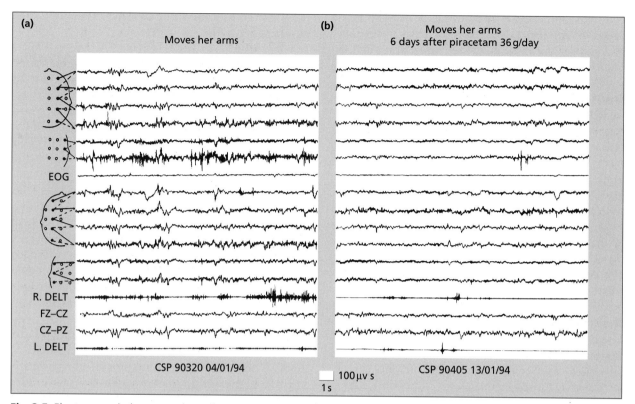

Fig. 3.5 Electroencephalogram-polygraphy. A 14-year-old girl with Unverricht–Lundborg disease of 6 years' duration. (a) On valproate and clonazepam, numerous sharp waves on the EEG and intense myoclonus appearing both as muscular potentials superimposed on the temporal EEG leads and as jerks in the deltoid muscles. (b) Eight days after addition of piracetam, 36 g per day, with clear abolition of cephalic and peripheral myoclonias and of EEG abnormalities. The patient was able to leave her wheelchair and walk freely. This effect was maintained over a 1-year follow-up.

disease, as indeed it does in some forms of subcortical myoclonus.

Surgical therapy is sometimes effective for myoclonus caused by focal cortical lesions, including focal cortical dysplasia and Rasmussen's encephalitis. Resective cortical surgery is discussed further in Chapter 6.

IDIOPATHIC GENERALIZED EPILEPSY

Idiopathic generalized epilepsy (IGE) is a genetic disorder; this much is agreed, although the exact genetic mechanisms are unclear, and nor is it known to what extent different mechanisms underlie the different phenotypes. Nowhere in the study of epilepsy is there more divergence of opinion about the extent to which subclassification is justified (Table 3.36). At one extreme, the conditions could be considered a 'biological continuance' possibly with a unitary genetic mechanism, and at the other extreme,

syndromic subclassification depending on minute clinical differences has been proposed. Where nosological reality exists is not currently known. The features shared by these syndromes include: onset in childhood or early adult life; a positive family history; a triad of seizure types – generalized absence (petit mal), generalized tonic–clonic seizures and myoclonus – the EEG signature of generalized 3 Hz

Table 3.36 Subtypes of idiopathic generalized epilepsy.

Benign neonatal convulsions

Benign myoclonus of infancy

Childhood absence epilepsy (pyknolepsy)

Juvenile absence epilepsy

Juvenile myoclonic epilepsy (impulsive petit mal)

Epilepsy with grand mal seizures on awakening

Epilepsy with eyelid myoclonia

Perioral myoclonia with absence

spike and wave discharges on a normal background, often exacerbated by overbreathing and photosensitivity; a diurnal pattern of seizure recurrence, especially on awakening and during sleep; normal intellect; the absence of underlying structural aetiology, although possibly minor developmental changes defined microscopically; and, finally, an excellent response in most cases to sodium valproate.

A number of overlapping syndromes have been described and these include the following.

Childhood absence epilepsy (pyknolepsy, pure petit mal)

This is a relatively well-defined syndrome with onset between the ages of 3–12 years and a peak age of onset of 6–8 years. Seizures take the form of absence attacks which can be daily and very frequent—sometimes hundreds a day. The absences are associated with bilateral, symmetrical, synchronous spike and wave EEG discharges at 3 Hz on a normal background, and are activated by hyperventilation. Marked photosensitivity is considered by some to be an exclusion criterion, and a positive family history is present in 15–44%.

Juvenile absence epilepsy

The age of onset is older than in childhood absence epilepsy, with a peak age of onset at 10–12 years (range 7–16 years). The absences do not manifest the same explosive daily frequency as in childhood absence epilepsy, and tend to be longer. Myoclonic seizures occur more frequently and 80% of patients develop generalized tonic–clonic seizures. These can precede or post-date the onset of absence attacks. Between 10 and 20% of cases of juvenile absence epilepsy are said to be photosensitive.

Juvenile myoclonic epilepsy

This is the most common syndrome and accounts for between 3 and 12% of all epilepsies. Seizure types include myoclonic jerks which are universal (defining the syndrome) and occur alone in 8% of cases, with absence attacks in 28% and with generalized tonic–clonic seizures in 90% of cases. There is a marked diurnal variation, with the myoclonus occurring particularly on awakening, and the seizures are exacerbated by sleep deprivation and alcohol intake. The myoclonic jerks vary in severity and range from what may be mistaken for tremor to severe jerks which result in a fall. They can sometimes be overlooked unless specific enquiry is made, if the patient is presenting with generalized tonic–clonic seizures. The myoclonic jerks sometimes occur in series and

can sometimes lead on to a generalized tonic–clonic seizure. The myoclonus persists into adult life, although also tends to diminish over time. Patients have normal intellect and are without additional neurological handicaps. The condition has a genetic basis, although the genetic mechanisms have not yet been elucidated. The EEG has a normal background with bursts of generalized 3 Hz spike and wave (the signature of the idiopathic generalized epilepsies) or fast polyspike discharges. Photosensitivity is found in between 20 and 50%. The response to treatment is usually excellent, and the epilepsy should not usually pose a serious handicap.

Epilepsy with grand mal seizures on awakening

Seizures occur shortly after awakening in this syndrome and are exacerbated by sleep deprivation and alcohol. Seizures may also occur after a period of relaxation in the evening. Absence and myoclonus are rare.

Epilepsies with eyelid myoclonias

Eyelid myoclonias can occur in certain patients with idiopathic generalized epilepsies. Whether or not these cases form a separate syndromic group is an arguable point, and eyelid myoclonia can coexist with generalized myoclonus and also absence and tonic–clonic attacks. The patients are usually photosensitive. Some children with this condition self-stimulate the attacks by photic stimulation, presumably because the attacks induce a pleasurable feeling. Therapy with valproate is usually successful in controlling the myoclonus.

Eyelid myoclonia with absence (Jeavon's syndrome) is a relatively specific entity. It presents in the first few years of life. The fast myoclonic jerks of the eyelids are frequently accompanied by upward deviation of the eyes and sometimes the head. The EEG shows generalized spike or polyspike and wave discharges with eye closure and with photic stimulation or hyperventilation.

Perioral myoclonia with absence

This is a much rarer condition and is treatment-resistant. The predominant seizure type is that of absence with rhythmic myoclonus and perioral facial muscles. Absence status also occurs.

Other syndromes related to idiopathic generalized epilepsy

These include myoclonic absence epilepsy which is a relatively rare condition characterized by myoclonic absences, age of onset peaking at 7 years and with a less favourable prognosis than childhood absence epilepsy. Other seizure types occur in two-thirds of cases. Intellectual function deteriorates and mental subnormality is common. Benign myoclonic epilepsy in infancy comprises generalized myoclonic jerks with generalized spikes or polyspike and wave on the EEG. There may be a family history of febrile convulsions and a positive family history of epilepsy and generalized tonic–clonic seizures develop subsequently in a proportion of patients. Benign familial myoclonus has an autosomal-dominant inheritance and an average age of onset of 10 years. The myoclonus is massive and symmetrical and often stimulus-sensitive. No other seizure types occur, there are no other neurological abnormalities and the EEG is normal.

Although it will be clear from the above that all these conditions overlap markedly and one can argue whether or not subdivision is valid, they all are clearly distinguished from other cryptogenic generalized epilepsies. It is quite wrong to allocate any case of cryptogenic generalized epilepsy to the category of idiopathic generalized epilepsy, and this confusion has bedevilled previous clinical studies.

Treatment

Lifestyle manipulation can be quite helpful in many cases of IGE, especially in adolescence. The avoidance of sleep deprivation and excessive alcohol intake can be very beneficial. Photosensitive patients should be counselled to avoid relevant stimuli. Some patients with established mild epilepsy can avoid drug treatment altogether by taking simple measures (Table 3.37).

Absence seizures

The first-line treatment of absence seizures in IGE (petit mal seizures) is with either ethosuximide or sodium valproate. For many years ethosuximide has been standard drug therapy and it is highly effective and in general well tolerated. However, the drug is relatively ineffective in controlling generalized tonic–clonic seizures. The main use of ethosuximide is therefore in childhood absence epilepsy, as it is in children that there is anxiety about the idiosyncratic effects of valproate. Sodium valproate is however considered a drug of choice by many people. It is as effective as ethosuximide, and indeed both drugs can be expected to fully control absence seizures in over 90% of patients. It has the added advantage of being useful against both generalized tonic–clonic and myoclonic seizures which commonly accompany absence seizures.

Phenobarbital is an effective second-line agent against absence seizures. Other drugs which have been used in the past but which are now hardly ever prescribed, largely because of their side-effect profiles, include methosuximide and trimethadone. The benzodiazepine drugs, particularly clonazepam, can also be effective against absence epilepsy although the drug-induced drowsiness caused by clonazepam can exacerbate absence seizures.

Occasionally, absence seizures will be resistant to monotherapy with either valproate or ethosuximide,

Table 3.37 Drug treatment in idiopathic generalized epilepsy.

Seizure type	First-line drugs	Main second-line therapy
Absence seizures	Valproate, ethosuximide	Acetazolamide Benzodiazepines Lamotrigine Phenobarbital/primidone
Myoclonus	Valproate	Benzodiazepines Ethosuximide Lamotrigine Phenobarbital/primidone Piracetam
Tonic–clonic seizures	Valproate	Acetazolamide Carbamazepine Clobazam/clonazepam Gabapentin Lamotrigine Levetiracetam Oxcarbazepine Phenobarbital Phenytoin Primidone Topiramate

and the combination of both drugs may be helpful. Lamotrigine and topiramate both have potential in the treatment of absence epilepsy, although their position in its treatment has not yet been fully established.

Myoclonic seizures

Sodium valproate is a drug of choice for the myoclonic seizures of IGE. Complete seizure control can be expected in four out of five cases with valproate used alone. Second-line treatments include the benzodiazepine drugs, particularly clobazam or clonazepam, which can be used alone or in combination with valproate. Phenobarbital and ethosuximide can be tried and again lamotrigine and topiramate show potential in at least some cases, but their exact place in therapy has not been established. Piracetam can be remarkably effective in pure myoclonus, although it has no effect in absence or generalized tonic–clonic seizures. Levetiracetam (LO59) is a drug currently in late clinical trials, which shows promise in being effective in all these seizure types.

Generalized tonic–clonic seizures

Typically in IGE, generalized tonic–clonic seizures occur in combination with myoclonic and/or absence seizures. The seizures occur predominantly shortly after wakening, when drowsy or while asleep. Most antiepileptic clinical trials have been seizure—rather than syndrome—orientated, it is therefore at present unclear whether the generalized tonic–clonic seizures of idiopathic generalized epilepsy respond to a different antiepileptic drug profile than the generalized seizures in other types of epilepsy. There is a strong clinical suspicion that valproate is more effective in treating tonic–clonic seizures when they are part of the syndrome of idiopathic generalized epilepsy than in other situations. Similarly, vigabatrin or tiagabine may be less effective than in secondarily generalized seizures, although there is no clinical trial evidence to back up this anecdotal clinical impression. Complete seizure control can be expected in at least two-thirds of patients with generalized tonic–clonic seizures alone or in combination with absence or myoclonic attacks. Any of the other major antiepileptic drugs are appropriate as second-line therapy.

SPECIAL ISSUES IN THE TREATMENT OF EPILEPSY IN WOMEN

Sexuality

Hyposexuality has long been recognized as a feature of epilepsy. Between 30 and 60% of men have reported lack of desire and impotence, and in one study 21% of men with chronic epilepsy had not experienced sexual intercourse. Amongst women, self reports of dyspareunia, vaginismus and arousal insufficiency are common, and also dissatisfaction with sexual experience. There are a number of potential mechanisms. Clearly, the psychosocial difficulties encountered by people with epilepsy could play a part, including stigmatization, lack of self-esteem, restricted lifestyles, parental overprotection, and depression and anxiety. Biological changes, including altered levels of sex hormones—especially free levels—are found in epilepsy, caused by the seizures and the drug therapy; these too could contribute to sexual difficulties. Seizures involving limbic structures too might be expected to alter sexual behaviour, and there is evidence, albeit inconclusive, that those with temporal lobe epilepsy have a greater degree of sexual dysfunction than those with generalized epilepsy. Antiepileptic drugs can alter the metabolism of sex steroid hormones and also affect their protein binding. There is a body of evidence demonstrating quite wide cultural differences which suggests that the social factors certainly have a role and, one suspects, are more important than the biological factors. Having said this, most people with epilepsy of course have quite normal and fulfilling sexual lives.

Treatment should begin with a careful analysis of potential causes, some of which may be quite independent of epilepsy or its treatment; psychosexual counselling can be very helpful. Control of seizures and reduction of antiepileptic therapy, including the withdrawal of sedative drugs, may improve sexual functioning, as may individual or couple sexual therapy.

Fertility

Fertility rates have been shown to be lower in women with treated epilepsy than in an age-matched control population. In one study of a general population of 2 052 922 persons in England and Wales, an overall fertility rate was 47.1 (95% CI 42.3–52.2) live births per 1000 women with epilepsy per year compared with a national rate of 62.6. The difference in rates was found in all age categories between the ages of 25–39 years. The reasons for these lower rates are probably complex. There are undoubtedly social effects: women with epilepsy have lower rates of marriage, marry later and suffer social isolation and stigmatization. Some avoid having children because of the risk of epilepsy in the offspring, and some

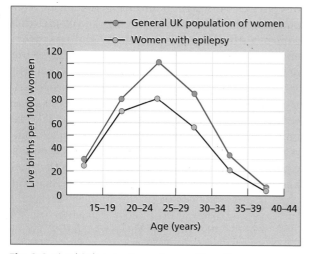

Fig. 3.6 Live birth rates in mothers with epilepsy on treatment compared to general population (study of a UK population of over 2 million persons).

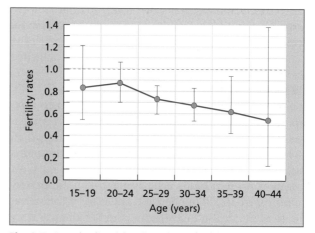

Fig. 3.7 Standardized fertility ratio of mothers with epilepsy.

because of the teratogenic potential of antiepileptic drugs. Other patients have impaired personality or cognitive development. There are other biological factors which could lead to reduced fecundity. These include genetic factors and adverse antiepileptic drug effects. The latter are discussed below. The lowering of fertility is a worrying finding which is another important disadvantage for women with epilepsy. If there are potentially preventable causes, these should be sought (Figs 3.6 and 3.7).

Oral contraception

Enzyme-inducing antiepileptic drugs, such as barbiturate, phenytoin and carbamazepine, increase the rate at which the steroid hormone content of the contraceptive pill is metabolized. These drugs have the potential, therefore, to inactivate the contraceptive action of low-oestrogen-containing preparations (< 50 μg of oestrogenic hormone). There is no risk with non-enzyme-inducing drugs, such as vigabatrin, valproate, benzodiazepines or gabapentin. Lamotrigine has some enzyme-inducing action but has not been shown to affect oral contraception. In spite of this risk, inappropriate prescribing of low-dose contraceptive with enzyme-inducing drugs is widespread, In a large UK general practice survey, 17% (390 of 2341) of all women with epilepsy were taking an oral contraceptive. Of these, 200 were comedicated·with an enzyme-inducing antiepileptic drug, and 44% (87 of the 200) were taking a contraceptive pill with less than 50 μg of oestradiol. That this is a real problem is shown in one study which found that

8.5% of pregnant epileptic women reported oral contraceptive failure.

If women taking enzyme-inducing antiepileptic drugs wish to take the oral contraceptive pill, a preparation with at least 50 μg of oestradiol is safe in most but not all women. Breakthrough bleeding (mid-cycle bleeding) is a useful sign of inadequate oestrogenic effect, but it is not invariable and contraceptive failure can occur without mid-cycle bleeding. Occasionally, 80 or even 100 μg oestradiol are needed for contraceptive effect. Alternatively, 'tricycling' a 50-μg oestradiol preparation can be employed, which entails taking three-monthly packets of the contraceptive without a break, followed by an interval of four days rather than the usual seven. Sixty, 80 or 100 μg can be administered by providing a double dose of a 30, 40 or 50 μg compound. Women should be advised that even using higher dose preparations, there is a risk of contraceptive failure, and figures of 3 failures per 1000 women years are quoted, compared to the 0.3 per 1000 rate in the general population. It is also worth pointing out that the higher dose contraceptives are prescribed simply to keep up with the increased metabolism, and the oestrogen levels attained are equivalent to those provided by lower dose contraceptives in non-epileptic women. There should therefore be no excess risk of oestrogen-induced complications, such as thrombosis.

Injectable contraception

The injectable contraceptives do not have the same problems. One hundred and fifty micrograms of Depo-Provera given every 12 weeks has a failure rate of about 0.5 per 1000 women years. The rate limiting step of Depo-Provera metabolism is hepatic blood flow and comedication with enzyme-inducing drugs does not affect hormonal levels.

Menstruation and catamenial epilepsy

There is no doubt that in a proportion of women with active epilepsy, seizures are more likely to occur in a pattern related to the menstrual cycle. Although studies have shown a positive association in less than 10%, it seems likely that this is an underestimate. Oestrogen is mildly epileptogenic, and the high oestrogen concentration in the follicular phase of the menstrual cycle is a possible underlying cause for the greater propensity for seizures. Premenstrual tension and water retention are other possible contributory factors.

Epilepsy in which the seizure pattern has a strong relationship to the menstrual cycle is referred to as catamenial epilepsy. There have been attempts to devise special treatment approaches to patients with catamenial seizures. Hormonal manipulation has been attempted with oral progesterone or norethisterone with only marginal benefit. Attempts to abolish the menstrual cycle by hormonal means or even oophorectomy have had surprisingly disappointing results. In most patients seizures tend to continue at much the same frequency, albeit with some loss of pattern regularity. Intermittent antiepileptic therapy taken around the risk period each month has also been tried. Five to seven days' therapy with acetazolamide has proved successful in a few cases. Clobazam, taken in the same manner, has shown more promise with improvement noted in one study in 78% of women. This approach though, in routine clinical practice, produces a worthwhile effect in only a small number of women. Reasons for these disappointing results include irregularities of the cycle, the fact that the catamenial exacerbation is seldom reliably linked to any particular day of the cycle and tolerance to the effects of clobazam.

Teratogenicity of antiepileptic drugs

The first report of an antiepileptic drug-induced malformation was in 1963 caused by methpenytoin. In 1968, Meadows conducted a pioneering enquiry and concluded that congenital malformations were twice as common in children exposed *in utero* to antiepileptic drugs as would be expected, and this has set the scene for numerous subsequent investigations.

There is now conclusive evidence that antiepileptics do cause malformations: animal testing has shown patterns of malformation similar to that seen in humans; malformation rates in the offspring of mothers with epilepsy on treatment are higher than those off treatment; mean antiepileptic drug levels are higher in the mothers of infants with malformations than in those without; and infants of mothers on polytherapy have higher malformation rates than those exposed to single-drug treatment. It had been argued that seizures themselves may be a confounding factor, but most investigations have shown that seizures during pregnancy do not increase the risk of congenital malformations (Table 3.38).

Table 3.38 Fetal abnormalities, attributable to phenytoin and other older antiepileptic drugs.*

Growth
Perinatal growth deficiency
Postnatal growth deficiency
Microcephaly
Craniofacial
Short nose, low cranial bridge
Hypertelorism
Epicanthic folds
Strabismus and other ocular abnormalities
Low set ears and other aural abnormalities
Wide mouth and prominent lips
Wide fontanelles
Cleft lip and cleft palate
Limbs
Hypoplasia of nails
Transverse palmar crease
Short fingers
Cerebral
Mild learning disability
Development delay
Systemic
Short neck, low hairline
Rib, sternal or spinal anomalies
Widely spaced hypoplastic nipples
Hernias
Undescended testicles
Neuroblastoma and neural ridge tumours
Cardiac and renal abnormalities

* This is a list of reported abnormalities, although many are uncontrolled observations and the frequency of these anomalies is unclear (indeed some may be no more frequent in patients with epilepsy than in the general population). The contribution of phenytoin is unclear and some authors prefer the term 'fetal anticonvulsant syndrome' to emphasize the lack of clarity about the role of phenytoin.

Malformations associated with antiepileptic drugs

The most common major malformations associated with traditional antiepileptic drug therapy (phenytoin, phenobarbital, primidone, benzodiazepine) are cleft palate, cleft lip and cardiac malformations. There is also a risk of neural tube and skeletal abnormalities. Unfortunately, because most studies were of women on multiple-drug therapy, the risks of individual drugs are not clearly established. Phenytoin therapy, however, has been clearly associated with an increased risk of neuroblastoma in the infant, although the absolute risk is very small.

The background population risk of spina bifida is approximately 0.2–0.5% with geographical variation. Valproate is associated with a 1–2% risk of spina bifida aperta, a risk which is strongly dosage-related. Carbamazepine carries a risk of spina bifida aperta of about 0.5–1%. Both carbamazepine and valproate have been associated with hypospadias. It is instructive to note that the induction of neural tube defects by valproate and carbamazepine were not noticed in animal toxicology. One study purported to demonstrate smaller head circumference in babies of mothers on carbamazepine, but the statistical basis of this observation was not well founded.

In addition to the major malformations, less severe dysmorphic changes (fetal syndromes) have been postulated, although there is little agreement about their frequency or even existence. The problem is further complicated by the confounding factor of genetic influence which is potentially of great importance. The fetal phenytoin syndrome was the first to be described, and is said to comprise a characteristic pattern of facial and limb disturbances (see Table 3.38). Most of these features though are minor and overlap with the normal variation seen in children born to healthy mothers. Recent prospective and blinded studies have failed, however, to confirm a clear-cut drug effect for most features. Only hypertelorism and distal digital hypoplasia occurred at any greater frequency than in the general population, and even this association is weak. Furthermore, the nail hypoplasia tends to disappear during childhood.

Case reports of primidone and phenobarbital 'syndromes' have been published, comprising facial changes and developmental delay. The complexity of the subject is shown by one report of four siblings with the classical 'hydantoin syndrome' born to a mother taking phenytoin and primidone for the first three pregnancies but only primidone during the fourth. A 'carbamazepine syndrome' has been claimed on the basis of a few case reports which are unconvincing. Finally, recent interest has focused on a 'valproate syndrome' said to occur in up to 50% of infants born to mothers on valproate; again, no blinded studies have been carried out and the true status of this syndrome is unclear.

Even greater controversy exists in relation to the question of whether maternal drug usage results in infantile developmental delay or learning disability. While there is no doubt that these occur at a higher frequency amongst infants born to epileptic mothers—between two- and sevenfold increases—the association could be caused by genetic factors, and population studies which have attempted to segregate drug effects have not demonstrated any significant associations. Small increases in pre- and postnatal growth retardation rates have been found in controlled studies of mothers taking antiepileptics, but the growth differences had disappeared by the time the offspring were 5 years old. One preliminary study suggests that the effect is greater with valproate.

When considering the teratogenic potential of the newer antiepileptic drugs, three lessons from the experience with the traditional therapies are worth making. First, even today the full range of their teratogenicity has not been not established. Secondly, the risk of major malformations were not noticed until the drugs had been in extensive use for decades. Thirdly, negative animal results are not a reliable indicator of safety. Any claims for safety for newer drugs should be seen in this context.

It is not clear whether or not the benzodiazepines have any teratogenic potential, although there are case reports of facial clefts, cardiac and skeletal abnormalities. Vigabatrin has caused cleft palate and fusion defects in the rabbit. Since its licensing 10 years ago, infants born to mothers taking vigabatrin with spina bifida, cleft palate, absent diaphragm and Siamese twins have been reported. Topiramate, in animal models, causes right-sided limb and rib and vertebral abnormalities, a pattern similar to that observed with acetazolamide, also a carbonic anhydrase inhibitor. No similar human abnormalities have been reported on carbonic anhydrase inhibitors, and none in the small number of pregnancies in woman taking topiramate. Gabapentin causes hydroureter and hydronephrosis in rabbits, but there have been no reported human pregnancy abnormalities. Lamotrigine has not been associated with any consistent animal or human abnormalities, although human experience is extremely limited. Currently, the advice has to be to avoid the use of any of these drugs in pregnancy until more definitive advice can be given.

Pregnancy

Effects of epilepsy on pregnancy

About 50 live births per 1000 women of childbearing age with epilepsy occur each year. Epilepsy has been reported, in retrospective and therefore biased investigations, to increase up to threefold the risks of various common complications (Table 3.39). The perinatal mortality rate has been found to be 1–2 times that of the general population. No large-scale prospective investigation has been carried out, but there seems little doubt that these pregnancies require special consideration. The potential reasons for any increased risk are several. The occurrence of convulsive seizures may lead to abdominal injury. The side-effects of the antiepileptic drugs can complicate many aspects of pregnancy. The obstetricians may be more likely to recommend intervention and to manage the case in a distinctive manner. The occurrence of seizures during delivery carries obvious risks, and home birth should not generally be contemplated.

Effects of pregnancy on epilepsy

Pregnancy has a random effect on seizure frequency. About one-third of women experience increased numbers of seizures, and this is especially likely in severe epilepsy. There are a number of potential causes, including hormonal effects, non-compliance with medication, inappropriate dosage reductions, changing drug disposition and serum levels, fluid reten-

tion, vomiting, stress anxiety and sleep deprivation. A similar number of women have fewer seizures during pregnancy.

The effect of seizures on the fetus is uncertain. Clearly, in the latter stages of pregnancy, a convulsion carries the risk of trauma to the placenta or fetus, especially if the woman falls. Seizures can result in maternal hypoxia for a few minutes and although this could theoretically affect the fetus, the risk does seem small. One study has suggested that first trimester seizures are accompanied by a higher risk of fetal malformation than seizures at other times, although methodological issues cloud the reliability of the conclusions. Stillbirth has been recorded after a single seizure or series of seizures, but this must be very rare. Status epilepticus during pregnancy results in significant maternal and infant morbidity.

About 1–2% of all women with epilepsy will have tonic–clonic seizures during delivery and this can clearly complicate labour. The fetal heart rate during labour can be dramatically slowed by a seizure, and fetal monitoring is recommended during vaginal delivery.

Folic acid supplementation

The fetus of an epileptic women is at a greater than expected risk of a neural tube defect. This is particularly true if the mother is taking valproate, but an association is also noted with the ingestion during pregnancy of other antiepileptics. A recent MRC trial of folic acid supplementation during pregnancy showed a 72% protective effect against neural tube defects in women who had conceived a fetus previously with neural tube defects. A positive primary preventative action of folic acid has also been demonstrated. Although there has been no specific study in epilepsy, it would seem reasonable for all epileptic women to be given folic acid supplementation during pregnancy, especially as many patients with epilepsy have low serum and tissue folate levels caused by enhanced drug-induced hepatic metabolism. This advice is given notwithstanding the weak evidence that folic acid may predispose to increased seizures. A dose of 4–5 mg per day is recommended on an empirical basis, as lower doses may not fully restore folate levels.

Table 3.39 Complications of pregnancy in epilepsy.*

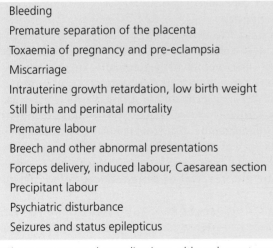

Bleeding

Premature separation of the placenta

Toxaemia of pregnancy and pre-eclampsia

Miscarriage

Intrauterine growth retardation, low birth weight

Still birth and perinatal mortality

Premature labour

Breech and other abnormal presentations

Forceps delivery, induced labour, Caesarean section

Precipitant labour

Psychiatric disturbance

Seizures and status epilepticus

*These are reported complications, although most are based on uncontrolled observations, and it is not clear to what extent some of these are more frequent in pregnancies in women with epilepsy than in general obstetric practice.

Reducing the risk of pregnancy to the mother and child

Pre-conception review and the principles of drug therapy during pregnancy. Most of the major malformations will have been established within the first trimester, many within the first 8 weeks. The mother's antiepileptic drug regimen should therefore be reviewed before conception. This is a counsel of perfection, often not realized, yet is of great importance. Referral of women for review of drug therapy when they are 10 weeks pregnant is too late to make changes which will minimize these teratogenic risks.

It is important to establish whether antiepileptic therapy is needed at all. This will be an individual decision, based on the estimated risk of exacerbation of seizures and their danger, remembering that tonic–clonic seizures can result in injury and occasionally death to both mother and fetus. The decision will balance risks of teratogenicity against the risks of worsening epilepsy. Some women with partial or non-convulsive seizures will elect to withdraw therapy, even if seizures are active or likely to become more frequent. Conversely, some women who are seizure-free will wish to continue therapy because of the social and physical risks of seizure recurrence.

In some patients it is reasonable to withdraw therapy for the first half of pregnancy and then to reinstate the drugs; this approach is based upon the fact that the teratogenic risk is greatest in the first trimester and the risk of seizures greatest in the later stages of pregnancy. The relative risks need to be carefully assessed, however, and a specialist review is needed before embarking upon this unusual course.

If the women elects to continue therapy, the appropriate regime in most cases is the minimally effective dose of the single antiepileptic which best controls the epilepsy. A few women with severe epilepsy will need combination therapy, but this should be avoided wherever possible.

It is useful to measure the serum drug concentrations that give optimal control of the epilepsy before contraception. These values form a useful starting point on which to base subsequent drug dosage adjustments.

Drug dosage during pregnancy. If a preconception review has not been made, relevant drug adjustments should be made as soon as practicable, according to the principles listed above. Teratogenic effects can occur throughout pregnancy, but it should be recognized that many of the major malformations will have been established within the first trimester, thus reducing the value of drug changes made at a later stage.

Once optimal therapy is established, the use of antiepileptic drugs is relatively straightforward. It is important to emphasize the need for compliance. Dosage

adjustments should be based upon serum levels which should be monitored regularly (at least three monthly) during pregnancy. Dose increases may be necessary as serum antiepileptic drug levels can fall especially in the last trimester. The mechanisms of the changing dose: serum level relationship include reduced drug absorption, reduced serum albumin, protein binding changes, increased clearance and fluid retention. Levels of ethosuximide may be halved, and levels of phenytoin, phenobarbital, carbamazepine and valproate can also be markedly reduced.

Folic acid. Folic acid supplementation should be initiated in all patients who are or have recently been taking antiepileptic drugs.

Drugs in pregnancy. Much of our information on this vital topic is incomplete and it is indeed difficult to advise patients wisely about these risks. Some general guidelines, however, can be given.

Overall risk. The baseline population risk of a noticeable fetal malformation is about 3%. This is increased to about 7% in the offspring of mothers taking a single antiepileptic and to 15% in those taking two antiepileptic drugs. Thus, antiepileptic drug intake should be reduced to the minimally acceptable level—prior to conception wherever possible—as major malformations are formed within the first 12 weeks of a pregnancy.

Drug dosage and regimen. Drug dosage should be reduced where possible. High peak levels should be avoided, and thus it has become customary to split the administration into three or four times daily dosage, especially of valproate, because blood levels swing widely.

Folic acid. The evidence in non-epileptic women that folic acid reduces the frequency of fetal neural tube defects is conclusive. Antiepileptic drug intake increases the risk of neural tube defects, and it seems sensible to prescribe folate supplements to all women on antiepileptics, especially those taking valproate or carbamazepine. Controversy about the dosage reflects lack of clinic trial evidence, but it seems sensible to use high dose folic acid (4–5 mg per day) to ensure the reversal of drug-induced folate deficiency.

Which drug should be used in pregnancy? As will be clear from what has been said above, advice is difficult.

Certain now seldom-used drugs are frequently teratogenic and are absolutely contraindicated in pregnancy; these include trimethadione. Other drugs are known to be associated with a definite but low risk of teratogenicity. In this category are carbamazepine, phenytoin, valproate, benzodiazepines, and phenobarbital. In many patients, the risks of seizures to the infant and mother outweigh the risks of teratogenicity and in these cases therapy should be continued. As information about the teratogenicity of the newer antiepileptic drugs is sparse, it is best to avoid these. This is particularly true of topiramate and gabapentin, both of which have demonstrable animal teratogenicity.

Carbamazepine is currently the drug considered safest in pregnancy for those with partial and secondarily generalized epilepsy. In idiopathic generalized epilepsy the choice is more difficult. Although valproate is the drug of choice in this syndrome, it is associated with a small but definite risk of spina bifida and a possibly greater risk of other features (valproate syndrome). Whether lamotrigine is a safer drug is quite unclear.

Screening for fetal malformations. Some malformations can be detected in the prenatal phase. If therapeutic termination of pregnancy is acceptable, screening procedures should include, where appropriate, a high quality ultrasound scan at 10, 18 and 24 weeks, measurement of alpha fetoprotein levels and amniocentesis. About 95% of significant neural tube defects can be detected prenatally in this manner, as well as cleft palate, major cardiac kidney and midline defects. However, the mother should be informed that not all malformations are detectable, even with the most sophisticated screening methods.

Vitamin K. When the mother is taking enzyme-inducing drugs, the infant may be born with a relative vitamin K deficiency. This predisposes to infantile haemorrhage, including cerebral haemorrhage. The neonate should therefore receive 1 mg of vitamin K i.m. at birth. In some units, it is also recommended that the mother take oral vitamin K (20 mg/day) in the last trimester. If there is evidence of neonatal bleeding, or if concentrations of factors II, VII, IX or X fall below 25% of normal, an emergency infusion of fresh frozen plasma is required.

New-onset epilepsy during pregnancy
The incidence of epilepsy at childbearing age is about 20–30 cases per 100 000 persons. In some cases, the association of epilepsy and pregnancy is probably coincidental. Occasionally, epileptic seizures occur only during pregnancy (gestational epilepsy). This rare pattern must reflect the lower seizure threshold for epilepsy in pregnancy in some women.

Certain underlying conditions have a propensity to present during pregnancy. Some meningiomas grow in size faster during pregnancy as a result of oestrogenic stimulation. Arteriovenous malformations are also said to present more commonly in pregnancy, although evidence for this is weak. The risk of ischaemic stroke increases 10-fold in pregnancy. The underlying causes of ischaemic stroke include arteriosclerosis, cerebral angiitis and moya-moya disease, Takayasu's arteritis, embolic disease from a cardiac or infective source, and primary cardiac disease. Haematological diseases can also present as stroke, including sickle cell disease, antiphospholipid antibody syndrome, thrombotic thrombocytopenic purpura, deficiencies in antithrombin, protease C and S, and factor V Leiden deficiency. There is also a higher incidence of subarachnoid haemorrhage and of cerebral venous thrombosis. Pregnancy can also predispose to cerebral infections caused by bacteria (including *Listeria*), fungi (*Coccidioides*), protozoa (*Toxoplasma*), viruses and human immunodeficiency virus (HIV) infection. Epilepsy can be the presenting symptom, or occur, in all these conditions. The extent of the investigation will depend on the clinical setting. X-radiation, including computerized tomography (CT), should be avoided wherever possible. The risks of MRI to the developing fetus are unknown; nevertheless MRI is the imaging modality of choice if urgent imaging is required. In the non-urgent situation, investigation should be deferred until the pregnancy is completed.

The treatment of new-onset epilepsy follows the same principles in the pregnant as in the non-pregnant woman. The underlying cause may also need specific therapy.

Eclampsia and pre-eclampsia
Most new-onset seizures in the late stages of pregnancy (after 20 weeks) are caused by eclampsia. Pre-eclampsia is characterized by hypertension, proteinuria, oedema, abnormalities of hepatic function, platelets and clotting parameters. About 5% of cases, if left untreated, progress to eclampsia. The eclamptic encephalopathy results in confusion, stupor, focal neurological signs, and cerebral haemorrhage as well as seizures. The epilepsy can be severe and progress rapidly to status epilepticus. The incidence of eclampsia in Western Europe is about one in 2000 pregnancies, but it is more common in some developing countries with rates as high as one in 100. It carries a maternal mortality rate of between 2 and 5% and significant infantile morbidity and mortality.

Traditionally, obstetricians have used magnesium sulphate for the treatment of seizures in eclampsia, and the superiority of magnesium over phenytoin and/or diazepam has been clearly demonstrated in recent randomized controlled studies. Not only does magnesium confer better seizure control, but there are fewer complications of pregnancy, the infant survival is better and magnesium seems also to lessen the chance of cerebral palsy in low birth weight babies and to decrease the secondary neuronal damage after experimental traumatic brain injury. The mechanism by which magnesium sulphate acts in eclampsia is unclear; it may do so via its influence on NMDA receptors or on free-radicals, prostacyclin, other neurochemical pathways or, more likely, by reversing the intense eclamptic cerebral vasospasm. It is possible that patients would benefit from magnesium and a conventional antiepileptic, but this has not been investigated. Magnesium should be administered as an intravenous infusion of 4 g, followed by 10 g IM, and then 5 g IM every 4 h as required.

Management of labour

Regular antiepileptic drugs should be continued during labour. If oral feeding is not possible, intravenous replacement therapy is possible for at least some drugs. Tonic–clonic seizures occur in about 1–2% of susceptible mothers and, if the risk is high, oral clobazam (10–20 mg) is useful given at the onset of labour as additional seizure prophylaxis. Fetal monitoring is advisable. Most women have a normal vaginal delivery, but sleep deprivation, overbreathing, pain and emotional stress can greatly increase the risk of seizures and elective Caesarean section should be considered if there is considered to be a particular risk. A history of status epilepticus or life-threatening tonic–clonic seizures are an indication for a Caesarean section. If a severe seizure or status epilepticus occurs during delivery, an emergency Caesarean section is often required. Intravenous lorazepam or phenytoin should be given during labour if severe epilepsy develops and the patient prepared for Caesarean section. It should not be forgotten that there is a maternal as well as infant mortality rate associated with severe seizures during delivery. The hypoxia consequent on a seizure may be more profound in the gravid than in nongravid women because of the increased oxygen requirements of the fetus, and resuscitation facilities should be immediately at hand in the delivery suite.

Puerperium

There is still an increased risk of seizures in the puerperium, and precautions may be necessary. It is sometimes helpful to prescribe clobazam for a few days after delivery to cover this period. If antiepileptic drug dosage had been increased because of falling levels during pregnancy, the dose should be returned during the first week to its previous levels; this is necessary as the pharmacokinetic changes of pregnancy are rapidly reversed in the puerperium.

Drugs circulating in the mother's serum cross the placenta. If maternal antiepileptic drug levels were high, the infant may experience withdrawal symptoms (tremor, irritability, agitation and even seizures) and neonatal serum levels should be measured in cases at risk.

Breast-feeding

Drug concentrations in breast-milk are generally low (Table 3.40). Breast-feeding is therefore acceptable unless the mother is taking high doses of phenobarbital, ethosuximide or benzodiazepine drugs. Particular caution is advised in the case of maternal phenobarbital ingestion as in neonates the half-life of phenobarbital is long (up to 300 h) and the free fraction is higher than in adults; neonatal levels can therefore sometimes exceed maternal levels. Neonatal phenytoin and valproate half-lives are also increased (Table 3.40). Neonatal lethargy, irritability and feeding difficulties have also been attributed to maternal antiepileptic drug intake, although evi-

Table 3.40 Neonatal pharmacokinetics of anticonvulsants.

Antiepileptic drugs	Breast milk/plasma concentration ratio	Elimination half-life (h)	
		Adult	**Neonate**
Carbamazepine	0.4–0.6	8–25	8–28
Ethosuximide	0.9	40–60	40
Phenobarbital	0.4–0.6	75–126	45–500
Phenytoin	0.2–0.4	12–50	15–105
Primidone	0.7–0.9	4–12	7–60
Valproic acid	0.01	6–18	30–60

dence is slight and symptoms do not seem to be correlated with maternal drug dosage or serum level.

FURTHER READING

Aicardi, J. (1991) The agyria–pachygyria complex: a spectrum of cortical malformations. *Brain Dev*, **13**, 1–8.

Aicardi, J. (1991) Myoclonic epilepsies in childhood. *Int Pediatr*, **6**, 195–200.

Aicardi, J. (1994) *Epilepsy in Children*, 2nd edn, p. 555. Raven Press, New York.

Aminoff, M.J. (ed) *Neurology and General Medicine*. Churchill Livingstone, New York 1989.

Andermann, F. & Rasmussen, T.B. (1991) Chronic encephalitis and epilepsy: an overview. In: *Chronic Encephalitis and Epilepsy*: *Rasmussen's Syndrome* (ed. F. Andermann), pp. 283–8. Butterworth, Boston.

Annegers, J.F., Baumgartner, K.B., Hauser, W.A. & Kurland, L.T. (1988) Epilepsy, antiepileptic drugs, and the risk of spontaneous abortion. *Epilepsia*, **29**, 451–8.

Annegers, J.F., Hauser, W.A. & Elveback, L.R. (1979) Remission of seizures and relapse in patients with epilepsy. *Epilepsia*, **20**, 729–37.

Annegers, J.F., Shirts, S.B., Hauser, W.A. & Kurland, L.T. (1986) Risk of recurrence after an initial unprovoked seizure. *Epilepsia*, **27**, 43–50.

Beghi, E., Tognoni, G. & The Collaborative Group for the Study of Epilepsy (1988) Prognosis of epilepsy in newly referred patients: a multicenter prospective study. *Epilepsia*, **29**(3), 236–43.

Berkovic, S.F., Anderman, F., Carpenter, S. & Wolfe, L.S. (1989) Progressive myoclonus epilepsies: specific causes and diagnosis. *N Engl J Med*, **315** (5), 296–305.

Chadwick, D. & Turnbull, D.M. (1985) The comparative efficacy of antiepileptic drugs for partial and tonic–clonic seizures. *J Neurol Neurosurg Psychiatry*, **48**, 1073–7.

Delgado-Escueta, A.V. & Janz, D. (1992) Consensus guidelines: preconception counselling, management, and care of the pregnant women with epilepsy. *Neurology*, **42** (Suppl. 5), 149–60.

Duncan, J.S. & Panayiotopoulos, C.P. (eds) (1995) *Typical Absences and Related Epileptic Syndromes*. Churchill Communications Europe, London.

Duncan, J.S., Patsalos, P.N. & Shorvon, S.D. (1991) Effects of discontinuation of phenytoin, carbamazepine, and valproate on concomitant antiepileptic medication. *Epilepsia*, **32**, 101–15.

Elwes, R.D.C., Johnson, A.L., Shorvon, S.D. & Reynolds, E.H. (1984) The prognosis for seizure control in newly diagnosed epilepsy. *N Engl J Med*, **311**, 944–7.

Engel, J. & Pedley, T.A. (1997) *Epilepsy: a comprehensive textbook*. Lippincott Raven, Philadelphia.

European Chromosome 16 Tuberous Sclerosis Consortium: Nellist, M., Janssen, B., Brook-Carter, P.T. *et al.* (1993) Identification and characterization of the tuberous sclerosis gene of chromosome 16. *Cell*, **75**, 1305–15.

First Seizure Trial Group (1993) Randomized clinical trial of the efficacy of antiepileptic drugs in reducing the risk of relapse after first unprovoked tonic–clonic seizure. *Neurology*, **43**, 478–83.

Foy, P.M., Chadwick, D.W., Rajgopalan, N., Johnson, A.L. & Shaw, M.D.M. (1992) Do prophylactic anticonvulsant drugs alter the pattern of seizures after craniotomy? *J Neurol Neurosurg Psychiatry*, **55**, 753–7.

Futrell, N., Schultz, L.R. & Millikan, C. (1992) Central nervous system disease in patients with systemic lupus erythematosus. *Neurology*, **42**, 1649–57.

Gilmore, R.L. (1988) Seizures and antiepileptic drug use in transplant patients. *Neurol Clin*, **6**, 279–96.

Hanly, J.G., Walsh, N.M.G. & Sangalang, V. (1992) Brain pathology in systemic lupus erythematosus. *J Rheumatol*, **19**, 732–41.

Hansten, P.D. (1985) *Drug Interactions. A Handbook for Clinical Use*, 5th edn. Lea and Febiger, Philadelphia.

Hart, Y.M., Sander, J.W., Johnson, A.L. & Shorvon, S.D. (1990) National general practice study of epilepsy: recurrence after a first seizure. *Lancet*, **336**, 1271–4.

Heller, A.J., Stewart, J., Hughes, E. *et al.* (1993) Comparative efficacy and toxicity of phenobarbital, phenytoin, carbamazepine, and valproate in adults and children with newly diagnosed previously untreated epilepsy: a randomized long-term trial. *Epilepsia*, **34** (Suppl. 2), 66.

Hopkins, A. (1995) The causes of epilepsy, the risk factors for epilepsy and the precipitation of seizures. In: *Epilepsy*, 2nd edn (eds A. Hopkins, S.D. Shorvon & G. Cascino), pp. 59–85. Chapman and Hall, London.

Janz, D. *et al.* (eds) (1982) *Epilepsy, Pregnancy and the Child*. Raven Press, New York.

Jennett, B. (1975) *Epilepsy After Non-missile Head Injuries*, 2nd edn, pp. 179. Year Book Medical, Chicago.

Kilpatrick, C.J., Tress, B.M., O'Donnell, C., Rossitor, C. & Hopper, J.L. (1991) Magnetic resonance imaging and late-onset epilepsy. *Epilepsia*, **32**, 358–64.

Levine, R.R. (1983) *Pharmacology: Drug Actions and Reactions*, 3rd edn. Little Brown, Boston.

Levy, R.H., Mattson, R., Medrum, B.S. *Antiepileptic Drugs*, 4th edn. Raven Press, New York.

Lockwood, A.H. (1992) Hepatic encephalopathy. In: *Metabolic Brain Dysfunction in Systemic Disorders* (eds A.I. Arieff & R.C. Griggs), pp. 167–82. Little Brown, Boston.

Mattson, R.H., Cramer, J.A., Collins, J.F. & The Department of Veteran Affairs Epilepsy Cooperative Study No. 264 Group (1992) A comparison of valproate with carbamazepine for the treatment of complex partial seizures and secondarily generalized tonic–clonic seizures in adults. *N Engl J Med*, **327**, 765–71.

Mattson, R.H., Cramer, J.A., Collins, J.F. *et al.* (1985) Comparison of carbamazepine, phenobarbital, phenytoin, and primidone in partial and secondarily generalized tonic–clonic seizures. *N Engl J Med*, **313**, 145–51.

McKusick, V.A. (1994) *Mendelian Inheritance in Man: Catalogs of Autosomal Dominant, Autosomal Recessive and X-linked Phenotypes*, 7th edn. Johns Hopkins Press, Baltimore.

Medical Research Council Vitamin Study Research Group (1991) Prevention of neural-tube defects: results of the Medical Research Council Vitamin Study. *Lancet*, **338**, 131–7.

Messing, R.O. & Simon, R.P. (1986) Seizures as a manifestation of systemic disease. *Neurol Clin*, **4**, 563–84.

MRC Antiepileptic Drug Withdrawal Study Group (1991) Randomised study of antiepileptic drug withdrawal in patients in remission. *Lancet*, **337**, 1175–80.

Patsalos, P.N. & Duncan, J.S. (1993) Antiepileptic drugs: a review of clinically significant drug interactions. *Drug Safety*, **9**, 156–84.

Raskin, N.H. (1989) Neurological aspects of renal failure. In: *Neurology and General Medicine* (ed. M.J. Aminoff), pp. 233–41. Churchill Livingstone, New York.

Roger, J., Bureau, M., Dravet, Ch. *et al.* (1992) *Epileptic Syndromes in Infancy, Childhood and Adolescence.* John Libbey, London.

Rosciszewska, D. (1987) Epilepsy and menstruation. *Epilepsia*, **12**, 373–8.

Rosenberg, I.H. (1992) Folic acid and neural-tube defects – time for action? *N Engl J Med*, **327**, 1875–6.

Salazar, A.M., Jabbari, B., Vance, S.C. *et al.* (1985) Epilepsy after penetrating head injury. I. Clinical correlates: a report of the Vietnam Head Injury Study. *Neurology*, **35**, 1406–14.

Sander, J.W.A.S., Hart, Y.M., Johnson, A.L. & Shorvon, S.D. (1990) National General Practice Study of Epilepsy: newly diagnosed epileptic seizures in general population. *Lancet*, **336**, 1267–70.

Schmidt, D., Canger, R., Avanzini, G. *et al.* (1983) Change of seizure frequency in pregnant epileptic women. *J Neurol Neurosurg Psychiatry*, **46**, 751–5.

Shorvon, S.D., Dreifuss, F., Fish, D., Thomas, D. (eds) (1996) *The Treatment of Epilepsy.* Blackwell Science, Oxford.

Shorvon, S.D., Gilliatt, R.W., Cox, T.C.S. & Yu, Y.L. (1984) Evidence of vascular disease from CT scanning in late onset epilepsy. *J Neurol Neurosurg Psychiatry*, **47**, 225–30.

Sibley, J.T., Olszynski, W.P., Decoteau, W.E. & Sundaram, M.B. (1992) The incidence and prognosis of central nervous system disease in systemic lupus erythematosus. *J Rheumatol*, **19**, 47–52.

Sila, C.A. (1989) Spectrum of neurologic events following cardiac transplantation. *Curr Concepts Cerebrovasc Dis Stroke*, **24**, 19–23.

Stafstrom, C.D. (1993) Epilepsy in Down syndrome: clinical aspects and possible mechanisms *Am J Ment Retard*, **98** (Suppl.), 12–26.

Sugimoto, T., Yasuhara, A., Ohta, T. *et al.* (1992) Angelman syndrome in three siblings: characteristic epileptic seizures and EEG abnormalities. *Epilepsia*, **33**, 1078–82.

Sung, C.Y. & Chu, N.S. (1990) Epileptic seizures in elderly people: aetiology and seizure type. *Age Ageing*, **19**, 25–30.

Tallis, R.C., Craig, I., Hall, G. & Dean, A. (1991) How common are epileptic seizures in old age? *Age Ageing*, **20**, 442–8.

Turnbull, D.M., Rawlins, M.D., Weightman, D. & Chadwick, D.W. (1982) A comparison of phenytoin and valproate in previously untreated adult epileptic patients. *J Neurol Neurosurg Psychiatry*, **45**, 55–9.

Volpe, J.J. (1989) Neonatal seizures: current concepts and classification. *Pediatrics*, **84**, 422–8.

Walker, R.W. & Brochstein, J.A. (1988) Neurologic complications of immunosuppressive agents. *Neurol Clin*, **6**, 261–78.

Wallace, H., Shorvon, S.D., Tallis, R. (1998) Age-specific incidence and prevalence rates of treated epilepsy in an unselected population of 2,052,922 and age-specific fertility rates of women with epilepsy. *Lancet*, **352**, 1970–3.

Wisnieski, S.M., Segan, C.M. & Miezejeski, E.A. (1991) The Fra-X syndrome: neurological, electrophysiological, and neuropathological abnormalities. *Am J Med Genet*, **38**, 476–83.

Wong, K.L., Woo, E.K.W., Yu, Y.L. & Wong, R.W.S. (1991) Neurological manifestations of systemic lupus erythematosus: a prospective study. *Quart J Med*, **81**, 857–70.

Yerby, M.S. (1987) Problems in the management of pregnant women with epilepsy. *Epilepsia*, **28** (Suppl. 3), S29–S36.

Zori, R.T., Hendrickson, J., Woolven, S. *et al.* (1992) Angelman syndrome: clinical profile. *J Child Neurol*, **7**, 270–80.

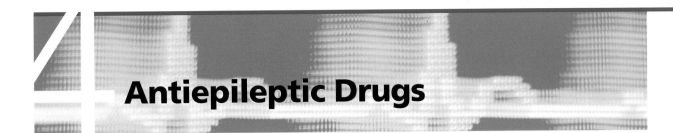

Antiepileptic Drugs

Carbamazepine

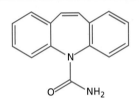

Primary indications	First-line or adjunctive therapy in partial and generalized seizures (excluding absence and myoclonus). Also in Lennox–Gastaut syndrome and childhood epilepsy syndromes
Usual preparations	Tablets: 100, 200, 400 mg; chewtabs: 100, 200 mg; slow-release formulations: 200, 400 mg; liquid: 100 mg/5 mL; suppositories: 125, 250 mg
Usual dosages	Initial: 100 mg at night. Maintenance: 400–1600 mg per day (maximum 2400 mg). (Slow-release formulation, higher dosage). Children: <1 year, 100–200 mg; 1–5 years, 200–400 mg; 5–10 years, 400–600 mg; 10–15 years, 600–1000 mg
Dosage intervals	2–3 times per day (2–4 times per day at higher doses or in children)
Significant drug interactions	Carbamazepine has a large number of interactions with antiepileptic and other drugs
Serum level monitoring	Useful
Target range	20–50 µmol/L
Common/important side-effects	Drowsiness, fatigue, dizziness, ataxia, diplopia, blurring of vision, sedation, headache, insomnia, gastro-intestinal disturbance, tremor, weight gain, impotence, effects on behaviour and mood, hepatic disturbance, rash, and other skin reactions, bone marrow dyscrasias, hyponatraemia, water retention and nephritis
Main advantages	Highly effective and usually well-tolerated therapy
Main disadvantages	Transient adverse effects on initiating therapy. Occasional severe toxicity
Mechanisms of action	Action on neuronal sodium-channel conductance. Also action on monoamine, acetylcholine and NMDA receptors
Oral bioavailability	75–85%
Time to peak levels	4–8 h
Metabolism and excretion	Hepatic epoxidation and then conjugation
Volume of distribution	0.8–1.2 L/kg
Elimination half-life	5–26 h (but very variable)
Plasma clearance	0.133 L/kg/h (but very variable)
Protein binding	75%
Active metabolites	Carbamazepine epoxide
Comment	A drug of first choice in tonic–clonic and partial seizures in adults and children

Carbamazepine is the veritable workhorse of the antiepileptic drugs. Initial open clinical trials were carried out in the 1950s, and since then it has become established as the major first-line antiepileptic drug for partial and some generalized seizures. It is the most commonly prescribed drug in Europe for epilepsy. It was originally developed in the search for new antipsychotic compounds and, as has been the case for most antiepileptics in current use, its value in epilepsy was discovered largely by chance. It is a tricyclic compound and is also widely used for the treatment of depression and of certain pain syndromes.

PHYSICAL AND CHEMICAL CHARACTERISTICS

Carbamazepine is a crystalline substance which is virtually insoluble in water, and therefore can only be taken orally. It is inherently not a very stable substance and so care needs to be taken with storage. The bioavailability of cabamazepine is reduced by up to 50% by storage in hot or humid conditions or when there has been absorption of moisture.

Mode of action

The exact mode of the antiepileptic action of carbamazepine has not been fully established. It stabilizes neuronal membranes pre- and postsynaptically by use- and frequency-dependent blockade of sodium channels. This is probably its main action, although a blockade of the NMDA (*N*-methyl-D-aspartate) receptor-activated sodium and calcium flux may also be contributory. The action on the sodium channel reduces the sustained high-frequency repetitive firing of action potentials which are a feature of epileptic activity. It has also been proposed that carbamazepine acts on other receptors, including the purine, monoamine and acetylcholine receptors.

PHARMACOKINETICS

Absorption

As there is no intravenous formulation, bioavailability measurements can be estimates only but it appears that, generally speaking, between 75 and 85% of the drug is absorbed following oral ingestion. Absorption can be slow and erratic, there is a marked intraindividual variation and different formulations may have different absorption characteristics. It does not appear to make any difference whether the drug is taken before or after food. Peak levels are reached between 4 and 8 h after absorption.

Distribution

Approximately 75–85% of the drug is bound to plasma proteins. The free fraction of carbamazepine usually ranges between 20 and 24% of the total plasma concentration, and cerebrospinal fluid carbamazepine levels vary in a range between 17 and 31%. There is, however, large inter- and intraindividual variability in the protein binding and the ratio of bound : unbound drug. Salivary levels bear a good and constant relationship to free blood levels, and can be a useful method of assaying drug concentrations. The apparent volume of distribution of carbamazepine is between 0.8 and 1.2 L/kg and of the 10,11-epoxide 0.59–1.5 L/kg. Epoxide and parent drug levels are found in approximately equal amounts in the brain.

Biotransformation and excretion

Carbamazepine is extensively metabolized in the liver. The major pathway is first epoxidation to carbamazepine 10,11-epoxide and then hydrolysis to carbamazepine 10,11-*trans*-dihydrodiol. There are also other conjugated and unconjugated metabolites and less than 1% of the drug is excreted unchanged in the urine. The drug induces its own metabolism and there is a marked increase in clearance and fall of about 50% in serum half-life during the first few weeks of carbamazepine therapy. This autoinduction is usually completed within a month.

In the postinduced state, a new steady state after changes in drug dosage will be achieved within 3 days. At steady state, epoxide levels are approximately 50% of carbamazepine plasma levels. The epoxide has antiepileptic action, and also contributes to the side-effects of carbamazepine and for this reason it is often useful to measure the serum levels both of carbamazepine and also its epoxide. There are marked variations in the ratio of carbamazepine : carbamazepine epoxide, and the rate of metabolism varies within individuals and between individuals. This rate is increased by age factors and comedication and varies with dosage regimens. There is a relatively low extraction ratio (less than 10%) which reflects the limited ability of liver to handle the plasma carbamazepine load. An average clearance value for carbamazepine is 0.133 L/kg/h but this is very variable. The volume of distribution is usually between 0.8–1.2. Because of the low intrinsic clearance and low extraction ratio, changes in hepatic blood flow do not alter carbamazepine clearance to any great extent.

Greater variations in serum levels are found during once daily, rather than during two or three times daily dosage regimens. One study showed a mean 79% change between peak and trough levels on a twice daily dosage which was reduced to 40% on a four times daily regimen. Peak-level side-effects are common in clinical practice, and these can be avoided by flattening out the diurnal blood-level swings. This can be achieved by more frequent dosage, or the use of the controlled-release formulation of carbamazepine which has been clearly shown to improve the tolerability of once or twice daily dosage. There are no significant differences between the absorption and steady-state concentrations, efficacy or tolerability between conventional or chewable tablets, and the suspension, syrup and tablets have been shown to have similar pharmacokinetics. Rectal administration of carbamazepine in a sorbitol-free gel is possible but not widely used.

There are no major difference between infants and adults in absorption, protein binding and distribution of carbamazepine and its epoxide. The volume of distribution is 1–1.5 times that of the adult level. In children, absorption, half-life and clearance show very marked intraindividual variations, although the mean population values are similar to those in adults. The diurnal variation in levels in children is greater than in adults, and to avoid peak dose side-effects it is often necessary to use twice or three times daily dosage and the slow-release formulation.

In gastrointestinal disease, the absorption of carbamazepine can be quite severely reduced and drug levels require careful monitoring. In the presence of severe liver disease, carbamazepine pharmacokinetics may be disordered and dose reductions needed, but moderate disease has little effect. Renal disease has no effect on carbamazepine kinetics. Dialysis does not have a marked effect on carbamazepine plasma levels. Severe congestive cardiac failure has been shown to result in abnormally slow absorption, and the drug is also cleared and metabolized at a slower rate. The water and sodium retention induced by the antidiuretic action of carbamazepine can aggravate cardiac failure. The absorption of carbamazepine is not modified during the first two trimesters of pregnancy. Data concerning the last 3 months are controversial, the unbound levels of carbamazepine and its epoxide are not changed, nor is their ratio, but as maternal plasma protein concentrations decline towards the end of pregnancy, the total levels fall. Dosage adjustments are only occasionally needed. If clinically indicated, measurement of free levels can be useful.

Because of the wide variation in the dosage–serum level relationship both at a inter- and intraindividual level, carbamazepine (and carbamazepine epoxide) levels are commonly measured. There is a relationship between carbamazepine level and therapeutic effectiveness, but no universal 'therapeutic range'. Thus, although levels are useful as a guide, particularly in long-term therapy, there is little point in adhering to any predetermined target range, and daily dosage should be tailored to individual need. Having said this, maximum effect is usually observed between 20 and 50 µmol/L.

Drug interactions

Carbamazepine is a potent hepatic enzyme inducer and is also highly susceptible to enzyme induction (including autoinduction). The first metabolite of carbamazepine (carbamazepine 10,11-epoxide) has antiepileptic action which complicates the clinical assessment of carbamazepine interactions.

Effect of other antiepileptic drugs on carbamazepine levels

Phenytoin, primidone and phenobarbital. All these drugs induce carbamazepine metabolism. The effect can be very marked, and indeed it is common clinical experience that satisfactory carbamazepine levels cannot be achieved in many patients comedicated with phenytoin without causing intoxication—presumably as the result of high epoxide levels. Serum carbamazepine levels in monotherapy have been shown to fluctuate by between 23 and 45% diurnally; this fluctuation will be greater in the presence of combination therapy and the use of the slow-release formulation is advised in any patient on moderate doses of carbamazepine in combination with other drugs.

Imidazole drugs. These include the experimental antiepileptics, denzimol and stiripentol, which can both double carbamazepine levels when added as comedication.

Valproate. Serum carbamazepine epoxide levels may be increased as much as fourfold without any marked change in carbamazepine levels, an interaction caused by valproate-induced inhibition of the enzyme epoxide hydrolase. The valproic acid pro-drug, valpromide, is associated with an even greater inhibition, with up to eightfold increases in epoxide levels.

Effect of other non-epileptic drugs on carbamazepine levels

Various drugs and classes of drug inhibit carbamazepine metabolism, and can result in marked increases in carbamazepine serum levels. These include the macrolide antibiotics, such as erythromycin, which can increase levels two- to threefold; the calcium-channel blockers, diltiazem and verapamil, which can double levels (nifedipine has no effect); cimetidine, which can cause a 20–30% increase in carbamazepine levels (ranitidine has no effect); imidazole drugs, such as nifimidone; propoxyphene which increases concentrations by 30–60%. Other drugs which markedly increase carbamazepine levels in comedication include danazol, fluoxetine, fluvoxamine and viloxazine.

Effect of carbamazepine on levels of other drugs

Carbamazepine induces the metabolism and hence lowers the concentrations of a wide variety of concurrently administered drugs. These include the anti-epileptic drugs: phenytoin, primidone, valproate, ethosuximide and clonazepam. Amongst the non-antiepileptic drugs where an interaction can compromise clinical effects are oral contraceptives, oral anticoagulants, beta-blockers, haloperidol and theophylline (Fig. 4.1, Tables 4.1 and 4.2).

SIDE-EFFECTS

Carbamazepine side-effects are experienced particularly on initiating treatment, or when the dose becomes too high (Table 4.3). Once a stable regimen is established, adverse effects are uncommon or mild. The most common side-effects on initiating therapy are sedation, headache, diplopia, dizziness and ataxia. These can be largely avoided by starting treatment at a very low dose and incrementing the dose slowly. When the drug dose is too high, typical side-effects include ataxia, dizziness and visual blurring

or diplopia. These side-effects tend to be manifest a few hours after dosage, and are caused by peak blood levels either of the carbamazepine itself or of its 10,11-epoxide. Peak level side-effects can be reduced in frequency and intensity by switching to the slow-release formulation of the drug, or by increasing the frequency of dosage. These reversible transient neurotoxic side-effects are more common in patients taking combination therapy and also in the elderly. The frequency of these common side-effects is similar in children. The tolerability of carbamazepine has been compared to other newer drugs in a variety of studies, sponsored usually by the manufacturers of the comparator drug. In these studies, carbamazepine has usually been up-titrated faster than in optimal clinical practice, and the differences in tolerability noted may be due to this study-design feature. This makes comparison difficult, but it seems likely to the author at least that carbamazepine is in

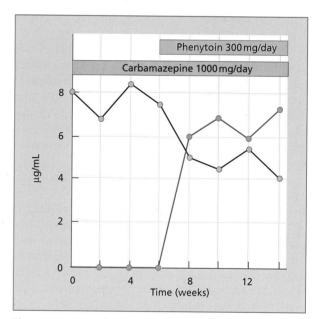

Fig. 4.1 Decline of plasma carbamazepine level following addition of phenytoin.

Increasing	Decreasing	Variable	No effect
Phenobarbital (from primidone)	Clonazepam	Phenytoin	Clobazam
	Ethosuximide	Phenobarbital	Gabapentin
	Felbamate		Levetiracetam
	Lamotrigine		Oxcarbazepine
	Tiagabine		Piracetam
	Topiramate		Vigabatrin
	Valproate		

Table 4.1 Effect of carbamazepine on plasma levels of other antiepileptic drugs.

Table 4.2 Effect of other antiepileptic drugs on carbamazepine plasma levels.

Increasing	Decreasing	No effect
Felbamate*	Clonazepam	Clobazam
Lamotrigine*	Felbamate	Ethosuximide
Valproate*	Phenobarbital	Gabapentin
Valpromid*	Phenytoin	Levetiracetam
	Primidone	Oxcarbazepine
		Piracetam
		Tiagabine
		Topiramate
		Vigabatrin

*Elevation of carbamazepine epoxide levels.

most patients as well (or badly) tolerated as are other newer antiepileptic drugs.

Rarer neurological effects include asterixis and dystonia. The drug can exacerbate atypical absence, tonic and myoclonic seizures and has been said to worsen the aphasia in occasional patients with the Landau–Kleffner syndrome. Carbamazepine has, in formal testing, little effect on cognitive function or behaviour. Having said this, complaints of slowing and memory disturbance are commonly encountered in the clinic, blamed on drug therapy, including carbamazepine, although usually a causative association

cannot be established. The reported frequency of side-effects in different studies has varied greatly, but overall between 30 and 50% of subjects taking carbamazepine will experience some side-effects, although these are usually mild and less than 5% of patients will need to withdraw the medication because of side-effects. Sporadic psychiatric disturbances have occurred in relation to carbamazepine therapy, but these are generally rare. It was claimed when the drug was first introduced that the drug had a 'positive psychotropic action' caused putatively by its tricyclic structure. Such claims are now not made. It is interesting to note that similar claims were made for phenytoin and phenobarbital when they were introduced, and are now being made for lamotrigine. One can muse on the extent that these effects reflect marketing enthusiasm, placebo effect or simply over-optimism on the part of the doctor or patient.

When carbamazepine was first introduced, a number of serious skin reactions were recorded. These included fatal cases of Stevens–Johnson syndrome, Lyell's syndrome and exfoliative dermatitis. It has been suggested that the rashes were caused by the incipient in the early formulations, although there seems no doubt that carbamazepine can cause severe skin reactions, and the lack of serious recent problems may be because of the slow incrementation of dose now recommended. Whatever the reason, serious skin reactions on carbamazepine are now extremely rare. About 5% of people will experience a mild

Table 4.3 Incidence and prevalence of adverse effects with use of carbamazepine.

Effect	Percentage of patients* (*n* = 231)	Percentage at 12-month visit† (*n* = 130)
Sedation	42	8
Weight gain	32	9
(Large weight gain)	8	3
Nystagmus	30	6
Gatrointestinal symptoms	29	6
Gait problems	25	4
Change in effect or mood	24	4
Tremor	22	5
Cognitive disturbances	18	3
Rash	11	1
Diplopia	10	0
Impotence	7	2

*Percentage of patients in whom each type of adverse effect occurred at any time during the trial (mean follow-up, 36 months).

† Percentage of patients in whom each type of adverse effect was noted at the 12-month visit.

rash on initiation of therapy and, should this develop, the drug should be withdrawn. The less severe forms of carbamazepine hypersensitivity seem to be caused by activation of the suppressor-cytotoxic subset of T cells and successful desensitization carried out by the reintroduction of the drug at very low doses has been carried out without complications. Systemic lupus erythematosus has very rarely been induced by carbamazepine, although less often than with phenytoin.

Elevated hepatic enzymes are found in up to 5–10% of patients taking carbamazepine, caused by induction of the hepatic enzyme systems; these changes are without clinical significance. There were about 20 cases of carbamazepine hepatotoxicity reported by the 1980s with a mortality rate of about 25%. This took the form either of a hypersensitivity-induced granulomatous hepatitis or acute hepatitis with hepatic necrosis. Most patients had been taking carbamazepine for less than 1 month and the hypersensitivity was associated with rash and fever.

Severe haematological complications have also been rarely associated with carbamazepine therapy. These include cases of thrombocytopenia, aplastic anaemia, agranulocytosis and pancytopenia. The risk of aplasmic anaemia is said to be 5.1 cases per million, of agranulocytosis 1.4 cases per million and for death as a result of marrow suppression 2.2 cases per million treated patients. These hypersensitivity reactions develop usually in the first few months of therapy, and carry an appreciable mortality rate. They seem to be more common in the elderly. As with other manifestations of severe hypersensitivity, serious haematological effects are, however, very rare. Not uncommonly, carbamazepine lowers the total white blood count and the neutrophil count, but this is usually of no clinical significance. Leucopenia develops in between 10 and 20% of adults or children, and does not seem to be dose-related. If the neutrophil count is below 1200 per mm^3 the measurements should be monitored carefully and if it falls below 900 per mm^3 the drug dosage should be reduced. If red blood cell counts are also reduced in the presence of normal iron and low reticulocyte counts, the drug should be stopped.

Carbamazepine has rarely induced brady-arrhythmia and atrioventricular conduction delay in susceptible subjects. Patients with underlying cardiac disease are most at risk, although heart block has been reported in otherwise healthy children and also patients with tuberous sclerosis. A few cases of cardiac arrest and death have been attributed to the initiation of carbamazepine, and the drug should be used with caution in those with pre-existing heart disease and especially those with prolonged QT or other A–V conduction defects.

About 5–10% of subjects develop mild gastrointestinal side-effects such as nausea, vomiting or diarrhoea.

Carbamazepine has a dose-related antidiuretic effect, resulting in low serum sodium and water retention. This effect is more frequent in the elderly. The mechanism is obscure, and evidence has been adduced for both a renal and also a pituitary effect. Usually, the mild hyponatraemia and water retention are asymptomatic and require no correction. Occasionally, a large fluid load—typically, pints of beer—will cause symptomatic hyponatraemia with nausea, weakness and dizziness. Caution is needed when prescribing carbamazepine to the elderly on low-sodium diets, and all patients should be monitored for symptoms of hyponatraemia.

Carbamazepine can induce a variety of biochemical changes in circulating pituitary and sex hormones, but the clinical significance of these effects is quite unclear. Free cortisol levels can be increased and free testosterone levels reduced. T4 levels are reduced but other thyroid hormone levels are normal and patients are generally euthyroid. Carbamazepine induces the metabolism of the oestrogen content of the oral contraceptive, carrying the risk of contraceptive failure (see p. 76). Mild hypocalcaemia and lowered vitamin D levels have been recorded, although frank osteomalacia has not. Carbamazepine may also elevate the high-density lipoprotein levels in the blood, which theoretically could lead to an increased risk of atherosclerosis.

Antiepileptic effect

Carbamazepine is one of the most widely used antiepileptic drugs in the world, and one of the most widely studied. It is the drug of first choice for partial and secondarily generalized seizures where its

Table 4.4 Patients with complex partial seizures who were seizure-free for 12-months in the VA Cooperative Study.

	n	Percentage
Carbamazepine	14	67
Phenobarbital	3	21
Phenytoin	12	43
Primidone	7	33

$P \leq 0.04$ for carbamazepine vs. phenobarbital or primidone.

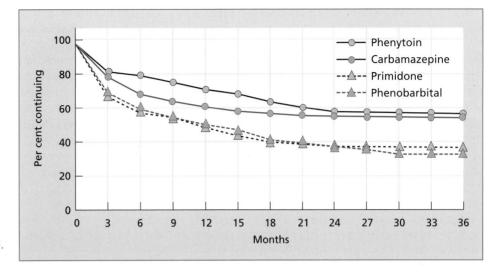

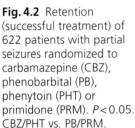

Fig. 4.2 Retention (successful treatment) of 622 patients with partial seizures randomized to carbamazepine (CBZ), phenobarbital (PB), phenytoin (PHT) or primidone (PRM). *P*<0.05. CBZ/PHT vs. PB/PRM.

effects are equal or superior to that of phenytoin and sodium valproate (Table 4.4 and Fig. 4.2). It is effective against the entire range of partial seizures and in the cryptogenic and symptomatic partial seizure syndromes. Carbamazepine is also useful in generalized tonic–clonic seizures associated with idiopathic generalized epilepsy. A huge number of open studies have shown effectiveness in adults and in children, in monotherapy and in combination with various other antiepileptics. As carbamazepine is the industry standard, there have been a range of blinded and controlled comparative studies comparing carbamazepine to other newer antiepileptic drugs. Carbamazepine has shown equal or superior efficacy when compared to clonazepam, lamotrigine, oxcarbazepine, phenytoin, phenobarbital, primidone, vigabatrin and valproate. In the large comparative veterans study 1-year remission rates were recorded in 58 and 44%, respectively, of patients with generalized seizures and with partial seizures. Patients were completely seizure-free with carbamazepine more frequently than with phenobarbital at 1, 2 and 3 years of follow-up. In primary generalized tonic–clonic seizures, another study found a >50% decrease in attacks in 80% of patients followed for up to 2 years.

The drug has been widely used in children as well as in adults. It is a first-line drug for any child with partial or secondarily generalized seizures, and in the partial epilepsy syndromes. It is the drug of choice in benign childhood epilepsy with centrotemporal spikes (rolandic epilepsy) and other benign syndromes. Its use in the generalized epilepsy syndromes of childhood is more controversial. It can exacerbate the non-convulsive generalized seizures of the Len-

nox–Gastaut syndrome even where controlling the convulsive attacks. It worsens generalized absence and myoclonic seizures in idiopathic generalized epilepsy, yet may control the tonic–clonic seizures of the same syndrome. Febrile convulsions are also resistant to carbamazepine therapy.

CLINICAL USE IN EPILEPSY

Carbamazepine is available in 100, 200 and 400 mg tablets, also chewable tablets for children at doses of 100 and 200 mg, and also slow-release formulations at 200 and 400 mg capsules and as liquid and suppositories.

It is usual in adults to start at 100 mg nocte and to double this dose every fortnight to a level of 400–800 mg per day in two divided doses. In adults, maintenance doses of between 400–1600 mg are commonly used, although higher doses (up to 2800 mg) are occasionally required. Starting at a higher initial dose often results in acute nausea, vomiting, diplopia, dizziness and drowsiness. Slow introduction at a low dose reduces the risk of this reaction. Once the maintenance dose is reached, the slow-release formulation should be prescribed if the drug is poorly tolerated, and this formulation should be used if high doses are required. Low doses and low blood levels will completely control seizures in many cases, and it is usual to aim initially for a low maintenance dose. It is usual to give the drug in a twice daily regimen, and the use of the slow-release formulation is a better option than higher dosage frequency in most situations.

In children the same principles apply. Children below 1 year of age require a maintenance dose of 100–200 mg, between 1 and 5 years a maintenance dose of 200–400 mg, between 5 and 10 years a maintenance dose of 400–600 mg, between 10 and 15 years a maintenance dose of 400–1000 mg. As the clearance of carbamazepine in children is faster, three times daily dosage is often required.

A 'therapeutic range' of serum levels has been defined, based on mean responses in populations of patients (20–50 µmol/L). Many patients are well controlled at lower levels and some patients do not suffer side-effects when the range is exceeded, so the range should be considered as a general guideline only. In combination therapy the blood levels are even more difficult to interpret.

Clobazam

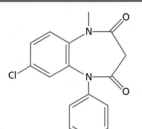

Primary indications	Adjunctive therapy for partial and generalized seizures. Also for intermittent therapy, one-off prophylactic therapy, and non-convulsive status epilepticus
Usual preparations	Tablet, capsule: 10 mg
Usual dosages	10–30 mg per day (adults); higher doses can be used. Children aged 3–12 years, up to half adult dose
Dosage intervals	1–2 times per day
Significant drug interactions	Minor interactions are common, but usually not clinically significant
Serum level monitoring	Not useful
Target range	–
Common/important side-effects	Sedation, dizziness, weakness, blurring of vision, restlessness, ataxia, aggressiveness, behavioural disturbance, withdrawal symptoms
Main advantages	Highly effective in some patients with epilepsy resistant to first-line therapy. Better tolerated than other benzodiazepines
Main disadvantages	Development of tolerance in as many as 50% of subjects within weeks or months
Mechanisms of action	$GABA_A$ receptor agonist. Also action on ion-channel conductance
Oral bioavailability	90%
Time to peak levels	1–4 h
Metabolism and excretion	Hepatic oxidation and then conjugation
Volume of distribution	–
Elimination half-life	10–50 h (clobazam); 50 h (*N*-desmethylclobazam)
Plasma clearance	–
Protein binding	83%
Active metabolites	*N*-desmethylclobazam
Comment	Excellent second-line therapy in some patients with resistant epilepsy

Clobazam is a remarkable drug whose role in epilepsy is underestimated. This is partly because it is a benzodiazepine and carries with it all the encumbrances of this drug class. There is also a surprising lack of promotion by its manufacturers, in a market place not generally characterized by reticence.

The drug has a 1,5 substitution instead of the usual 1,4-diazepine structure. It is unique in this regard, and this structural change results in an 80% reduction in its anxiolytic activity and a 10-fold reduction in its sedative effects, when compared with diazepam in animal studies. The drug was introduced as an anxiolytic, its potent antiepileptic effects were demonstrated later and its human antiepileptic effect was first reported a decade after its introduction. It has been licensed in Europe since 1975 and Canada since 1988 but is unavailable in the USA. It is widely used in specialist epilepsy clinics, where this underdog of a drug has many champions.

PHYSICAL AND CHEMICAL CHARACTERISTICS

Clobazam is relatively insoluble in water and therefore cannot be given by intravenous or intramuscular injection. It is a weak organic acid. It is also relatively lipid-insoluble, about 40% of that of diazepam. It is also insoluble in water, throughout the range of physiological pH.

Mode of action

Presumably clobazam works at the benzodiazepine binding site of the γ-aminobutyric acid (GABA$_A$) receptor complex, thus enhancing the inhibitory neurotransmitter action of GABA. Quite why its action is distinct from other benzodiazepine drugs is not clearly known, but this could reflect differential binding to the various GABA$_A$ receptor subunits; at least 16 have already been identified. The drug may also exert an action away from the GABA receptor, affecting voltage-sensitive calcium-ion conductance and sodium-channel function.

PHARMACOKINETICS

Absorption

Clobazam has an oral bioavailability of about 90%. It is absorbed rapidly and the time to peak plasma concentrations (T_{max}) is 1–4 h. Absorption is relatively unaffected by age or by gender. The rate of absorption is reduced when the drug is taken with or after meals, but the extent of absorption is unaffected. For the epilepsy patient the timing of ingestion is seldom critical.

Distribution

The plasma protein binding of clobazam has been found to be 83%, and the proportion of bound:unbound drug is independent of clobazam concentrations. There is a higher free (unbound) proportion though in situations where the protein content is greatly lowered, for instance in advanced hepatic or renal disease. Clobazam is distributed widely, but the concentration in the brain is proportional to the concentration of the unbound drug in the serum, as is the drug concentration in saliva. There is a good correlation also between plasma concentration and dosage in an individual patient, but there are large interindividual variations.

Biotransformation and excretion

Clobazam is extensively oxidized in the liver to N-desmethylclobazam (otherwise known as norclobazam) (Fig. 4.3). This is an important fact, as N-desmethylclobazam could be responsible for much of the antiepileptic effect of the drug. Arguing against this are the facts that the lipid solubility of the metabolite is lower than that of the parent drug, and that its affinity for the benzodiazepine receptor is 10-fold less than that of clobazam. However, the half-life of norclobazam is very much longer, about 50 h in healthy volunteers but less in patients on other enzyme-inducing drugs, and its plasma concentration considerably higher than that of the parent drug. This is a case of swings and roundabouts, and the exact role of the metabolite is not fully established. The elimination half-life of clobazam is variable, from 11 to 77 h in one investigation. It is usually in the 10–50 h range. The longest half-lives are in the elderly. In patients receiving other antiepileptic drugs the half-life is reduced to approximately 12 h. Desmethylclobazam is itself conjugated in the liver and excreted in the bile as glucuronate and in the urine as a sulphate. At normal clinical dosage the plasma concentration of the metabolite is between 300 and 3500 ng/mL, about 10-fold higher than the usual clobazam concentrations (20–350 ng/mL).

Drug interactions

Clobazam usually causes no clinically significant change in the blood in phenytoin or carbamazepine drug levels, although some patients on high phenytoin doses have developed phenytoin toxicity when clobazam is added. Carbamazepine epoxidation can also be enhanced by clobazam comedication. A rare but unpredictable increase in sodium valproate lev-

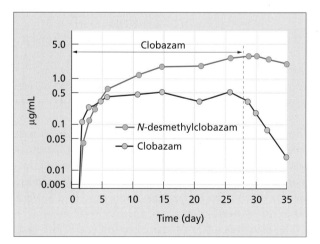

Fig. 4.3 Clobazam (grey) and N-desmethylclobazam (blue) levels after 10 mg twice daily for 28 days (means of 10 subjects).

els has also been reported. Desmethylclobazam levels can be raised and clobazam levels lowered in patients on combination therapy with phenobarbital, phenytoin or carbamazepine. In the great majority of patients, however, the clinical effects of these interactions are slight and in normal practice problems are rare.

SIDE-EFFECTS

Because clobazam has been so widely used in psychiatric practice as an anxiolytic, its side-effect profile is well known. The side-effects are essentially similar to those of other benzodiazepines. The frequency of side-effects in clinical trials of clobazam's anxiolytic effect has been reported to lie between 20–85%, but in only 5–15% were the side-effects of a severity sufficient to change dosage or terminate treatment. In clinical practice, it must be said, side-effects are seemingly less common, possibly reflecting the different patient group. The most common are sedation, dizziness, ataxia, blurred vision and diplopia. Occasionally, behavioural disturbances, irritability, depression and disinhibition are reported, especially in institutionalized populations. Muscle fatigue and weakness occur, as with other benzodiazepines, caused by disorderly recruitment of motor units, and for this reason the drug should not be given to patients with myasthenia gravis. Of all these side-effects, sedation is the most important, but the measured effects of normal dosage of clobazam on cognitive tests has been shown to be slight.

Undoubtedly, clinically the most problematic phenomenon is the tendency for clobazam to lose its beneficial effect (the development of tolerance). This is a property shared by all benzodiazepines but, in animal studies, tolerance developed more frequently with clobazam than with clonazepam. At least 50% of patients treated with clobazam can expect to develop tolerance, yet despite its frequency and importance the mechanisms underlying benzodiazepine tolerance are quite unknown. Better news is that tolerance to the sedative effects are much more prominent than tolerance to the antiepileptic effects, and if a patient develops sedation on starting treatment, it is well worthwhile carrying on therapy as the sedative effects usually wear off within a week or so.

Idiosyncratic allergic reactions are very rare and, as far as this author is aware, no fatal side-effects have been reported.

ANTIEPILEPTIC EFFECT

The drug was introduced before double-blind placebo-controlled clinical trials had become a fundamental requirement. Nine trials in refractory partial epilepsy, however, have been carried out with striking benefit. In one study, over 50% of patients showed a greater than 50% reduction of seizures, and in another the mean seizure reduction was 30%. As the trials were all carried out in patients with long-standing chronic and previously refractory epilepsy, this is an impressive result—and certainly better than observed with many other currently available drugs. The patients in these clinical trials all had partial epilepsy, and all were taking other antiepileptic drugs.

The drug has also been the subject of numerous open studies, often with a wider range of patients, and some reported quite remarkable effects. It has been claimed that the patient who typically obtains the most worthwhile benefit from clobazam has partial seizures without secondarily generalization and is without learning disability. Patients with secondarily generalized seizures also respond, however, as do those with the Lennox–Gastaut syndrome, startle epilepsy, non-convulsive status epilepticus, electrical status during slow-wave sleep (ESES), reflex epilepsies, alcohol withdrawal seizures and also those with benign childhood partial epilepsies.

There have been no large-scale trials of clobazam in monotherapy in adults, but in drug-naïve children with new onset epilepsy, a recent multicentre Canadian study found the drug to be equally as effective as monotherapy with phenytoin or carbamazepine.

No clear relationship has been found between serum level and seizure control, but this is confused by the development of tolerance. An optimum range of serum levels in chronic epilepsy has not been established.

The development of tolerance is the major clinical problem. Manoeuvres such as intermittent therapy, drug holidays, initiation at very low dose, and the use of very high doses have all failed to circumvent this problem.

Clobazam exerts a mild antianxiolytic effect which is also useful in some patients with epilepsy.

CLINICAL USE IN EPILEPSY

Clobazam should be considered as adjunctive therapy whenever treatment with a single first-line antiepileptic drug has proved ineffective. In the author's practice, clobazam is often the first adjunctive drug to be tried. It is effective in a wide range of epilepsies, although perhaps best in those with partial seizures alone. It can be used in patients with Lennox–Gastaut syndrome and other primary and secondarily generalized epilepsies. It is effective in a broad spectrum of other types of epilepsy and non-convulsive status syndromes.

Clobazam also has a particularly useful role as one-off prophylactic therapy on special occasions when it is particularly important to prevent a seizure (e.g. on days of travel, interview, examinations, etc.). Although there are no formal studies of the drug used in this way, the effect is often rapid and reliable, and the low incidence of side-effects makes it an ideal choice for such therapy.

Clobazam can also be used in intermittent therapy (i.e. in catamenial epilepsy; see p. 77). It is administered orally at a dose of 10–20 mg per day usually taken at night or in a twice daily regime. The only available preparation is a 10 mg tablet or capsule. Higher dosage is seldom effective and should be avoided. The rectal administration of the drug has been explored experimentally, but is not used in clinical practice. There are no parenteral formulations. It is advisable to observe the same precautions with clobazam as with other benzodiazepine drugs.

Clonazepam

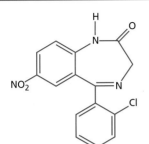

Primary indications	Adjunctive therapy in partial and generalized seizures (including absence and myoclonus). Also, Lennox–Gastaut syndrome and status epilepticus
Usual preparations	Tablets: 0.5, 2 mg, liquid: 1 mg in 1 mL diluent
Usual dosages	Initial: 0.25 mg. Maintenance: 0.5–4 mg (adults); 1 mg (children under 1 year), 1–2 mg (children 1–5 years), 1–3 mg (children 5–12 years). Higher doses can be used
Dosage intervals	1–2 times per day
Significant drug interactions	Minor interactions are common, but usually not clinically significant
Serum level monitoring	Not useful
Target range	–
Common/important side-effects	Sedation (common and may be severe), cognitive effects, drowsiness, ataxia, personality and behavioural changes, hyperactivity, restlessness, aggressiveness, psychotic reaction, seizure exacerbations, hypersalivation, leucopenia, withdrawal symptoms
Main advantages	Useful add-on action, especially in children
Main disadvantages	Side-effects are sometimes prominent, particularly sedation, tolerance and a withdrawal syndrome
Mechanisms of action	$GABA_A$ receptor agonist. Also action on sodium-channel conductance
Oral bioavailability	>80%
Time to peak levels	1–4 h
Metabolism and excretion	Hepatic reduction and then acetylation
Volume of distribution	2.0 L/kg
Elimination of half-life	20–80 h
Plasma clearance	0.09 L/kg/h
Protein binding	86%
Active metabolites	Nil
Comment	A wide antiepileptic effect, use limited by side-effects, but helpful particularly in children with severe epilepsy

Clonazepam was one of the earliest benzodiazepine drugs used for epilepsy. It was licensed in Europe in 1975 and is also licensed in North America and throughout the world. It is a 1 : 4 substituted benzo-diazepine, a structure shared with diazepam and all the other antiepileptic drugs of this class, with the notable exception of clobazam. It has in the past been widely used, although now is largely superseded by other drugs with fewer side-effects.

PHYSICAL AND CHEMICAL CHARACTERISTICS

Clonazepam is a crystalline powder with pKa values of 1.5 and 10.5, and is virtually undissociated throughout the physiological pH range. It is highly lipid-soluble.

Mode of action

Clonazepam, like all other benzodiazepines, is an agonist at the $GABA_A$ receptor. The benzodiazepines increase channel opening frequency at the $GABA_A$ receptor, resulting in enhanced chloride uptake into the neurone and neuronal hyperpolarization. Clonazepam has higher affinity binding to the benzodiazepine receptor than diazepam or other benzodiazepines and, furthermore, clonazepam binds to subgroups of the $GABA_A$ receptor which do not bind the other benzodiazepine drugs. In the rat, clonazepam alone binds in the spinal cord and striation and has a high concentration in the cerebellum. The drug also appears to have some action on sodium-channel conductance.

PHARMACOKINETICS

Absorption

Clonazepam is well and reliably absorbed, with an oral bioavailability of 80% or more. It reaches a peak plasma level within 1–4 h of oral administration in most people, although this can be delayed up to 8 h.

Distribution

Clonazepam is 86% bound to plasma proteins. It has a volume distribution of between 1.5 and 4.4 L/kg in normal volunteers (in most about 2.0 L/kg), reflecting its lipid solubility. It rapidly crosses into the brain and has a consistent brain : plasma concentration ratio.

Biotransformation and excretion

Clonazepam is metabolized in the liver first by acetylation, a process greatly influenced by the patient's genetic acetylator status. The acetylated compound is then reduced and nitrated. There are a variety of metabolites, none of which have clinically important pharmacological activity. The half-life of clonazepam is quite variable, in most patients falling between 20 and 80 h. In studies in neonates half-lives have been recorded of 20–43 h and in children of 22–33 h. There seems to be no correlation between antiepileptic efficacy and plasma level. The clearance of clonazepam is low; in adults approximately 100 mL/min. Less than 0.5% of the parent drug is recovered unchanged in the urine.

Drug interactions

It is rare for clonazepam to alter levels of other drugs in any clinically relevant manner. Clonazepam levels, however, are lowered by coadministration with carbamazepine or phenobarbital and presumably other enzyme-inducing drugs. However, this effect is seldom of clinical importance.

SIDE-EFFECTS

The most common important side-effect of clonazepam is sedation. There is no doubt that, even at small doses, a significant number of patients experience unacceptable levels of drowsiness and this limits the use of the drug in normal clinical practice. This adverse effect seems to be less frequent in children than in adults, and this might explain the greater popularity of clonazepam amongst paediatricians than adult neurologists.

Other side-effects are much less troublesome and are typical of those expected from all benzodiazepine drugs. These include ataxia, incoordination, hyperactivity, restlessness, irritability, depression and other neuropsychiatric effects. This list may be long, but the side-effects are not usually dose-limiting. Hypersecretion and hypersalivation may be troublesome in infants and children. Cardiovascular and respiratory depression have also been observed in infants. Like other benzodiazepines, clonazepam may occasionally increase certain seizure types (e.g. tonic seizures). Occasional idiosyncratic allergic reactions, including marked leucopenia, have been observed.

ANTIEPILEPTIC EFFECT

Clonazepam is a potent antiepileptic drug. However, because of its potential to cause sedation and the problem of tolerance, it is usually prescribed as second-line adjunctive therapy after other antiepileptics have proved ineffective. It has a wide spectrum of activity, although its effects are usually modest. Early reports suggested that it was useful in partial seizures, although a recent literature review concluded that its effect was slight. It has been used in benign rolandic epilepsy and also epilepsia partialis continua. In the generalized epilepsies, its effectiveness in absence epilepsy is well documented and it has some effect in tonic–clonic seizures. It can be useful in Lennox–Gastaut syndrome. It is an effective therapy in myoclonic seizures, and is indeed one of the drugs of choice for this indication. It is effective in myoclonus caused by primary generalized epilepsy, and also the symptomatic secondary myoclonic epilepsies. It is frequently used by specialists in movement disorders for subcortical myoclonus. Clonazepam has also been shown to be relatively safe in acute intermittent porphyria. Intravenous clonazepam is effective in controlling neonatal convulsions.

Clonazepam is still used widely in the treatment of various forms of status epilepticus. Its indications are exactly the same as for diazepam, and its effectiveness is similar. It can be given intravenously or rectally in the emergency setting (see Chapter 5).

Tolerance to the anticonvulsant effects of clonazepam is less prominent than tolerance to the motor and sedative effects, but nevertheless remains a common clinical problem. Exactly how frequently this occurs is uncertain, and certainly tolerance can develop after weeks or months of therapy in some patients and after only days of therapy in others. The brain mechanisms underlying tolerances are not clearly understood. Down-regulation of the GABA$_A$ receptor is said to occur; this is descriptive rather than explanatory.

Withdrawal of clonazepam can also be problematic. In spite of its long half-life, if clonazepam is suddenly withdrawn there is a serious risk of seizure exacerbation and of status epilepticus. The drug should be withdrawn very cautiously, and the author's practice is usually to do this at a rate not exceeding 1 mg per month. Withdrawal seizures in animal models are also well documented, but the mechanism of rebound seizures is not understood. Psychiatric withdrawal reactions also occur, such as rebound insomnia, anxiety, tremor and psychosis. In one study in children, discontinuation symptoms occurred in about half of cases.

CLINICAL USE IN EPILEPSY

Although clonazepam is a potent antiepileptic drug, it is rarely used as first-line therapy in the treatment of epilepsy because of its strong tendency to cause sedation and also the problem of tolerance. It is more commonly used in children than in adults and usually given as second-line adjunctive therapy. It is used in a wide range of generalized and partial epilepsies. It also has a particular role in myoclonus, where it is a drug of choice. It has also been a staple drug in convulsive and non-convulsive status epilepticus, although its use has been substantially superseded by its close relations lorazepam, midazolam and diazepam.

It is available as 0.5 mg and 2 mg tablets and also as an intravenous solution. The initial dose in adults is usually 0.25 mg and this is increased slowly to between 0.5 and 4 mg per day in a single or twice daily regimen. In children the usual maintenance dose is between 1–3 mg per day.

Ethosuximide

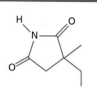

Primary indications	First-line or adjunctive therapy in generalized absence seizures
Usual preparations	Capsules: 250 mg; syrup: 250 mg/5 mL
Usual dosages	Initial: 250 mg (adults); 10–15 mg/kg per day (children). Maintenance: 750–2000 mg per day (adults); 20–40 mg/kg per day (children)
Dosage intervals	2–3 times per day
Significant drug interactions	Ethosuximide levels are increased by valproate. Levels may be reduced by carbamazepine, phenytoin and phenobarbital
Serum level monitoring	Useful
Target range	300–700 µmol/L
Common/important side-effects	Gastrointestinal symptoms, drowsiness, ataxia, diplopia, headache, sedation, behavioural disturbances, acute psychotic reactions, extra-pyramidal symptoms, blood dyscrasia, rash, systemic lupus erythematosus
Main advantages	Well-established treatment for absence epilepsy without the risk of hepatic toxicity carried by valproate
Main disadvantages	Side-effects common
Mechanisms of action	Effects on calcium T-channel conductance
Oral bioavailability	<100%
Time to peak levels	<4 h
Metabolism and excretion	Hepatic oxidation then conjugation
Volume of distribution	0.65 L/kg
Elimination half-life	30–60 h
Plasma clearance	0.010–0.015 L/kg/h
Protein binding	Nil
Active metabolites	Nil
Comment	Drug of first choice in absence seizures

Ethosuximide is the only widely used drug of the succinimide family. Other succinimides have been licensed, but of these only mesuximide is still prescribed (albeit in a very small number of patients). All the other compounds in this family have been supplanted by more modern antiepileptics. Ethosuximide was introduced into clinical practice in 1958 and is widely available around the world. Its primary indication is as a drug of first choice in the treatment of generalized absence seizures.

Physical and chemical characteristics
Ethosuximide is a crystalline substance soluble in water and in chloroform.

Mode of action
Ethosuximide has a highly selective effect on generalized absence seizures, and their EEG signature the 3-Hz spike and wave discharge. The drug inhibits low-threshold calcium currents in the thalamus and this is almost certainly the mechanism by which

spike wave discharges are inhibited. The drug has other effects at other brain sites, and also acts at the GABA receptor.

PHARMACOKINETICS

Absorption

Ethosuximide is rapidly absorbed with an oral bioavailability approaching 100%. Peak plasma levels are reached within 4 h of single-dose administration. The syrup formulation tends to be more rapidly absorbed than the capsules.

Distribution

The apparent volume of distribution following oral administration is approximately 0.65 L/kg body weight in adults. There is negligible plasma protein binding. Plasma concentrations are equivalent to concentrations in saliva and in cerebrospinal fluid and tears. The drug readily crosses the placenta and also into breast milk.

Biotransformation and elimination

Ethosuximide is extensively metabolized in the liver; first by oxidation and then conjugation by the subgroup CYP3A of the hepatic cytochrome P450 system. The metabolites have no significant antiepileptic action. About 20% of the drug is excreted unchanged in the urine. Ethosuximide is cleared slowly, with a mean half-life in adults of 50–60 h and 30–40 h in children, although there is considerable interindividual variability. The elimination half-life is unaffected by drug dosage, but the clearance does seem to be slightly lower in women than in men. Ethosuximide does not induce hepatic microsomal enzymes, nor is there autoinduction.

Drug interactions

Ethosuximide does not affect serum levels of other antiepileptic or non-antiepileptic drugs. Comedication with sodium valproate can result in an increase of up to 50% in ethosuximide levels because of valproate-induced inhibition of ethosuximide metabolism. Comedication with carbamazepine can result in a significant decrease in ethosuximide plasma concentrations, because of the hepatic enzyme-inducing properties of carbamazepine. Rifampicin, a well-known inducer of CYP3A enzymes, has been shown to increase the clearance of ethosuximide by 90%. Other drugs acting on this enzyme system can be expected to have a similar effect.

SIDE-EFFECTS

Idiosyncratic reaction

Skin rashes, which can be severe and include erythema multiforme and Stevens–Johnson syndrome, are not uncommon with ethosuximide. Occasional blood dyscrasias have occurred, although mild leucopenia and marrow depression are common occurrences. Other immunologically mediated reactions include the occasional development of systemic lupus erythematosus, pericarditis, myocarditis and thyroiditis.

Dose-related side-effects

Other most commonly reported side-effects are gastrointestinal symptoms, such as nausea, abdominal discomfort, anorexia and hiccups. Headache may be troublesome and can be severe. Sedation may also be a problem, and is not uncommon following the increase in plasma level of ethosuximide in patients in whom valproate has been added. There is little other effect on cognition in most patients, although an occasional severe encephalopathy can be induced by ethosuximide, as it can by other succinimide drugs. The evaluation of cognitive function is complicated by the effects of the drug on spike wave EEG disturbances, and striking improvements can sometimes occur when ethosuximide is given to children with frequent spike wave bursts. Ethosuximide can cause severe behavioural change, particularly irritability, depression and anxiety and occasionally a psychotic reaction. The drug should be used with caution in patients with a history of psychiatric disturbance. Other rare side-effects include bradykinesia and parkinsonism.

ANTIEPILEPTIC EFFECT

Ethosuximide, like valproate, is a drug of first choice in the treatment of children with generalized absence seizures. Its effect in this condition can be remarkable, with almost all patients showing some improvement and with over half showing a >90% reduction in EEG spike wave discharges. The effectiveness of the drug is equal to that of valproate and, furthermore, the drugs in combination can have a synergistic effect in patients who have not responded adequately to either drug alone. Tolerance does not develop with ethosuximide. Although ethosuximide does not generally control tonic–clonic seizures, a gratifying effect is occasionally encountered in resistant idiopathic generalized epilepsy. The usual lack of effect in tonic–clonic seizures is a disadvantage compared with valproate which has a broader spectrum action. Plasma level measurements of ethosuximide are useful in defining dosage, and there is a clear relationship between plasma level and clinical effectiveness. The target range of drug levels is between 300 and 700 µmol/L.

CLINICAL USE IN EPILEPSY

Ethosuximide is a first-line drug in the treatment of childhood absence seizures. Its use has been supplanted in older children and adults by valproate, because of the latter drug's superior action against tonic–clonic seizures, which often also occur in idiopathic generalized epilepsy, and also because of the risks of serious idiosyncratic hepatic or haematological reactions on valproate are less than in young children.

The drug is available as a capsule and as a syrup. The commonly recommended starting dose is 10–15 mg/kg per day with incremental rises to a dose of between 20 and 40 mg/kg per day. Adults start with a dose of 250 mg per day and increase fortnightly by 250–500 mg to a maintenance dose of between 750 and 2000 mg per day, in two divided doses. The generally accepted plasma range is 300–700 µmol/L. It takes about one week in children to reach steady state, and two weeks in adults; blood levels should not be measured before steady state is reached.

Felbamate

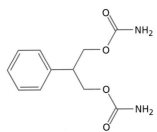

Primary indications	Adjunctive therapy in refractory partial and secondarily generalized epilepsy. Also in Lennox–Gastaut syndrome
Usual preparations	Tablets: 400, 600 mg; syrup: 600 mg/5 mL
Usual dosages	Initial: 1200 mg per day (adults); 15 mg/kg per day (children). Maintenance: 1200–3600 mg per day (adults); 45–80 mg/kg per day (children)
Dosage intervals	3–4 times per day
Significant drug interactions	Felbamate increases the concentration of phenobarbital, phenytoin, carbamazepine epoxide and valproate. Felbamate lowers the concentration of carbamazepine. Phenytoin, phenobarbital and carbamazepine lower felbamate levels; valproate increases felbamate levels
Serum level monitoring	Value not established
Target range	200–460 µmol/L
Common/important side-effects	Severe hepatic disturbance and aplastic anaemia are rare but serious side-effects. Insomnia, weight loss, gastrointestinal symptoms, fatigue, dizziness, lethargy, behavioural change, ataxia, visual disturbance, mood change, psychotic reaction, rash, neurological symptoms
Main advantages	Highly effective novel antiepileptic drugs for refractory patients
Main disadvantages	Severe hepatic and aplastic anaemia in occasional patients. Other side-effects also frequent on initial therapy, and in patients on polytherapy
Mechanisms of action	Probably by effect on NMDA receptor (glycine recognition site) and sodium-channel conductance
Oral bioavailability	90%
Time to peak levels	1–4 h
Metabolism and excretion	Hepatic hydroxylation and then conjugation (60%); renal excretion as unchanged drug (40%)
Volume of distribution	0.75 L/kg
Elimination half-life	20 h (13–30 h; lowest in patients comedicated with enzyme inducers)
Plasma clearance	0.027–0.032 L/kg/h (but variable)
Protein binding	20–25%
Active metabolites	Nil
Comment	Highly effective novel anticonvulsant in severe resistant epilepsy, but use limited by rare but severe hepatic and haematological toxicity

Felbamate was granted a licence in the USA as adjunctive and monotherapy in adults with partial seizures with or without generalization and as adjunctive therapy in children with the Lennox–Gastaut syndrome in 1993. It was subsequently approved in European countries, but following the occurrences of aplastic anaemia and hepatic failure, approval for general use was withdrawn. It is now available only on a very limited basis.

Mode of action

The specific site of felbamate action is not known, but a number of possible mechanisms have been explored. It seems likely that it blocks the N-methyl-D-aspartate (NMDA) receptor, and also modulates sodium-channel conductance. Interestingly, felbamate has no effect on GABA or benzodiazepine receptor binding.

Its protective index in various animal models compares favourably with other drugs (Table 4.5). In addition to its activity against seizures, felbamate has been shown to have a neuroprotective effect in models of hypoxic–ischaemic injuries, such as the rat hippocampal slice, kainic acid and bilateral carotid ligation in rat pups.

Absorption and distribution

In humans, orally administered felbamate is well absorbed. In patients with epilepsy, time to peak plasma concentration has been found to be from 1 to 4 h after the dose.

Felbamate is distributed rapidly into a number of tissues, including brain. Lipid-mediated blood–brain barrier penetration of felbamate is similar to that of phenytoin and phenobarbital. In humans, 20–25% of the total concentration is bound, primarily to albumin, and this degree of binding is not clinically significant.

Biotransformation and excretion

Felbamate is extensively metabolized by the liver via hydroxylation and conjugation. The hepatic elimination creates the potential for a number of drug–drug interactions. In human volunteers, 40–49% of a felbamate dose is recovered in the urine as the par-ent compound. The major identified metabolites of felbamate are p-hydroxy-felbamate, 2-hydroxy-felbamate, a monocarbamate and 3-carbamoyloxy-2-phenylpropionic acid.

The half-life of felbamate in normal male volunteers is approximately 20 h and ranges from 13 to 30 h as monotherapy. Multiple dosing does not alter the elimination half-life. In patients with epilepsy receiving either phenytoin or carbamazepine, the half-life of felbamate was shorter, approximately 13–14 h with a range of 11.4–19.6 h. Conversely, when phenytoin was decreased or eliminated in patients comedicated with felbamate, felbamate concentrations increased and its apparent clearance decreased by 21%. Similarly, decreasing or eliminating carbamazepine led to an additional decrease of the apparent clearance of 16.5%. Valproate has the opposite effect, and felbamate concentrations are significantly higher than expected in the presence of valproate. Felbamate also increases phenytoin levels in comedication, and reduces carbamazepine and increases carbamazepine-epoxide levels. These complex interactions of felbamate can be important clinically, and can require dosage changes. The potential for interactions with other newer antiepileptic drugs exists but has not been fully studied.

Side-effects

Felbamate is usually well tolerated by patients with epilepsy. The most common side-effects of felbamate have been insomnia, weight loss, nausea, decreased appetite, dizziness, fatigue, ataxia and lethargy. In clinical trials, 12% (120 of 977 adults) discontinued felbamate because of side-effects. These were anorexia (1.2%); nausea (1.4%); skin rash (1.2%); weight loss (1.1%); and various neurological (1.4%) or psychological symptoms (2.2%). Side-effects are much more common in patients treated with other antiepileptic drugs but, with monotherapy, few adverse experiences have been reported and were mild and self-limited. After the drug had been licensed in both the USA and

Table 4.5 The protective index (median toxic dose : median effective dose) of felbamate and standard antiepileptic drugs.

Drug	Maximal electroshock	Pentylenetetrazol	Picrotoxin	NMDA	Kindling
Felbamate	16.3	5.51	5.2	146	>35.8
Carbamazepine	8.1	NP	37.2	16	>17.3
Ethosuximide	NP	3.4	1.8	4	NP
Phenytoin	6.9	NP	NP	71	NP
Valproate	1.6	2.9	1.1	5.8	7.3

NMDA, N-methyl-D-aspartate; NP, not protected.

some European countries, cases of aplastic anaemia and hepatic failure occurred. A total of 14 cases of fatal hepatic failure have been reported. These occurred in a population of approximately 110 000 patients. By mid-July 1995 there have been 31 cases of aplastic anaemia and 10 deaths. Both of these idiosyncratic effects seem to occur within 6 months of the initiation of therapy and in patients taking polytherapy. No other risk factors have been identified.

Antiepileptic effect

There have been a variety of studies of felbamate efficacy, some with very novel designs. All showed felbamate to be highly effective. Studies in partial seizures have included several placebo-controlled and blinded evaluations of felbamate as adjunctive therapy. In one study, for instance, 64 adult patients with partial seizures were randomized to felbamate or placebo in addition to the antiepileptic drugs used at the conclusion of the presurgical evaluation. Felbamate doses were increased rapidly, 1800 mg on day one, 2400 mg on day two and 3600 mg on day three. The efficacy variable, the time to fourth seizure, was statistically significant ($P = 0.028$) in favour of felbamate. All the published trials demonstrated the ability of felbamate quickly and safely to reduce the occurrence of frequent partial-onset seizures after reductions in the dosages of standard antiepileptic drugs, and the lack of significant side-effects even with rapid titration in patients whose other antiepileptic drugs had been withdrawn.

Two studies of felbamate monotherapy using an 'active placebo' consisting of low-dose valproate have formed the basis of its recommended use as the sole antiepileptic drug in refractory patients. Both showed a highly significant difference in effectiveness in favour of felbamate.

Efficacy of felbamate in the Lennox–Gastaut syndrome was evaluated in a double-blind add-on parallel study involving 73 patients, mostly in the paediatric age-range. Felbamate or placebo was added to standard antiepileptic drugs. The dosage of felbamate was titrated to a maximum of 45 mg/kg of body weight per day or 3600 mg per day, whichever was less. Patients treated with felbamate had a 34% decrease in the frequency of atonic seizures ($P = 0.01$), and a 19% decrease in the frequency of all seizures ($P = 0.002$). A 'quality of life' measure, the global-evaluation scores, was significantly higher in the felbamate group as compared to the placebo group.

Clinical use in epilepsy

The use of felbamate is restricted to patients with severe partial epilepsy or the Lennox–Gastaut syndrome who have not responded to other medication. This limited usage is because of the small but definite risk of aplastic anaemia and hepatic failure. The drug is highly effective (indeed more so than most other antiepileptic drugs) and this restriction is regrettable but necessary.

A 'therapeutic range' has not yet been determined for felbamate concentrations, but levels between 30 and 100 µg/mL have been observed to be effective and non-toxic in various studies. Some patients may need higher doses.

In outpatient adults, felbamate can be initiated at 1200 mg per day in three or four divided doses, with increases to 2400 and 3600 mg per day in weekly or biweekly increments of 600 or 1200 mg steps, as tolerated. In inpatient settings, felbamate can be titrated over a few days, especially if the other antiepileptic drugs have been or are eliminated or reduced. In the clinical environment, the doses of other antiepileptic drugs should be reduced, generally by 20–33% upon initiation, and by further reductions as felbamate dose is increased. Most side-effects can be eliminated by reducing doses of concomitant antiepileptic drugs, especially if the goal is to attain monotherapy with felbamate. Some patients have tolerated doses as high as 7200 mg per day as monotherapy.

In children, recommended starting doses have been 15 mg/kg per day with weekly incremental increases to 45 mg/kg per day. Again, concomitant antiepileptic drugs should be reduced by 20% or more upon initiation and reduced further on the basis of symptoms and blood levels. Doses for children usually need to be higher than those for adults, and doses of up to 80 mg/kg have been used.

Felbamate is available as 400 mg tablets useful for children; 600 mg tablets and 600 mg/5 mL suspension.

Gabapentin

Primary indications	Adjunctive therapy or monotherapy in adults with partial or secondarily generalized epilepsy
Usual preparations	Capsules: 100, 300, 400 mg
Usual dosages	Initial: 300 mg per day. Maintenance: 900–3600 mg per day
Dosage intervals	2–3 times per day
Significant drug interactions	None
Serum level monitoring	Not useful
Target range	–
Common/important side-effects	Drowsiness, dizziness, seizure exacerbation, ataxia, headache, tremor, diplopia, nausea, vomiting, rhinitis
Main advantages	Lack of side-effects (especially at low doses) and good pharmacokinetic profile
Main disadvantages	Lack of therapeutic effect in severe cases. Seizure exacerbation
Mechanisms of action	Not known. Possible action on calcium channels
Oral bioavailability	<60%
Time to peak levels	2–4 h
Metabolism and excretion	Renal excretion without metabolism
Volume of distribution	0.9 L/kg
Elimination half-life	5–9 h
Plasma clearance	0.120–0.130 L/kg/h
Protein binding	Nil
Active metabolites	Nil
Comment	Novel anticonvulsant of uncertain relative efficacy, but easy to use and few side-effects

Gabapentin was a drug developed to have a close structural relationship to gamma-aminobutyric acid (GABA). Although designed as a GABA agonist, clinical and experimental evidence showed that gabapentin has in fact little or no action at the GABA receptor. It was first studied as an antispasmodic, and also has effectiveness as an analgesic. Early clinical trials into its antispastic action proved disappointing and attention then turned to its antiepileptic action. It is now licensed widely in the UK, USA, Europe and other countries as an antiepileptic, although most of its use is currently unlicensed as an analgesic in certain pain syndromes.

PHYSICAL AND CHEMICAL CHARACTERISTICS

Gabapentin is a highly soluble crystalline substance, with a pKa of 3.7 and 10.7. It is chemically very similar to GABA.

Mode of action

The mode of action of gabapentin is uncertain. It appears to bind to a calcium channel receptor in the cerebral neocortex and hippocampus. In experimental models it has a profile of action which differentiates it from other antiepileptics.

PHARMACOKINETICS

The drug has a generally trouble-free kinetic profile; the main difficulty relates to its variable absorption.

Absorption and distribution

Gabapentin's bioavailability is less than 60% and, furthermore, is quite variable particularly at higher doses, where absorption can be significantly reduced. It is actively transported across the gut wall by an L-amino acid transporter. What few data there are suggests that age has little effect on absorption nor does food. Because absorption is incomplete and relies on an active transport system, caution should be exercised when gabapentin is used in those clinical circumstances in which absorption might be expected to be compromised. The drug readily crosses the blood–brain barrier and the plasma : cerebrospinal fluid concentration ratio is approximately 0.1. Peak serum levels are achieved within 2–4 h of oral dosage. The volume of distribution in adults is about 50 L at steady state. Gabapentin is not bound to plasma proteins at all.

Biotransformation and elimination

The drug is not metabolized and is entirely excreted in an unchanged form. This lack of hepatic metabolism is a great advantage, and there are no pharmacokinetic drug interactions. The drug does not induce hepatic enzyme systems. The renal clearance is 120–130 mL/min and is linearly correlated with creatinine clearance. There is potential for interaction at renal sites (e.g. with felbamate) but there are no specific studies of this point. There is a linear relationship between dose and 2 h post-dose concentration in volunteers, but this relationship has not been studied in patients in normal clinical practice. The elimination half-life of the drug is only 5–9 h, and because of this twice or three times daily dosage is usually recommended. Steady-state levels are achieved within a few days, and the half-life does not change on chronic administration nor is it influenced by co-medication. The serum levels of gabapentin are not routinely measured and there are few data on the correlation between serum level and effectiveness.

SIDE-EFFECTS

In the early double-blind studies, 44% of patients reported adverse effects on gabapentin 900 mg. Similar levels of side-effects were recorded in later studies on 1200 mg. In a US study of patients taking 1800 mg per day, somnolence was recorded in 36%, dizziness in 24%, ataxia in 26%, nystagmus in 17%, headache in 9%, tremor in 15%, fatigue in 11%, diplopia in 11%, rhinitis in 11% and nausea or vomiting in 6%. Most of these effects were mild (Table 4.6).

There have been very few potentially serious side-effects reported. The incidence of rash is 0.5% and neutropenia 0.2%. Electroencephalogram changes and/or angina were found in 0.05%. No cases of hepatotoxicity have been recorded. There are no consistent changes in any other clinical or laboratory measure, and no serious idiosyncratic or hypersensitivity reactions. Pancreatic carcinoma was reported in the animal toxicology, but there have been no clinical reports of pancreatic disease. At the time of writing, no cases of visual field constriction have been reported.

ANTIEPILEPTIC EFFECT

Gabapentin has been studied in a variety of open and double-blind investigations. A large multicentre study carried out in the UK randomized patients to add-on therapy with either gabapentin 1200 mg or placebo. Twenty-eight per cent of the patients given gabapentin showed a 50% or more reduction in partial seizures compared with 9.8% of placebo. In a similar study from the USA, patients were randomized to 600, 1200 or 1800 mg of gabapentin or placebo. The percentage of patients who had a 50% or more reduction in seizures ranged from 18 to 26% with gabapentin and 8% on placebo. Similar findings were obtained from an international study of 272 patients, which showed responder rates of 21% on 900 mg and 28% on 1200 mg. Gabapentin has been used in childhood epilepsy, with rather mixed results. A double-blind study in children with partial epilepsy showed a responder rate of 17% on gabapentin

Table 4.6 Frequency of adverse events reported in controlled clinical trials with the addition of either gabapentin or placebo (all side-effects occurring more frequently in gabapentin and in more than 5% of cases).

	Gabapentin (%)	Placebo (%)
Somnolence	20	9
Dizziness	18	7
Ataxia	13	6
Fatigue	11	5
Tremor	7	3
Diplopia	6	2

vs. 7% on placebo. A pair of double-blind placebo controlled studies in childhood absence showed no effect. These trials showed that the drug has an antiepileptic action. However, the number of responders is disappointingly low and, at the dosage tested, the drug seems rather weak. Large postmarketing open studies have been carried out. In the STEPS trial, over 2000 persons were entered into the study of gabapentin as adjunctive therapy. A responder rate of 45% was found at doses over 1800 mg/day compared to 18% at lower doses. A similarly better response to high doses (3600–4800 mg/day) has been consistently found in other postmarketing studies, and since licensing, it has become customary to prescribe much higher doses. Although the drug has not been subjected to double-blind controlled trials at these higher doses, there is a clinical impression of greater effectiveness at higher doses, at least in some patients. The side-effects at higher doses are also more prominent.

CLINICAL USE IN EPILEPSY

Gabapentin is a useful drug in the treatment of partial and secondarily generalized tonic–clonic seizures. It has an excellent pharmacokinetic profile and its lack of protein binding, its lack of metabolism and its lack of drug interactions are attractive properties. It is particularly useful in renal or hepatic disease or for patients on complicated drug regimens. It is relatively well tolerated although it does have some side-effects, particularly at higher doses, but these are usually relatively minor. Certainly, severe behavioural or psychiatric disturbances are not commonly reported nor idiosyncratic or serious systemic side-effects. There are, however, disadvantages. The drug appears to have only a rather modest efficacy, particularly at lower doses, and it is unusual for patients with severe epilepsy to derive much benefit. Furthermore, a substantial minority of patients treated with gabapentin suffer a worsening rather than a lessening of seizure frequency and occasionally this deterioration can be marked. Also, the drug is ineffective in most generalized seizure disorders and in myoclonus. Its absorption is also erratic, particularly at higher doses.

Gabapentin is available as 300 or 400 mg capsules and it is common practice to titrate this dose up at weekly intervals to a maximum of 3200 mg per day. Although all the trials used three times daily dosage, a twice daily regimen seems equally effective. In routine practice withdrawal can be carried out at weekly decremental rates of 400 mg.

Lamotrigine

Primary indications	Adjunctive or monotherapy in partial and generalized epilepsy. Also in Lennox–Gastaut syndrome
Usual preparations	Tablets: 25, 50, 100, 200 mg; chewtabs: 5, 25, 100 mg
Usual dosages	Initial: 12.5–25 mg per day. Maintenance: 100–200 mg (monotherapy or comedication with valproate); 200–400 mg (comedication with enzyme-inducing drugs)
Dosage intervals	2 times per day
Significant drug interactions	Autoinduction. Lamotrigine levels are lowered by phenytoin, carbamazepine, phenobarbital and other enzyme-inducing drugs. Lamotrigine levels increased by sodium valproate
Serum level monitoring	Value not established
Target range	4–60 µmol/L
Common/important side-effects	Rash (sometimes severe), headache, blood dyscrasia, ataxia, asthenia, diplopia, nausea, vomiting, dizziness, somnolence, insomnia, depression, psychosis, tremor, hypersensitivity reactions
Main advantages	Effective and well tolerated
Main disadvantages	High instance of rash (occasionally severe) and other side-effects
Mechanisms of action	Blockage of voltage-dependent sodium conductance
Oral bioavailability	<100%
Time to peak levels	1–3 h
Metabolism and excretion	Hepatic glucuronidation (without phase I reaction)
Volume of distribution	0.9–1.3 L/kg
Elimination half-life	29 h (monotherapy approx.); 15 h (enzyme-inducing comedication); 60 h (valproate comedication)
Plasma clearance	0.044–0.084 L/kg/h (but variable)
Protein binding	55%
Active metabolites	Nil
Comment	A useful medication in a wide variety of epilepsies

The recent history of epilepsy treatment has seen many drugs developed on the basis of incorrect mechanistic premises, and lamotrigine is a good example. In the 1960s, it was postulated—wrongly—that the antiepileptic effects of phenytoin and phenobarbital could be mediated through their antifolate properties. Lamotrigine was then developed, but found to have weak antifolate effects only; a pronounced antiepi-

leptic effect was, however, noted. By 1998, over 1.3 million patients worldwide had received lamotrigine.

PHYSICAL AND CHEMICAL CHARACTERISTICS

The drug is a triazine compound unrelated chemically to any other antiepileptic. It is poorly soluble in water or in ethanol.

Mode of action

In its short life a whole range of mechanisms of action have been postulated, only to be subsequently discounted. It seems now that the most likely major antiepileptic action is by the stabilization of neuronal membranes by blocking voltage-dependent sodium channel conductance. In this sense its action is similar to that of carbamazepine or phenytoin. Whether or not the drug has any more direct neurotransmitter action is uncertain, although antifolate, antiglutamate and antiaspartate actions have been suggested. In experimental seizure models, lamotrigine has a rather similar profile of action to that of phenytoin and carbamazepine.

PHARMACOKINETICS

Absorption and distribution

The drug is well absorbed orally with a bioavailability approaching 100%. Peak concentrations occur within 1–3 h after dosage. Linear relationship between dose and concentration has been observed in the dosage ranges normally used clinically but there is a second lamotrigine peak after oral administration, attributed to intestinal reabsorption of the drug sequestered in the stomach. Lamotrigine is 55% bound to plasma proteins and has a volume of distribution of between 0.9 and 1.3 L/kg body weight.

Metabolism and elimination

The drug undergoes extensive metabolism in the liver, largely to the inert glucuronide conjugate, most of which is renally excreted. A small percentage can be recovered unchanged in the urine. The elimination half-life of lamotrigine in healthy volunteers ranges from 24 to 41 h. Elderly patients require lower doses than younger persons.

Drug interactions

Lamotrigine does not induce or inhibit hepatic enzymes and consequently will not influence the metabolism of other lipid-soluble drugs, including the contraceptive pill and warfarin.

Unfortunately, the concomitant administration of other antiepileptic drugs does have a profound effect on the metabolism of lamotrigine. Enzyme inducers reduce half-life from a mean of 29 h to 15 h. Sodium valproate lengthens the half-life, by mechanisms which are unclear, to 60 h or more. In chil-

dren, the half-life falls to less than 10 h in those comedicated with enzyme-inducing antiepileptics and is between 15 and 27 h in monotherapy or when valproate is given with inducers, and 44–94 h in valproate monotherapy. As a result of these major interactions, lamotrigine dosage needs to be modified according to concomitant therapy and, conversely, when the dosage of comedication is altered, lamotrigine levels will also change.

SIDE-EFFECTS

The most common side-effects of lamotrigine are headache, nausea and vomiting, diplopia, dizziness, ataxia and tremor. Sedation can occur but is usually not prominent, and there are also reports of aggression, irritability, agitation, confusion, hallucinations and psychoses. In general, the side-effects are not a particular problem, although in individual patients severe reactions do occur. Diplopia and unsteadiness seem particularly common when the drug is used in combination with carbamazepine and whether this is a pharmacodynamic or pharmacokinetic interaction is not known. Certainly, lowering either the carbamazepine or the lamotrigine dosage in this situation will usually reverse the visual disturbance.

Immunologically related adverse effects occur with lamotrigine (Table 4.7). Rash is the most common, with an incidence of up to 5%. Usually the rash is mild, but occasionally a severe rash amounting to a Stevens–Johnson syndrome or bullous erythema multiforme develops, which can be severe and debilitating and has been fatal. There can be an accompanying systemic illness with fever, arthralgia, lymphadenopathy and eosinophilia. A small number of deaths have been reported following disseminated intravascular coagulation and multiorgan failure. The severe rash seems to be more common in children. The incidence of rash seemed also to be higher when valproate is used as comedication, and this may reflect the higher levels of lamotrigine in patients comedicated with valproate. Initiating the drug at very low doses and incrementing the dose very slowly is said to lower the incidence of rash.

ANTIEPILEPTIC EFFECT

There have been 10 placebo-controlled trials exploring the use of lamotrigine as add-on therapy in refractory epilepsy. Nine of the 10 demonstrated lamotrigine to be significantly better than placebo,

Table 4.7 The adverse events reported in the randomized placebo controlled trials comparing lamotrigine and placebo carried out in the US. (Only those adverse events occurring at a frequency of 3% or more are included.)

| Side-effects | Number (%) of patients reporting side-effects | |
	Lamotrigine (*n* = 711)	Placebo (*n* = 419)
Dizziness	38	13
Headache	29	19
Diplopia	28	7
Ataxia	22	6
Nausea	19	10
Blurred vision	16	5
Rhinitis	14	9
Somnolence	14	7
Pharyngitis	10	9
Rash	10	5
Vomiting	9	4
Cough	8	6
Flu syndrome	7	6
Fever	6	4
Diarrhoea	6	4
In-coordination	6	2
Insomnia	6	2
Abdominal pain	5	4
Dyspepsia	5	2
Depression	4	3
Anxiety	4	3
Tremor	4	1
Irritability	3	2
Pruritis	3	2
Constipation	3	2
Vision abnormality	3	1
Speech disorder	3	0
(Female patients only)	(*n* = 365)	(*n* = 207)
Dysmenorrhea	7	6
Vaginitis	4	1

with a total decrease in seizures on lamotrigine of between 17 and 59%, and a responder rate between 7 and 17%. Most trials showed a seizure reduction of approximately 25–30%, and a 20–30% responder rate. There is also strong anecdotal, and limited clinical trial, evidence that lamotrigine is helpful in generalized seizures, including primary generalized tonic–clonic seizures, typical and atypical absence, atonic and myoclonic seizures. The drug can have a marked effect on seizures in the Lennox–Gastaut syndrome. There is now extensive experience with lamotrigine in children, and in monotherapy. In open studies in previously treated or untreated patients with epilepsy, monotherapy with lamotrigine has been shown to be of comparable efficacy to that with carbamazepine, phenytoin and valproate.

CLINICAL USE IN EPILEPSY

The drug is available in 25, 50, 100 and 200 mg tab-lets. Dispersible formulations of 5, 25 and 100 mg tablets are also available. There is no parenteral preparation. The drug is usually prescribed on a twice daily basis, although a single daily dose can be used if the drug is taken with valproate alone.

A low slow introduction regimen will reduce the likelihood of rash. The starting dose and titration rate will depend on comedication. In adults taking valproate alone, lamotrigine should be given at a dose of 25 mg on alternate days for 2 weeks increasing to 25 mg daily for a further 2 weeks and thereafter the dose can be increased on clinical criteria to an average of 100 or 200 mg twice a day as a maintenance dose. Patients comedicated with enzyme-inducing drugs should start on 25 mg per day increasing after 2 weeks to 25 or 50 mg twice a day, with further 2 weekly increments to an average maintenance dose of 200–400 mg taken twice a day. In monotherapy, the starting dose of 25 mg per day is advised, increasing to 50 mg per day for 2 weeks and then with further 2 weekly increments of 50 or 100 mg per day to a total dose of 200 mg per day.

For children aged between 2–12 years, recommended doses depend considerably on comedication. For those comedicated with valproate, the following dose schedules are recommended: for the first 2 weeks, 0.15 mg/kg, for weeks 3 and 4, 0.3 mg/kg, and then 0.3 mg/kg increments every 1–2 weeks to achieve a maintenance dose of 1–5 mg/kg. For those comedicated with enzyme inducing drugs (e.g. phenytoin, carbamazepine, phenobarbital, primidone), the following regime is recommended: the first two weeks, 0.6 mg/kg, for weeks 3 and 4, 1.2 mg/kg, and then 1.2 mg/kg increments every 1–2 weeks to achieve a maintenance dose of 5–15 mg/kg.

The drug is usually given twice a day, although where the total dose is less than 50 mg (100 mg or less in conjunction with valproate), it can be taken once a day. The monotherapy dose for children is initially 0.5 mg/kg per day rising to 1 mg/kg after 2 weeks with a maintenance dose ranging between 2 and 8 mg/kg.

The drug is useful as a second-line treatment for primary generalized epilepsy or partial and secondarily generalized seizures. It has the advantage of being licensed also for monotherapy, and is generally well tolerated. If a rash develops, the drug should be stopped immediately and it seems sensible to avoid using the drug in patients with severe hepatic impairment. Although its plasma level can be measured, and a therapeutic range has been postulated, there has been no significant relationship found between serum concentrations and anticonvulsant effect. Routine measurement of blood levels is therefore unnecessary.

Levetiracetam

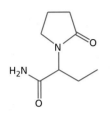

Primary indications	Adjunctive therapy in partial with or without secondarily generalized seizures
Usual preparations	Tablets: 250, 500, 750, 1000 mg
Usual dosages	Initial: 1000 mg per day. Maintenance: 1000–3000 mg per day
Dosage intervals	2 times per day
Significant drug interactions	None
Serum level monitoring	Value not established
Target range	–
Common/important side-effects	Somnolence, asthenia, infection, dizziness, headache
Main advantages	A recently licensed drug which, on the basis of clinical trial evidence, is well-tolerated and highly effective
Main disadvantages	Limited experience in routine clinical practice, as it is recently licensed
Mechanism of action	Not known
Oral bioavailability	<100%
Time to peak levels	0.6–1.3 h
Metabolism and excretion	Partially hydrolysed in the blood to inactive compound
Volume of distribution	0.5–0.7 L/kg
Elimination half-life	6–8 h
Plasma clearance	0.6 mL/min/kg
Protein binding	Nil
Active metabolites	Nil
Comment	A novel antiepileptic drug with promise in the therapy of partial-onset seizures (with or without secondarily generalization)

Levetiracetam (ucb-L059) is a novel antiepileptic drug, developed by UCB. It is an S-enantiomer pyrrolidone derivative. It was first investigated in the 1980s as a drug with cognitive enhancing and anxiolytic effects. More than 1500 patients were included in these early studies, the majority receiving doses ranging from 250 to 1000 mg per day, but the findings in these indications were inconclusive. Pharmacodynamic studies were then initiated in epilepsy, with excellent results, and clinical trials of the drug as adjunctive therapy in the treatment of partial-onset seizures began in 1991. These early studies showed a strong antiepileptic potential which has been confirmed in subsequent investigations. It is a powerful antiepileptic compound which shows promise.

PHYSICAL AND CHEMICAL CHARACTERISTICS

Early studies in other indications used the racemic mixture, etiracetam. Levetiracetam is the S-enantiomer of etiracetam (the R-enantiomer being an inactive substance in models of epilepsy). Levetiracetam provides potent protection in a broad range of animal models of epilepsy in a pattern which is distinctive and not shared by the other commonly used antiepileptic drugs. Furthermore, its effects on kindling suggest potential antiepileptogenic properties. The mode of action of levetiracetam is unknown, and its cerebral binding is to a selective stereospecific site.

PHARMACOKINETICS

Absorption and distribution

Levetiracetam is rapidly absorbed following oral administration. The peak concentration is reached at about 0.6–1.3 h after ingestion and oral bioavailability approaches 100%. The speed of absorption is slowed by food, but not its extent. There is no protein binding. The volume of distribution is approximately 0.5–0.7 L/kg. Preclinical studies indicated that levetiracetam crossed the placenta and that fetal concentrations were similar to maternal levels.

Metabolism and elimination

The major metabolic pathway is to an acidic compound, ucb-L057, by hydrolysis of the acetamide group. This metabolic pathway does not involve the enzymes of the cytochrome P450 system, but metabolism occurs in a number of different tissues and in blood but not plasma. The half-life of levetiracetam in young healthy people ranges between 6 and 8 h and does not vary either with dose within the usual dosage ranges, with different routes of administration or after multiple dosage. The principal metabolite (ucb-L057) is inactive. Levetiracetam and its metabolites are excreted renally, with cumulative urinary excretion of unchanged levetiracetam and of ucb-L057 of 66 and 24%, respectively, after 48 h. The renal clearance of levetiracetam is about 0.6 mL/min/kg. Renal elimination is proportional to the renal clearance, and the half-life increases in renal insufficiency and in situations where renal function can be impaired. The half-life of levetiracetam is increased from 7.6 h in the control group to 24.1 h in severely impaired renal patients. Both the drug and its principal metabolite are removed from the plasma during haemodialysis. In severe hepatic impairment, the half-life and the exposure to both levetiracetam and ucb-L057 were increased, but this is probably a result of coexistent renal disease, and hepatic impairment *per se* does not seem to affect the kinetics of the drug. The half-life in children (6–12 years of age) is about 6 h, the clearance 1.43 mL/min/kg and the C_{max} about 30% lower than in adults. In elderly persons, the half-life increases to 10–11 h, because of the decrease in renal function.

No significant drug interactions have been identified with other antiepileptic drugs, with the exception of inconsistent changes in phenytoin level in some cases where the phenytoin level is close to saturation levels. No clinically significant drug interactions have been observed in interaction studies with the oral contraceptive, warfarin or digoxin. *In vitro* studies of levetiracetam and ucb-L057 with the major human microsomal enzymes have failed to show any inhibition, even at high concentrations.

SIDE-EFFECTS

Pooled safety data are available on 1393 adult epilepsy patients and 1559 non-epilepsy patients. The total exposure in all studies was about 2500 patient-years, and in the placebo-controlled epilepsy studies in 672 patients was over 278 patient-years. These data show that levetiracetam is exceptionally well tolerated. In the placebo-controlled studies, the only adverse events recorded at a frequency above 3% are shown in Table 4.8. Significant differences between drug and placebo were noted only for somnolence, asthenia, infection and dizziness. The incidence of all three central nervous system-related adverse events is higher in the patients treated with either 2000 or 3000 mg compared to 1000 mg. The complaints of 'infection' seemed usually related to upper respiratory tract symptoms. In none of the patients was the drug discontinued and it was not associated with changes in white blood cell count. Most of the adverse events

Adverse events	Levetiracetam (*n* = 672) Percentage of patients	Placebo (*n* = 351) Percentage of patients
Dizziness	9.2	4.3
Infection	13.2	7.4
Asthenia	14.1	9.7
Somnolence	14.9	9.7

Table 4.8 Adverse events occurring in at least 3% of patients and with a difference in incidence between the levetiracetam group and the placebo group of at least 3%, in four placebo-controlled add-on studies in epilepsy.

were mild, and in Table 4.9 those side-effects leading to withdrawal of treatment, or dose reduction, are listed. Few patients withdrew from the studies because of adverse events and there were few differences between withdrawal in the treatment and placebo arms (Table 4.9). No patient withdrew because of infection. Overall, 58 (8.6%) of 672 levetiracetam-treated patients in the controlled trials had at least one serious adverse event compared to 25 (7.2%) of 351 placebo-treated patients. These are reassuring findings. Furthermore, the results from the other studies of the drug are very similar. There have been no serious acute idiosyncratic reactions recorded, and there is no evidence of visual field disturbance. Levetiracetam has no strong tendency to exacerbate seizures, in contrast to this paradoxical effect recorded in some patients with other antiepileptics.

In all epilepsy studies including the phase II and open extension studies, which represent exposure to levetiracetam of approximately 2258 patient-years, the adverse events reported in over 10% of cases were: headache (25%), accidental injury (25%), convulsion (23%), infection (23%), asthenia (22%), somnolence (22%), dizziness (18%), pain (15%), pharyngitis (11%), and a flu-like syndrome (10%). Given the long duration of therapy in these studies, this frequency of symptoms is not exceptional, and in most instances the drug may not have been the causal agent.

ANTIEPILEPTIC EFFECT

In the early phase of development of the drug, there were a number of small pilot studies which demonstrated antiepileptic efficacy. Following these, four placebo-controlled studies of 1023 persons were carried out. Three of these had a similar parallel group randomized placebo-controlled design and were designated the pivotal studies. These studies were performed in a fairly homogeneous group of 904 patients with refractory partial epilepsy. Efficacy was measured over a 12–14-week evaluation period at a daily

dose of between 1000 and 3000 mg of levetiracetam or placebo. The three studies showed a consistent statistically significant reduction in weekly seizure frequency compared to baseline of between 18 and 33% on 1000 mg, 27% on 2000 mg and 37–40% on 3000 mg (compared to a placebo rate of 6–7%). In all three studies, the trend towards a larger improvement was seen in the highest dosage group. The responder rate (defined as the proportion of patients that had a reduction of partial seizure frequency of at least 50%) was between 23 and 33% on 1000 mg, 32% on 2000 mg, and 40–42% on 3000 mg, compared to placebo rates of 10–17%. The difference was statistically significant for each dosage within each individual study when compared to placebo. In one study, 3% of the treated patients were rendered seizure-free on 1000 mg and 8% on 3000 mg, compared to 0% of the placebo group, during the entire 14-week evaluation period. Antiepileptic effect was noted against all types of partial seizures. The 'number needed to treat analysis' of the pivotal trials was 4.5 (95% CI: 3.6–5.9). The proportion of patients entering two long-term extension studies and the 1-year retention rates in these studies were high (>90 and >70%, respectively), indicating the favourable effects of the drug without loss of efficacy. The duration of exposure has been up to 7 years. In the long-term extension studies, concomitant antiepileptic drugs have been withdrawn in some patients and the favourable effect maintained on monotherapy with levetiracetam.

Efficacy as monotherapy was confirmed in a recently completed double-blind placebo-controlled conversion-to-monotherapy study. Out of 69 responders to add-on treatment with 3000 mg levetiracetam, 36 (52%) could be successfully converted to and maintained on monotherapy with the same dose of levetiracetam. During the 3-month monotherapy with levetiracetam, these patients had an average seizure reduction of 74% over their previous monotherapy with a classic antiepileptic drug.

The antiepileptic activity of levetiracetam has also been studied in humans either by measuring photo-

Table 4.9 Adverse events leading to dose reduction or discontinuation. Only events leading to withdrawal in >1% of cases and occurring more frequently on levetiracetam than on placebo are listed.

Adverse events	Levetiracetam (n = 672) Percentage of patients	Placebo (n = 351) Percentage of patients
Rash	0.0	1.4
Headache	1.2	0.6
Asthenia	1.3	0.9
Dizziness	1.6	0.0
Somnolence	4.6	1.7

paroxysmal response in patients with photosensitive epilepsy or by counting the abnormal epileptiform discharges on the EEG, including intracranial recordings in a small number of refractory and presurgical patients. In the photosensitive model, levetiracetam diminished or abolished the photosensitivity in more than 50% of the patients. All six patients receiving either 750 or 1000 mg showed a complete elimination of their photoparoxysmal response, with duration of action of more than 6 h in all patients and more than 24 h in two patients. Two patients with frequent daily myoclonic jerks reported a clear reduction of the jerks after taking levetiracetam. In the EEG model, levetiracetam induced a decrease in the number of frequent epileptiform discharges in most patients. In another open study, six of nine patients with juvenile myoclonic epilepsy refractory to valproate and/or lamotrigine became seizure-free on levetiracetam.

These results suggest that levetiracetam might have a useful effect in the generalized epilepsies, although formal controlled studies have not been carried out.

CLINICAL USE IN EPILEPSY

Levetiracetam is clearly a highly effective new antiepileptic drug with, to date, an excellent safety and tolerability profile. The mode of action of the drug is not known. The pharmacokinetics of the drug are generally felicitous, and there are few if any drug interactions. The efficacy and safety of levetiracetam have been established as add-on therapy for refractory partial onset seizures with or without secondarily generalization and there is also evidence of its value in monotherapy. The drug may also be effective in the generalized epilepsies, and further studies in this area are required. There were remarkably few adverse effects reported in the clinical trials, and few withdrawals from the studies because of adverse effects. The most common side-effects were somnolence, asthenia and dizziness, which were usually mild, dose-dependent and decreased over time. The limited data available suggest also that the effect of the drug is maintained over long-term follow-up.

Levetiracetam is available in 250, 500, 750 and 1000 mg tablets. In the clinical trials, antiepileptic effect was noted at 1000–3000 mg per day, and currently this is the recommended maintenance dosage range. There is some positive experience with patients maintained on long-term treatment increasing to 4000 mg per day. Experience above and below this dose range is slight, however. The starting dose can be 500 mg twice a day, with weekly increments of 500–1000 mg per day to 3000 mg if required. The drug is best given twice a day. In patients with severe renal impairment and in the elderly, clearance is lowered and the dose should be reduced. The value of serum level measurements has not been established.

Levetiracetam is a compound of potential in epilepsy and, if the promise from the clinical trials is maintained in routine clinical practice, it is likely to be an important addition to the current range of antiepileptic drugs.

Oxcarbazepine

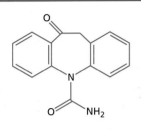

Primary indications	Adjunctive or monotherapy in partial and secondarily generalized seizures
Usual preparations	Tablets: 150, 300, 600 mg
Usual dosages	Initial starting dose: 600 mg per day. Titration rate of 600 mg per week. The usual maintenance dose is 900–2400 mg per day
Dosage intervals	2 times per day
Significant drug	Fewer than with carbamazepine
Serum level monitoring	Value not established
Target range	50–125 µmol/L
Common/important side-effects	Somnolence, headache, dizziness, rash, hyponatraemia, weight gain, alopecia, nausea, gastrointestinal disturbance
Main advantages	Better tolerated and fewer interactions than with carbamazepine
Main disadvantages	25% cross-sensitivity with carbamazepine. Higher incidence of hyponatraemia than with carbamazepine
Mechanisms of action	Sodium-channel blockade. Also affects potassium conductance and modulates high-voltage activated calcium-channel activity
Oral bioavailability	<100%
Time to peak levels	4–5 h
Metabolism and excretion	Hydroxylation then conjugation
Volume of distribution	0.3–0.8 L/kg
Elimination half-life	8–10 h (MHD)
Plasma clearance	–
Protein binding	38%
Active metabolites	MHD
Comment	Close structural similarity to carbamazepine but better tolerated and with fewer drug interactions. Licensed in some countries only, and for use for partial and secondarily generalized seizures

Oxcarbazepine is the 10-keto analogue of carbamazepine, recently developed in an attempt to avoid the autoinduction and potential for drug interactions of carbamazepine. The drug is licensed in over 50 countries, including the UK. Its clinical development had been initially slow and irregular, although since 1991 there have been six new well-controlled studies. The drug is now considered to be a first-line therapy in certain countries. Although it shares many characteristics with carbamazepine, it has a unique molecular structure which endows upon the drug a number of striking advantages. Because of its long usage in some countries, there has been a very wide experience with the drug. At the time of writing, nearly 200 000 patient years of epilepsy treatment has been recorded. The biotransformation of oxcarbazepine does not produce an epoxide metabolite. As it is the epoxide of carbamazepine which is responsible for many of the carbamazepine side-effects, the favourable tolerability of oxcarbazepine may be due to this lack of an epoxide derivative.

PHYSICAL AND CHEMICAL CHARACTERISTICS

Chemically speaking, oxcarbazepine is very similar to carbamazepine. It is a neutral lipophilic compound and, like carbamazepine, insoluble in water. It is not clear whether it is as unstable in humid conditions as carbamazepine.

Mode of action

The pharmacological action of oxcarbazepine is exerted primarily through its 10-monohydroxy metabolite. The mechanism of action in experimental models is identical to that of carbamazepine. It blocks voltage-sensitive sodium channels resulting in stabilization of hyperexcited neural membranes, inhibition of repetitive neuronal firing and inhibition of the spread of discharges. It also increases potassium conductance and modulates high-voltage activated calcium-channel activity.

PHARMACOKINETICS

Absorption and distribution

Oxcarbazepine is absorbed almost completely after oral ingestion, which is an advantage over carbamazepine. Absorption is not affected by food. Oxcarbazepine is rapidly metabolized to the biologically active 10-monohydroxy metabolite (MHD) 10,11-dihydro-10-hydroxy-5H-dibenzol[b,f]azepine-5-carboxamide, and its pharmacological action is caused by this metabolite. MHD is widely distributed to brain and other lipid tissues. The volume of distribution is 0.3–0.8 L/kg. Oxcarbazepine is about 67% and MHD about 38% bound to plasma proteins. Both oxcarbazepine and MHD rapidly cross the blood–brain barrier. There is a linear relationship of dose with both oxcarbazepine and MHD serum levels at the usual clinical dose ranges. Fetal and maternal plasma concentrations of the drug are similar, as judged by the neonatal and maternal levels in one case, and the plasma : breast milk ratio of oxcarbazepine is 0.5.

Biotransformation and excretion

Oxcarbazepine is rapidly and extensively metabolized in the liver, and less than 1% of the drug is excreted unchanged in the urine. The drug is converted first to MHD which is responsible for the antiepileptic action of the compound and this is then conjugated to a glucuronide compound. The hydroxylation is rapid and almost complete, and only trace amounts of oxcarbazepine are found in the blood; in this sense, oxcarbazepine can be considered a prodrug of MHD. Peak serum concentrations of MHD are reached in 4–6 h. It is not subject to epoxidation as is the case with carbamazepine. The lack of epoxidation could be the reason for the better tolerability of the drug, and also renders the drug metabolism immune to impairments in liver function. MHD is excreted by the kidneys and the dose of oxcarbazepine may need to be reduced in the presence of severe renal impairment. The plasma half-life is about 8–10 h, and is not altered by concomitant antiepileptic drug therapy. There is no autoinduction and far fewer interactions with other drugs than with carbamazepine. Most cytochrome p450 enzymes are unaffected by the drug, including CYP1A2, CYP2A6, CYP2C (CYP2D6, CYP2E1, CYP4A9, CYP4A11), although CYP2C19, CYP3A4 and CYP3A5 can be inhibited. Thus, as is the case with carbamazepine, oral contraceptive levels may be lower on comedication with oxcarbazepine (CYP3A family enzymes). Because of this potential interaction, women medicated with oxcarbazepine who require the contraceptive pill should take a formulation with a high (50 μg) oestrogen content. Oxcarbazepine has been shown not to induce the metabolism or interact with warfarin, cimetidine, erythromycin, verapamil or dextropropoxyphene.

SIDE-EFFECTS

The side-effect profile of oxcarbazepine is generally similar in nature to that of carbamazepine, although the frequency and severity of side-effects is less. In the comparative randomized controlled trials in both adults and children, the side-effect profile of the drug was better than with carbamazepine or phenytoin, and oxcarbazepine scored better on patients and physicians rating scales than carbamazepine, valproate or phenytoin. The withdrawal rates from side-effects in the published monotherapy studies of oxcarbazepine, compared to published studies of carbamazepine, valproate and phenytoin, are shown in Table 4.10.

Of the acute adverse effects, skin rash is relatively common (about 5% of all patients) and was the main reason for discontinuation of the drug in the

Table 4.10 Withdrawals due to adverse events from published monotherapy trials.

Adverse event	Oxcarbazepine (n = 482) % (n)	Carbamazepine (n = 100) % (n)	Valproate (n = 121) % (n)	Phenytoin (n = 240) % (n)
Allergy	3.1 (16)	16 (16)		5.8 (14)
Alopecia		2 (2)	3.3 (4)	
Diarrhoea		2 (2)		
Dizziness	0.6 (3)			
Drowsiness/sedation/fatigue	0.6 (3)	3 (3)		0.42 (1)
Gum hyperplasia/hirsutism				5.8 (15)
Nausea	0.2 (1)		1.6 (2)	
Pregnancy	0.4 (2)		1.6 (2)	
Other*	2.2 (10)†	4 (4)‡	1.6 (2)§	
Total discontinuations	7.3 (35)	28 (28)	8.3 (10)	15.5 (30)

*Other refers to all adverse events with only one patient experience.

†Includes 1 patient on methotrexate with toxic megacolon and reversible bone marrow suppression, 1 patient with raised intracranial pressure (an astrocytoma was diagnosed after enrolment), 2 pregnancies, 1 suicide attempt, and 1 report each of abdominal pain, psychosis, tongue ulceration, and psychic lability.

‡Includes 1 report each of abnormal vision, headache, leucopenia, raised liver parameters.

§Includes 1 report each of embolism and abdominal pain.

comparative monotherapy studies. The rash is similar to that caused by carbamazepine, although cross-reactivity with carbamazepine is present in only about 25% of cases, and so oxcarbazepine is a useful drug in patients who show carbamazepine hypersensitivity. Furthermore, the overall risk of idiosyncratic reactions is less than with carbamazepine. In comparative studies, there are less withdrawals because of rash from oxcarbazepine than from carbamazepine. The most common dose-related side-effects are fatigue, headache, dizziness and ataxia, and are very similar to those of carbamazepine. Other side-effects include weight increase, alopecia, nausea and gastrointestinal disturbance. The monotherapy studies of oxcarbazepine have shown better tolerability with fewer side-effects and fewer withdrawals (Table 4.10). Two studies have shown no impairment of cognitive function after 4–12 months of therapy with oxcarbazepine. Oxcarbazepine, like carbamazepine, results in hyponatraemia because of an alteration of regulation of antidiuretic hormone. The effect seems to be greater with oxcarbazepine (in about 20% of patients, the serum sodium falls to below 135 µmol/L) but the hyponatraemia is usually asymptomatic and mild, and not of clinical importance. In the regulatory data-

base, the incidence of marked hyponatraemia (below 125 mmol/L) was only 2.7%, and only 0.4% of patients recorded two consecutive measurements of levels below 125 mmol/L. There is no need to monitor the sodium levels regularly, unless there are special risks (e.g. in patients taking diuretics or in the elderly). Low sodium levels are reversed by lowering the dose of oxcarbazepine or by fluid restriction. It is sensible for patients taking oxcarbazepine to avoid large fluid loads. Other chronic side-effects are slight. As oxcarbazepine results in less liver enzyme induction than carbamazepine, it has fewer effects on thyroid or sex hormones, and cholesterol levels are lower. There have been no comparisons of the tolerability of oxcarbazepine and slow-release carbamazepine. As the slow-release formulation of carbamazepine is so well tolerated, this comparison would be of interest.

ANTIEPILEPTIC EFFECT

Oxcarbazepine has been subjected to four randomized double-blind trials in monotherapy, including one short-term study of patients being evaluated for epilepsy surgery, one study in new patients and two monotherapy substitution studies in refractory cases. All four studies demonstrated that high dosage of the drug was either superior to placebo or to low dosage. Two randomized double-blind add-on studies have also been carried out in refractory patients with partial seizures. Superiority of oxcarbazepine over placebo was demonstrated in both. In the add-on trials, the medium reduction in partial seizure frequency was between 26.4% (600 mg per day) and 50% (2400 mg per day). Postmarketing data includes a report of a large retrospective analysis of 10 years experience with oxcarbazepine in 947 patients. Eighty-two per cent substituted oxcarbazepine for other drugs and it was given in monotherapy in 63%. In different seizure types, between 32 and 48% showed a decrease in seizure frequency. In a study substituting carbamazepine with oxcarbazepine, 32% of patients experienced a >50% reduction in seizures and 79% showed improved tolerability. In a variety of monotherapy studies in patients with established epilepsy and in newly diagnosed epilepsy, oxcarbazepine was found to have similar efficacy to carbamazepine, phenytoin and valproate. A therapeutic range of MHD of 50–125 μmol/L has been suggested. Recent randomized controlled studies show a linear dose–response relationship in both partial and secondarily generalized seizures in children and adults.

CLINICAL USE IN EPILEPSY

The indications for oxcarbazepine are similar to those of carbamazepine. Its efficacy is similar to that of other first-line drugs, and it is generally well tolerated. It has a particular use in patients requiring carbamazepine who have proven hypersensitivity, or who are intolerant to the older drug. There is also evidence, however, that oxcarbazepine can be added to carbamazepine, and that the combination has additive effects. It has less enzyme-inducing effects than many other antiepileptic drugs, including carbamazepine, and fewer interactions with other drugs would be expected. If the drug is being substituted for carbamazepine, care is needed, as the removal of the carbamazepine enzyme-inducing effects could alter levels of the concomitant medication. Oxcarbazepine does, however, interact with the contraceptive pill, and low-dose oestrogen contraceptives should not be used. It is said that when carbamazepine is to be substituted by oxcarbazepine that the substitution can be made abruptly, at a carbamazepine : oxcarbazepine dose ratio of 200 : 300, without the need for up-titration of the oxcarbazepine or down-titration of the carbamazepine. The most common chronic effect is hyponatraemia, but this is usually mild and of no clinical significance, and need not be routinely monitored. The hyponatraemia is a result of a marked antidiuretic effect, and the consumption of large fluid volumes, including large quantities of beer, should be discouraged. It is only available orally. It can be introduced more quickly than carbamazepine, started initially at a dose of 10 mg/kg per day in children increasing in 10 mg/kg steps to 30 mg/kg per day. In adults a starting dose of 600 mg per day can be increased weekly in 600 mg increments to a maintenance dose of between 900 and 2400 mg per day in two daily dosage intervals; most patients are on 900–1200 mg/day, and thus a therapeutic dose is reached very quickly after initiation of therapy.

Phenobarbital

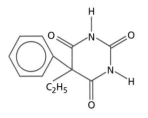

Primary indications	Adjunctive or first-line therapy for partial or generalized seizures (including absence and myoclonus). Also for status epilepticus, Lennox–Gastaut syndrome, childhood epilepsy syndromes, febrile convulsions and neonatal seizures
Usual preparations	Tablets: 15, 30, 50, 60, 100 mg; elixir; 15 mg/5 mL; injection: 200 mg/mL
Usual dosages	Initial: 30 mg per day. Maintenance: 30–180 mg per day (adults); 3–8 mg per day (children); 3–4 mg per day (neonates)
Dosage intervals	1–2 times per day
Significant drug interactions	Phenobarbital has a number of interactions with antiepileptic and other drugs
Serum level monitoring	Useful
Target range	40–170 µmol/L
Common/important side-effects	Sedation, ataxia, dizziness, insomnia, hyperkinesis (children), mood changes (especially depression), aggressiveness, cognitive dysfunction, impotence, reduced libido, folate deficiency, vitamin K and vitamin D deficiency, osteomalacia, Dupuytren's contracture, frozen shoulder, connective tissue abnormalities, rash
Main advantages	Highly effective and cheap antiepileptic drug
Main disadvantages	CNS side-effects
Mechanisms of action	Enhances activity of $GABA_A$ receptor, depresses glutamate excitability, affects sodium, potassium and calcium conductance
Oral bioavailability	80–100%
Time to peak levels	1–3 h (but variable)
Metabolism and excretion	Hepatic oxidation, glucosidation and hydroxylation, then conjugation
Volume of distribution	0.42–0.75 L/kg
Elimination half-life	75–120 h
Plasma clearance	0.006–0.009 L/kg/h
Protein binding	45–60%
Active metabolites	Nil
Comment	Highly effective antiepileptic, now not used as first-line therapy because of potential CNS toxicity, especially in children

Phenobarbital is a remarkable drug. It was introduced into practice in 1912 and is still, in volume terms, the most commonly prescribed antiepileptic drug in the world. It is highly effective, and its introduction opened a new chapter in the history of epilepsy treatment. It is by far the cheapest of the antiepileptic drugs commonly available.

PHYSICAL AND CHEMICAL CHARACTERISTICS

Phenobarbital is a crystalline substance which is a free acid, soluble in non-polar solvents but relatively insoluble in water. The pKa of phenobarbital is 7.2. Changes in pH, common in active epilepsy, can result in substantial shifts of phenobarbital between compartments. The sodium salt is soluble in water, but can be unstable in solution.

Mode of action

Phenobarbital seems to act in a relatively non-selective manner, both limiting the spread of epileptic activity and also elevating the seizure threshold. It has profound effects in a wide variety of experimental models. Its major action is probably via its ability to reduce sodium and potassium conductance. It also reduces calcium influx and has direct actions at the GABA receptor enhancing postsynaptic chloride conductance. It also depresses glutamate excitability and enhances postsynaptic GABAergic inhibition.

PHARMACOKINETICS

Absorption and distribution

Phenobarbital has a bioavailability of 80–100% in adults after oral or intramuscular administration. Peak plasma concentrations occur 1–3 h after oral administration, but can be significantly delayed in patients with poor circulation or reduced gastrointestinal mobility. After intramuscular administration, peak serum concentrations occur within 4 h, and peak plasma concentrations are similar to that after oral administration. Absorption is slowed by the presence of food, and the presence of ethanol in the stomach or the blood can increase the rate of phenobarbital absorption. Absorption occurs mostly in the small intestine because of its larger surface area and longer intraluminal dwell time, and disease at this site can markedly reduce absorption. The apparent volume of distribution has been found to be in the range between 0.42 and 0.75 L/kg after oral administration and 0.54 L/kg after intravenous administration. The distribution of phenobarbital is very sensitive to variations in the plasma pH and acidosis results in an increase of the transfer of phenobarbital from plasma into tissue. This is of potential importance in the treatment of status epilepticus for instance. Following intravenous administration, phenobarbital first distributes rapidly to highly vascular organs, such as liver, kidney and heart, but not into the brain and then, in the second phase, achieves a fairly uniform distribution throughout the body. Phenobarbital penetration into the brain has been reported to occur 12–60 min after intravenous administration, but in status epilepticus, because of local acidosis and increased blood flow, the uptake of phenobarbital is much faster. In physiological conditions, phenobarbital is 45–60% bound to plasma protein. Binding in newborns is lower (35–45%). The concentration of phenobarbital in cerebrospinal fluid in adults is about 50% of that in plasma, and correlates well with the unbound phenobarbital plasma concentrations. Maternally derived phenobarbital serum concentrations in neonates is similar to those in the mother. Breast milk concentrations are about 40% of those in the serum.

Metabolism and elimination

Phenobarbital has the longest half-life of any of the commonly used antiepileptic drugs, with an average half-life found in various studies of between 75 and 120 h. Its elimination can be further reduced when the urine has acidified, and by age and genetic factors, nutritional status and drug interactions. Phenobarbital half-life is longer in infants, typically 110 h, although ranges up to 400 h have been reported and rapid changes occur in the first weeks of life. Infants also eliminate maternally derived phenobarbital with a similar half-life. By the time the child is 6 months, however, the half-life has fallen to 21–75 h. Phenobarbital is subject to extensive biotransformation in the liver. p-hydroxyphenobarbital is the major metabolite of phenobarbital and approximately 8–34% of the daily dose is converted to this metabolite which is then largely excreted as the glucuronide conjugate. N-glucosidation is another important metabolic pathway, inactive at birth but becoming effective only after about 2 weeks of life, and this delay may contribute to the much longer phenobarbital half-life observed in newborns. Other metabolites include an epoxide, a high dihydrodiol catechol and methylcatechol derivative, but these are of less clinical significance. Although phenobarbital is a powerful inducer of hepatic microsomal enzymes, it does not exhibit autoinduction in humans.

The total renal clearance of phenobarbital is very variable but is considerably less than the glomerular filtration rate, indicating extensive resorption. Acidification of the urine increases resorption and a combination of sodium bicarbonate administration to increase plasma pH in urine coupled by forced diuresis can increase clearance by up to fivefold. There is no enterohepatic recirculation.

Drug interactions

Phenobarbital is involved in a number of drug interactions, the magnitude of which varies greatly from person to person depending on genetic factors and concomitant medication. Phenytoin, valproate, felbamate and dextropropoxyphene inhibit phenobarbital metabolism leading to elevation of phenobarbital levels. Rifampicin is a powerful enzyme inducer and may lower phenobarbital levels. Phenobarbital is a potent inducer of hepatic enzyme activity and increases metabolism of other drugs, such as oestrogen in the oral contraceptive pill, steroids, warfarin, aminophylline and valproate. The conversion of carbamazepine, diazepam and clonazepam is also accelerated by phenobarbital. The effect on phenytoin is complex and not reliably predictable in any individual because of the combined effects of inhibition and induction. A particular pharmacodynamic interaction between phenobarbital and valproate seems to occur in the occasional patient, resulting in profound drowsiness without very large effects on the drug levels of the serum levels of either medication.

SIDE-EFFECTS

The most important side-effects are impairment of cognitive function and alteration of behaviour; the latter is particularly prominent in children. Central nervous system effects include motor slowness, memory disturbance, loss of concentration, sedation and paradoxical hyperkinetic activity in children. To what extent these problems are common is uncertain but it is a clinical impression that in adults, at least, these deficiencies are usually of minor importance.

Sedation, particularly at the initiation of therapy, commonly subsides during chronic therapy. Behavioural changes include depression, irritability and occasional aggressiveness—the latter being said to be particularly common in children or those with cerebral damage. During chronic therapy, other side-effects include nystagmus, ataxia and decreased libido. Elderly patients with organic cerebral disease may also become confused and irritable rather than sedated. Chronic medication is also associated with coarsening of the facial features and a Dupuytren's contracture. Deficiency in vitamin D, leading to osteomalacia and rickets, can occur rarely and can be prevented by administration of supplementary vitamin. Folate deficiency is not uncommon, but is usually mild and asymptomatic. Very occasionally, a megaloblastic anaemia develops requiring folate

supplementation. Idiosyncratic skin reactions occurring in less than 3% of patients are usually mild and transient. Generalized hypersensitivity is very rare, and may include exfoliative dermatitis. An immunologically mediated hepatitis has also been reported. Phenobarbital, like other barbiturates, when used chronically can cause physical dependence and abrupt cessation can lead to withdrawal seizures. Withdrawal seizures can also be a problem in neonates of a mother receiving phenobarbital.

ANTIEPILEPTIC EFFECT

Phenobarbital has been extensively used in a wide variety of epileptic seizure types for many years. Because of its venerable age, the drug has not been subjected to the usual panoply of prelicensing controlled trials, and there are very few controlled data to document the extent of its self-evident effectiveness. In a multicentre double-blind trial comparing the efficacy of four antiepileptic drugs in the treatment of partial and secondarily generalized seizures, however, phenobarbital produced overall seizure control equal to phenytoin or carbamazepine. The proportion of patients with tonic–clonic seizures controlled was similar for all three drugs, but control rates of partial seizures were somewhat lower on phenobarbital than with carbamazepine. Interestingly, phenobarbital was associated with the lowest incidence of motor side-effects, gastrointestinal side-effects or idiosyncratic side-effects. There have been a handful of other open studies confirming the equivalence of effect, and also largely of side-effects, of phenobarbital compared with carbamazepine or valproate. Studies in partial and generalized seizures in children show similar effects, and the drug has been widely used.

In primary generalized epilepsy, phenobarbital is also an effective drug, probably more so than phenytoin or carbamazepine. Although valproate remains the drug of choice for this syndrome, phenobarbital is a useful second-line therapy.

The drug is also effective against other generalized seizure types, including atonic and tonic seizures, although clinical trial evidence of its value in the syndromes is largely lacking.

Serum level measurement of phenobarbital are widely used, and for most patients concentrations between 40 and 170 µmol/L are associated with optimal seizure control. Some patients, however, will experience good seizure control above or below this limit. Although side-effects are usually not too troublesome when levels are maintained in this range, there is a relatively inconsistent relationship between side-effect and level even on a statistical basis. This is possibly because of the tendency for tolerance of the side-effects of phenobarbital to develop over time.

Phenobarbital is also useful in neonatal seizures, in febrile seizures and in status epilepticus.

CLINICAL USE IN EPILEPSY

There is no large pharmaceutical company promoting or marketing phenobarbital and, as a result, its value is underestimated. It has a strikingly low cost and ease of use, which renders phenobarbital an important and valuable antiepileptic drug, especially in the developing world. Its efficacy is not in question, but its general use as a first-line drug is limited by its perceived potential to cause sedation and mental slowness. To what extent this is actually better or worse than other antiepileptics has really not been very clearly established. Nevertheless, its use is now largely confined to second-line therapy in patients intractable to other more modern first-line alternatives. Particular indications are in primary generalized epilepsy where valproate has failed, first-line therapy for neonatal seizures and as second-line therapy for severe secondary generalized seizure disorders. The drug is valuable in status epilepticus.

The drug is available in a large number of formulations and preparations. Tablet sizes include 15, 30, 50, 60 and 100 mg sizes, elixirs (15 mg/5 mL) and injections (200 mg in 1 mL) or propylene glycol and water. In adults, the starting dose of 30–60 mg per day. A dosage interval of once a day (occasionally twice per day for higher doses) is recommended. The dose can be increased in 15 or 30 mg increments to a maintenance dose of between 60 and 240 mg per day, with the most common dose for adults being between 90 and 120 mg per day. Too rapid an initiation of therapy can produce drowsiness which may persist for several weeks, and it is usually better to introduce the drug slowly. Many patients are well controlled on low serum levels and low doses.

In children, the usual starting dose is 3 mg/kg per day with maintenance doses in the range 3–8 mg/kg per day. Twice daily dosage may be necessary in younger children, because of the shorter half-life. The drug is widely used in neonatal seizures where rapid seizure control is needed and intravenous administration is used. Loading doses of 15–20 mg/kg intravenously followed by maintenance dose of 3–4 mg/kg per day are usually used.

The side-effects are more severe in children than in adults—particularly behavioural change and hyperkinetic behaviour—and these effects need to be particularly monitored. In the elderly, paroxysmal agitation and irritability can also occur, as they can also in patients with learning difficulty or cerebral damage. The use of the drug in these patient groups should therefore be circumspect.

Phenytoin

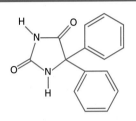

Primary indications	First-line or adjunctive therapy for partial and generalized seizures (excluding myoclonus and absence). Also for status epilepticus, Lennox–Gastaut syndrome and childhood epilepsy syndromes
Usual preparations	Capsules: 25, 50, 100, 200 mg; chewtabs: 50 mg; liquid suspension: 30 mg/5 mL, 125 mg/50 mL; injection: 250 mg/5 mL
Usual dosages	Initial: 100–200 mg per day (adults); 5 mg/kg (children).Maintenance: 100–300 mg per day (adults), higher doses can be used guided by serum level monitoring; 4–8 mg/kg (children)
Dosage intervals	1–2 times per day
Significant drug interactions	Phenytoin has a large number of interactions with antiepileptic and other drugs
Serum level monitoring	Useful
Target range	40–80 μmol/L
Common/important side-effects	Ataxia, dizziness, lethargy, sedation, headaches, dyskinesia, acute encephalopathy, hypersensitivity, rash, fever, blood dyscrasia, gingival hyperplasia, folate deficiency, megaloblastic anaemia, vitamin K deficiency, thyroid dysfunction, decreased immunoglobins, mood changes, depression, coarsened facies, hirsutism, peripheral neuropathy, osteomalacia, hypocalcaemia, hormonal dysfunction, loss of libido, connective-tissue alterations, pseudolymphoma, hepatitis, vasculitis, myopathy, coagulation defects, bone marrow hypoplasia
Main advantages	Highly effective and cheap antiepileptic drug
Main disadvantages	CNS and systemic side-effects
Mechanisms of action	Blockade of sodium channels and action on calcium and chloride conductance and voltage-dependent neurotransmission
Oral bioavailability	95%
Time to peak levels	4–12 h
Metabolism and excretion	Hepatic oxidation and hydroxylation, then conjugation
Volume of distribution	0.5–0.8 L/kg
Elimination half-life	7–42 h (mean, 20 h: dependent on plasma level)
Plasma clearance	0.003–0.02 L/kg/h (dependent on plasma level)
Protein binding	70–95%
Active metabolites	Nil
Comment	Well-established first-line therapy whose use is limited by side-effects

Phenytoin was introduced into clinical practice in 1938; 'a year of jubilee' for epileptics as Merritt and Putnam put it. Since then phenytoin has been a major first-line antiepileptic drug in the treatment of partial and secondarily generalized seizures. When it was introduced, only potassium bromide and phenobarbital showed equal effectiveness, but phenytoin was found to cause less sedation. Although phenobarbital continues to be used, the introduction of phenytoin meant that bromides were, after nearly 100 years of prescription, finally redundant.

PHYSICAL AND CHEMICAL CHARACTERISTICS

Phenytoin is a crystalline powder which is lipid-soluble. It is a weak acid with a pKa of 8.3–9.2 and is relatively insoluble in water at physiological pH but soluble in alkaline solution.

Mode of action
Phenytoin exerts its antiepileptic effect largely by blocking ionic movements in the sodium channel during the depolarization process. It suppresses the build-up of paroxysmal electrical activity, blocks post-tetanic potentiation and prevents spread of epileptic seizures. The drug also has an inhibiting effect on calcium and the sequestration of calcium in nerve terminals thereby inhibiting voltage-dependent neurotransmitter release at the synapse. It also inhibits the action of calmodulin and second messenger systems, although how these contribute to phenytoin's antiepileptic action, if indeed they do, is unclear.

PHARMACOKINETICS

Absorption and distribution
Phenytoin is usually given to patients as a sodium salt. This is a crystalline preparation which is absorbed rather slowly from the gastrointestinal tract. Absorption through the stomach is relatively poor because phenytoin is very insoluble at the pH of gastrointestinal juice. The high pH of the small intestine, however, allows phenytoin to go into solution and absorption occurs. The presence of food alters phenytoin absorption as do diseases of the small bowel. In an average healthy person, the oral bioavailability is about 95%, and the time to peak levels following oral administration is 4–12 h. Any factors which interfere with the dissolution of phenytoin in the gastrointestinal tract will retard or prevent absorption. There is a wide intra- and interindividual variability in absorption, and occasional patients have very unusual patterns for no obvious reason. Pregnancy reduces absorption, occasionally to extreme levels. Neonates absorb the drug poorly and erratically. The difference in formulation of some generic preparations of phenytoin can result in altered absorption, and so it is usually recommended that the same formulation of phenytoin is dispensed—this is particularly important in patients where metabolism is close to saturation levels. Phenytoin can also be given intravenously. Intramuscular phenytoin must not be given, as the drug precipitates in muscle resulting in a profound delay in absorption and sometimes in muscle necrosis. Phenytoin is between 70–95% bound to plasma proteins. Binding is lower in neonates and in the elderly. It is rapidly distributed to body tissues and its volume of distribution is 0.5–0.8 L/kg. The brain : plasma ratio is between 1 and 2. The cerebrospinal fluid levels of phenytoin are equal to the free plasma fraction, as are the salivary levels. The phenytoin breast milk : plasma ratio is about 0.2.

Metabolism and excretion
Phenytoin is extensively metabolized by the hepatic P450 mixed oxidase system (isoform CYP2C9). The first step involves a zero-order kinetic accounting for the non-linear dose : serum level relationship (see below). The para-hydroxylation step is mainly followed by glucuronidation, although there are a range of other minor metabolites. None of the phenytoin metabolites have anticonvulsant activity, and all are excreted via the kidney.

Because the first step in the enzymic degradation of phenytoin is rate limited, the dose : serum level ratio is not linear. As the dose is increased, plasma levels rise linearly initially until the point of enzymic saturation, and then in a much steeper fashion (Fig. 4.4). There is marked interindividual variability. The clearance and half-life of phenytoin therefore both vary considerably within populations, and also depend on the plasma level. At higher plasma concentrations, the half-life is much longer and the clearance much reduced because of saturation of the enzyme systems. The time to steady state will also vary non-linearly with dose—but linearly with plasma level—and up to 28 days may need to elapse before steady state is reached after certain dose changes.

Neonates eliminate phenytoin more slowly and young children more rapidly than adults. In the elderly, metabolism is less rapid than in younger adults.

Total plasma levels of phenytoin fall during pregnancy, especially in the last trimester, although free levels are often relatively maintained. Phenytoin doses need to be reduced in severe hepatic failure. In renal failure, phenytoin levels fall although those of its major metabolite rise. Haemodialysis has little effect on phenytoin plasma concentrations.

Drug interactions

Phenytoin is probably the antiepileptic drug with the most problematic interaction profile. This is partly caused by the saturable kinetics of phenytoin itself, which results in different interaction behaviour at different dose and serum levels. Phenytoin is also highly protein bound and metabolized by hepatic P450 enzymes.

Effect of other antiepileptic drugs on phenytoin levels

Carbamazepine and phenobarbital. There is a complex pattern of interactions between phenytoin and these two drugs. Phenytoin levels can be raised or lowered by carbamazepine or phenobarbital comedication, as both induce and compete for hepatic enzyme metabolism. The overall effect on phenytoin levels is thus variable and unpredictable.

Valproate displaces phenytoin from its protein-binding sites and also inhibits its metabolism. There is a transient rise in free levels but within weeks, as a result of redistribution, free levels return to previous values although total levels may be somewhat lower, and doses should not be increased. When levels are near saturation, through the combination of protein-binding displacement and metabolic inhibition, small dose changes can result in marked rises in phenytoin levels and toxicity. Care needs to be taken therefore particularly when high doses of phenytoin are used, or when pre-interaction serum levels are near the top of the therapeutic range.

Vigabatrin leads to an approximately 25% fall in phenytoin levels in most patients when introduced as comedication. The mechanism of this interaction is not known.

Phenytoin levels are affected by a wide range of other drugs. These are all more marked when phenytoin is close to the top of its therapeutic level. Amiodarone increases serum phenytoin concentrations by as much as 100–200%. Antacids can reduce the bioavailability of phenytoin, although the effect is variable, reflecting the complex effects on phenytoin dissolution, chelation and gastrointestinal motility; doses should be separated by at least 2 h. Cimetidine is a potent inhibitor of phenytoin metabolism and can rapidly cause phenytoin toxicity if phenytoin metabolism is close to saturation. Some nutritional formulas can reduce phenytoin absorption by up to 75%; Isocal and Osmolite are the main culprits, but Ensure apparently does not have a marked effect. Azapropazone, diazoxide, phenylbutazone, salicylate, sulphafurazole, sulphanethoxypyrine and

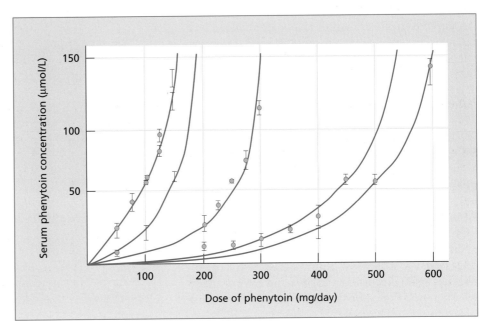

Fig. 4.4 Relationship between serum phenytoin concentration and daily dose in five patients. Each point represents the mean (± SD) of three to eight measurements of serum phenytoin concentration at steady state. The curves were fitted by computer using the Michaelis–Menten equation.

tolbutamide displace phenytoin from its protein-binding sites—in the same way as valproate—and will affect phenytoin dosage only when levels are close to saturation. Isoniazid markedly inhibits phenytoin metabolism, and symptoms of phenytoin intoxication are common within days of the introduction of isoniazid as comedication. The effects are greatest in those individuals who are slow acetylators of isoniazid, who thereby have higher isoniazid levels.

Effect of phenytoin on levels of other drugs

Phenytoin is a potent hepatic enzyme-inducing agent, and this results in a wide range of common and important interactions. The addition of phenytoin as comedication can lower the levels of carbamazepine, ethosuximide, felbamate, lamotrigine, primidone, tiagabine, topiramate and have a variable effect on valproate and phenobarbital levels. At times these effects can have marked clinical consequences. The metabolism of warfarin is inhibited and that of dicoumarol induced and clotting times need to be monitored frequently with both if phenytoin dosage changes are made. Corticosteroid metabolism (including dexamethasone) is induced, and doses may need to be twice normal to obtain the desired therapeutic effects. The levels, and thus effectiveness, of busulfan and possibly other antimitotic agents can also be significantly affected by phenytoin comedication. Theophylline levels can be lowered by as much as 35–75% by phenytoin comedication. Frusemide (furosemide) clearance can be increased by as much as 50%. Cyclosporin clearance is increased by 75%. Serum folate levels are reduced in about 50% of patients receiving phenytoin. Praziquantel levels are reduced by a mean of 75% by phenytoin comedication; this compares to a 10% reduction by carbamazepine, which may therefore be the drug of first choice in treating active cysticercosis. Levels of chloramphenicol and quinidine can be elevated by phenytoin.

SIDE-EFFECTS

Phenytoin has now been in constant use for over 60 years, and this very extensive experience has resulted in a large body of information about adverse effects. This having been said, many patients taking phenytoin suffer no or only minimal side-effects even after decades of therapy; an important point to emphasize when discussing the pros and cons of therapy. Phenytoin side-effects can be divided into acute

dose-related effects, acute idiosyncratic effects and chronic effects.

The acute dose-related effects of phenytoin are usually seen at serum levels above 80 μmol/L, although there is individual variation, and some patients have no side-effects at much higher levels. These effects (phenytoin intoxication) consist of nystagmus, ataxia, dysarthria, motor slowing, lethargy and sedative mental changes. A reversible encephalopathy can occur at high doses, with mental changes, confusion and a paradoxical exacerbation of seizures. Other dose-related symptoms include confusional states, ophthalmoplegia, an acute reversible peripheral neuropathy and involuntary movements including dystonia, orofacial dyskinesia and chorea (Table 4.11).

Idiosyncratic side-effects comprise hypersensitivity and immunologically mediated reactions. Skin rash is the most common, occurring in up to 5% of patients started on phenytoin, and is most common in the first 4 weeks of treatment. Occasionally, the rash is associated with fever, leucopenia and lymphadenopathy. The rash is usually minor, and serious skin reactions (exfoliative dermatitis, Stevens–

Table 4.11 Signs and symptoms in 38 cases of phenytoin hypersensitivity reaction.

Sign or symptom	Percentage of patients
Rash	
Morbilliform or licheniform	66
Erythema multiforme	18
Stevens–Johnson syndrome	13
Total	74
Fever	13
Abnormal liver function tests	29
Lymphoid hyperplasia	24
Eosinophilia	21
Blood dyscrasias	
Leucopenia	16
Thrombocytopenia	5
Anaemia	16
Increased atypical lymphocytes	3
Total	31
Serum sickness	5
Albuminuria	5
Renal failure	3

Johnson syndrome) are reported but are extremely rare. A mild leucopenia is common, but serious agranulocytosis, thrombocytopenia or red cell aplasia, although recorded, are fortunately rare.

Lymph node enlargement is not uncommon. There is controversy about the relationship of phenytoin therapy and malignant lymphoma. Cases of pseudolymphoma have been reported, which resolve when phenytoin therapy is withdrawn. A small number of persisting lymphomas have also been recorded in patients on phenytoin therapy, but it is not clear to what extent this is a chance association. An illness similar to systemic lupus erythematosus has also been reported in patients taking phenytoin. The immunological markers of drug-induced cases differ from those of the idiopathic form. Phenytoin exacerbates myasthenia gravis, and has been recorded to precipitate the condition. Acute hepatitis and hepatic necrosis have been rarely caused by phenytoin, usually in the context of an acute hypersensitivity reaction. A 'serum sickness'-like syndrome of rash, fever, arthralgia and atypical lymphocytes has also been recorded, as has a single case of autoimmune nephritis.

Phenytoin also has chronic effects on a variety of body systems. Usually these are asymptomatic and in most cases of no clinical significance.

Connective tissue effects

Gum hypertrophy occurs in up 20% of adult patients on phenytoin and there is possibly a higher incidence in children. In the past, before the widespread availability of plasma level monitoring, gum hypertrophy was often severe. Nowadays, however, the effects are usually relatively mild because of the avoidance of high phenytoin levels. Gum hypertrophy usually develops within 3 months of commencing phenytoin therapy and will regress within 6 months of discontinuing the drug, and can be reduced by good dental hygiene and periodic gingivectomy. Facial changes including coarsening, enlargement of the lips and nose, hirsutism, acne and pigmentation can result from chronic phenytoin therapy. These effects too have become much less prominent since the introduction of drug level monitoring.

Neurological side-effects

The most common neurological side-effects are the acute dose-related side-effects discussed above, and these reverse when the blood levels of phenytoin are lowered. Animal experimentation suggests that phenytoin can, in addition, cause loss of cerebellar Purkinje cells. Whether or not a chronic phenytoin-induced cerebellar syndrome occurs in clinical prac-

tice is controversial. Other uncommon neurological effects include a reversible neuropathy associated with phenytoin intoxication, and a mild usually asymptomatic sensorimotor neuropathy on chronic therapy. Phenytoin has been reported clinically to cause chronic motor slowing or mental dulling, although rigorous studies have failed to detect any clear-cut effects.

Immunological side-effects

Phenytoin can suppress both humoral and cellular mechanisms. Production of IgA is reduced, and antinuclear antibodies and lymphocytotoxins of the IgM class have been found. However, there is no clear evidence that patients taking phenytoin are more prone to infection, and these immunological effects are largely subclinical. Very rarely, pulmonary fibrosis has occurred in patients taking phenytoin and may be caused by an immune complex disorder.

Haematological side-effects

Mild leucopenia is very common in patients taking phenytoin, and does not require attention unless the neutrophil count falls below $1500/mm^3$. Macrocytosis occurs in up to one-third of patients on chronic therapy, a subnormal folate level in at least half the patients, and low cerebrospinal fluid folate levels in up to 45%. Despite this, less than 1% develop a frank megaloblastic anaemia. The mechanism of the folate deficiency is uncertain, but may reflect impaired absorption. Folate supplementation is not usually required unless the patient develops a megaloblastic anaemia, or in pregnancy. In up to 10% of patients, low serum B_{12} levels are also noted. It has been suggested that the folate deficiency results in depression or cognitive impairment, but the supporting evidence is sparse and inconclusive.

Endocrine side-effects

Phenytoin affects a range of endocrine measurements, but these changes are in most cases of no clinical significance. The drug impairs the absorption of vitamin D and calcium, and increases the hepatic metabolism of vitamin D. Biochemical abnormalities include an elevated plasma alkaline phosphatase and reduced plasma calcium and plasma 2-hydroxycholecalciferol. This can result in loss of bone density and occasionally in frank osteomalacia, especially in institutionalized patients and in Asian immigrants to northern climates—reflecting the contribution of dietary factors and sunlight exposure. There may also be secondary hyperparathyroidism. The metabolic bone disease can lead to repeated fractures, and the osteomalacia sometimes presents with a painful proximal myopathy and may require specific therapy. Asymptomatic patients, however, with biochemical changes only do not require active treatment. Osteomalacia or rickets reverse with appropriate therapy. Phenytoin can displace thyroxine from its plasma globulin binding. This can result in a decrease in total thyroxine levels, but triiodothyronine (T_3) and thyroid-stimulating hormone (TSH) levels are usually normal and the patients are euthyroid. The acute administration of phenytoin can increase adrenocorticotropic hormone (ACTH) and cortisol levels but this reverses on chronic administration. Phenytoin can affect the result of the dexamethasone suppression test. Free testosterone levels are lowered by chronic phenytoin therapy, and follicle-stimulating hormone (FSH), luteinizing hormone (LH) and prolactin levels are raised. Phenytoin treatment in experimental models does not affect fertility, but there is a higher than expected incidence of hyposexuality and sperm abnormalities recorded in patients taking phenytoin.

ANTIEPILEPTIC EFFECT

Phenytoin was introduced for the treatment of partial and tonic–clonic seizures on the basis of open experience (in few patients) and was not subjected to the type of controlled add-on clinical trial required nowadays. In the past decade, blinded controlled comparisons of new drugs with phenytoin, phenobarbital and carbamazepine have been carried out. In none of these were any significant differences in antiepileptic effect between the drugs found. There is consensus therefore that phenytoin is as effective as any other first-line drug in partial and in tonic–clonic seizures especially when secondarily generalized. Dispute exists about its tolerability. Some studies find similar levels of significant side-effects with phenytoin as with other newer drugs, and others higher levels with phenytoin. This is an area where marketing pressures by the manufacturers of the newer drugs interfere with objective scientific assessment, and the picture is confused. If significant side-effects are more common with phenytoin than with its competitors, as seems likely, the difference is not great.

The effectiveness of phenytoin in partial and secondarily generalized seizures is clearly serum-level-dependent. In any individual, better control is consistently obtained at higher serum levels. The concept of a therapeutic range was established on the basis of experience with phenytoin, and applies more to phenytoin than any other antiepileptic drug.

The upper limit of the target range is 80 µmol/L, although there are patients who respond better to higher levels without serious side-effects. Equally, there are large numbers of patients with low serum levels that are quite adequate for seizure control. At least 70% of patients with newly diagnosed epilepsy (partial or tonic–clonic seizures) will be controlled by phenytoin monotherapy.

The drug has no effect in generalized absence seizures nor in myoclonus, and probably a less consistent effect than valproate in primary generalized tonic–clonic seizures, or atonic or tonic seizures. In some of these seizure types, phenytoin can cause a paradoxical exacerbation of seizures, although this is unusual. The drug is also said to worsen seizures in patients with progressive myoclonic epilepsy.

CLINICAL USE IN EPILEPSY

Phenytoin is one of the most commonly used antiepileptics in the world. Fashions differ in different countries, and in North America, for instance, until recently it accounted for nearly 50% of all new prescriptions and 45% of the total antiepileptic drug market, eclipsing carbamazepine and valproate. In the UK and Scandinavia, phenytoin is used less commonly than carbamazepine or valproate, but in other European countries it remains a drug of first choice. As the efficacy of the major antiepileptic drugs in partial and secondary generalized epilepsy has not been shown to differ, the rational choice of a drug will depend largely on the side-effect and pharmacokinetic profile. Although phenytoin can cause many side-effects, in most patients none are experienced. The marketing of newer antiepileptic drugs has eclipsed that of phenytoin and other older antiepileptics, and the marketing pressures can exert an influence on prescribing choice beyond scientific evidence.

In the author's practice, phenytoin is a drug of second choice in partial and secondary generalized seizures, and also in primary generalized tonic–clonic seizures. The difficult pharmacokinetics of the drug, rather than its side-effects profile, weigh against its first-line use. Phenytoin is well tolerated by most patients of all ages. The potential for drug interaction remains a problem when other drugs are used in comedication. Because of the non-linear kinetics of phenytoin, blood level monitoring is essential. It is also often recommended after head trauma or neurosurgical procedures, although the frequency of rash and immunologically mediated side-effects seems greater in these acute situations than in routine therapy. Phenytoin is, after phenobarbital, a drug of choice in neonatal seizures when administered parenterally. The drug also has a major role in the treatment of status epilepticus.

Phenytoin is available in tablets and capsules of 25, 50, 100 and 200 mg. It is also available as a solution for intravenous injection and as a suspension and chewable tablet. In most patients it is given on a once- or, more commonly, twice-daily basis. A typical starting dose in an adult is 100–200 mg per day and this is increased up to 300 mg as initial maintenance therapy. The maintenance dose can be very variable, and serum level measurements are often needed to guide dosage choice. Serum concentrations usually take about a week to reach steady state after a change in dose, but occasionally steady state may not be reached for up to 4 weeks. In children the usual starting dose is 5 mg/kg per day and the drug given twice daily. The usual maintenance in children is between 4–8 mg/kg. Phenytoin can also be loaded intravenously or orally in emergency situations, the oral loading dose being 15 mg/kg in three oral doses at 1-h intervals. A low therapeutic range serum is usually achieved 12 h following such an oral loading dose. Intravenous loading is discussed in Chapter 5. Wherever possible, phenytoin should be used in monotherapy. Combination therapy complicates its therapeutics but, if required, it would be wise to avoid drugs with additive adverse effects or those with significant drug interactions.

Piracetam

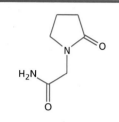

Primary indications	Adjunctive therapy for myoclonus
Usual preparations	Tablets: 800, 1200 mg; sachets: 1.2, 2.4 g; ampoules: 1, 3 g; baxter: 12 g; solution: 20, 33%
Usual dosages	Initial: 7.2 g per day. Maintenance: up to 24 g per day
Dosage intervals	2–3 times per day
Significant drug interactions	None
Serum level monitoring	Not useful
Target range	–
Common/important side-effects	Dizziness, insomnia, nausea, gastrointestinal discomfort, hyperkinesis, weight gain, tremulousness, agitation, drowsiness, rash
Main advantages	Well tolerated and very effective in some resistant cases
Main disadvantages	Not effective in all cases
Mechanisms of action	Unclear
Oral bioavailability	<100%
Time to peak levels	30–40 min
Metabolism and excretion	Renal excretion without metabolism
Volume of distribution	0.6 L/kg
Elimination half-life	5–6 h
Plasma clearance	–
Protein binding	Nil
Active metabolites	Nil
Comment	Useful drug for some patients with refractory myoclonus

Piracetam is a drug with an unusual clinical history. It was developed in 1967 in Belgium and deployed in clinical practice as a 'memory enhancing drug'. Its efficacy in this role has been contentious and the drug has not been licensed for this indication, either in the USA or the UK, although it is widely used in other countries, particularly in the developing world; the manufacturers report over a million prescriptions. Recent controlled trials do show a small but definite effect in improving memory. In 1978 its antimyoclonic effect was first noted in a case of post-anoxic myoclonus after cardiac arrest, where it was being given as a neuroprotective agent. In the last 10 years or so the remarkable effectiveness of this drug in cortical myoclonus of various aetiologies has been confirmed by controlled trial. It has recently received a licence in the UK and elsewhere for its use in this indication. Interestingly, levetiracetam (see p. 113), which is closely related to the L-isomer of piracetam, has a more marked broad-spectrum antiepileptic action, and is an antiepileptic drug in partial-onset seizures with or without secondarily generalization.

PHYSICAL AND CHEMICAL PROPERTIES

Piracetam is a white crystalline powder. Its mechanism of action is completely unexplained. It has effects on brain vasculature, but these are probably not related to its antimyoclonic effects. Piracetam appears to have no effect on brain GABAergic function, ionic channel function nor to affect cerebral serotonin or dopamine levels.

PHARMACOKINETICS

Absorption and distribution
The drug has an oral bioavailability of about 100%. The time to peak levels is between 30 and 40 min. Absorption of the drug is not affected by food. Piracetam has a distribution volume of 0.6 L/kg, but it may be preferentially concentrated in the brain and the elimination of piracetam from the cerebrospinal fluid seems slower than that from the blood. Piracetam is not bound to plasma proteins.

Metabolism and elimination
The drug does not undergo metabolism and is completely excreted by the kidneys with an elimination half-life of 5–6 h and almost complete elimination from the body after 30 h. There are no drug interactions. The elimination from cerebrospinal fluid occurs with a half-life of about 7 h.

SIDE-EFFECTS

The drug is very well tolerated and there is a low incidence of reported side-effects. Those that do occur, at a frequency of less than 10%, include dizziness, insomnia, nausea, gastrointestinal discomfort, hyperkinesis, weight gain, drowsiness, tremulousness and agitation. Rash occurs at a frequency of less than 1% and there have been no serious idiosyncratic reactions. In a placebo-controlled double-blind crossover study, the only adverse effects were a sore throat and headache in one patient and single seizures in two, and these side-effects may well not have been treatment-related. At the very high doses used in the treatment of myoclonus, most patients report few side-effects, although there are no formal studies of side-effects at these very high doses.

CLINICAL USE IN MYOCLONUS

Piracetam is useful in cortical myoclonus of a variety of types and causes. The drug has been shown to be effective in postanoxic action myoclonus, some cases of progressive myoclonic epilepsy, myoclonus caused by carbon monoxide poisoning, some cases of primary generalized epilepsy with myoclonus, post-electrocution myoclonus, myoclonus in Huntington's disease and in other symptomatic metabolic disorders (e.g. sialidosis). Initial case reports and then case series were followed by a well-conducted double-blind placebo-controlled study in 21 patients with severe myoclonus. A median 22% improvement was noted on piracetam on global rating scales of disability, and some patients became seizure-free. The results were impressive in this severe condition and, on this basis, the drug was licensed for use in myoclonus in the UK. There are now numerous reported cases of complete 'cure' of severe myoclonus by the drug, often in cases where all other therapy had failed, and indeed it may be the only drug which improves myoclonus in some patients.

Cortical myoclonus may produce profound disabilities. The jerks are often exacerbated by actions and patients may be bed-bound and immobile, unable to move without severe jerking which disrupts all motor activity. In some cases, but not all, piracetam can have a truly remarkable effect, suppressing the myoclonus and reversing completely even severe disability (see Fig. 3.5, p. 72). There does not seem to be tolerance of the antimyoclonic effect. It has been said that the drug works best in combination, say with clonazepam, although there is no doubt that monotherapy with piracetam can be highly efficacious.

CLINICAL USE IN EPILEPSY

Piracetam is indicated only for myoclonus in epilepsy, and is given usually as a second-line for patients resistant to treatment with valproate or benzodiazepine drugs. It is usually prescribed in combination therapy. Its remarkable effectiveness in some patients, even with severe and disabling myoclonus, combined with its almost complete lack of side-effects give the drug a special place in the therapy of myoclonus.

It is available as 800 and 1200 mg tablets, 1.2 and 2.4 g sachets, 1 and 3 g ampoules, 12 g baxter, and 20 and 33% drinkable solution. The initial dose is 7.2 g per day and this may be rapidly increased by 4.8 g every three days up to 24 g per day, according to clinical efficacy. Some patients require up to 32 g per day. The drug can be given in two or three divided doses. The major drawback at these higher doses is the number of tablets taken and their bulk. Serum level monitoring is neither necessary nor available. Dosage reductions in patients with moderate or severe renal disease are recommended and the drug is contraindicated in patients with creatinine clearances below 20 mL/min. There is no published experience of the drug in children with myoclonus, but there are published data in dyslexic children. Withdrawal needs to be gradual (two-weekly decrements of 800 or 1600 mg), and abrupt cessation has been associated with a severe exacerbation of myoclonus.

Primidone

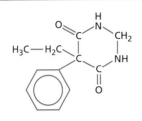

Primary indications	Adjunctive therapy in partial and secondarily generalized seizures (including absence and myoclonus). Also Lennox–Gastaut syndrome
Usual preparations	Tablets: 250 mg; oral suspension: 250 mg/5 mL
Usual dosages	Initial: 125 mg per day. Maintenance: 500–1500 mg per day (adults), 250–500 mg (children under 2 years), 500–750 mg (children 2–5 years), 750–1000 mg (children 6–9 years)
Dosage intervals	1–2 times per day
Significant drug interactions	Primidone has a large number of interactions with antiepileptic and other drugs
Serum level monitoring	Primidone, not generally useful. Derived phenobarbital, useful
Target range	<60 µmol/L primidone, 40–70 µmol/L derived phenobarbital
Common/important side-effects	Acute dizziness and nausea on initiation of therapy. Other side-effects as for phenobarbital
Main advantages	Highly effective and cheap antiepileptic drug
Main disadvantages	CNS side-effects. Also acute reaction on initiation of therapy
Mechanisms of action	Enhances activity of GABA$_A$ receptor, depresses glutamate excitability and affects sodium, potassium and calcium conductance
Oral bioavailability	<100%
Time to peak levels	3 h
Metabolism and excretion	Metabolized to phenobarbital and phenylmethylmalonamide
Volume of distribution	0.6–1.0 L/kg (derived phenobarbital)
Elimination half-life	5–18 h primidone; 75–120 h derived phenobarbital
Plasma clearance	0.006–0.009 L/kg/h (derived phenobarbital)
Protein binding	25% primidone; 45–60% derived phenobarbital
Active metabolites	Phenobarbital
Comment	Primidone is converted in the body to phenobarbital, and its antiepileptic effect is due to phenobarbital. It is therefore doubtful whether primidone carries any antiepileptic advantages over phenobarbital, but in many countries it is not subject to controlled drug restrictions which apply to phenobarbital

Primidone was introduced into clinical practice in 1952.

PHARMACOKINETICS

Primidone is rapidly metabolized into phenobarbital which is its primary metabolite and into phenylethylmalonamide. The main antiepileptic action of primidone is due to the derived phenobarbital, and whether either primidone itself or phenylethyl-malonamide add anything to its antiepileptic properties is controversial; if there is any effect, it is likely to be very minor. The efficacy of primidone is therefore usually assumed to be identical to that of phenobarbital, and it is doubtful whether there is any advantage at all in prescribing primidone rather than phenobarbital in routine clinical practice.

Primidone is well absorbed orally, with a bioavailability approaching 100%. Peak levels are obtained after about 3 h. The drug is 25% bound to proteins and concentrations in fluids, including cerebrospinal fluid, saliva and breast milk, approach those in plasma. The elimination half-life of primidone is between 5 and 18 h and the half-life of the derived phenobarbital is between 75 and 120 h. As it is metabolized by the cytochrome oxidase system, there is a potential for drug interactions, not only between primidone and other drugs but also phenobarbital. Phenytoin and carbamazepine increase the rate of conversion of primidone to phenobarbital, and primidone lowers carbamazepine levels. There is a complex interaction with valproate which usually elevates the phenobarbital : primidone ratio.

SIDE-EFFECTS

The side-effects of primidone are largely those of phenobarbital. Primidone, however, has one additional side-effect which can be troublesome. This is the occurrence of intense dizziness, nausea and sedation which occur commonly at the onset of therapy, sometimes after only one tablet. This reaction which is not uncommon is probably caused by the initially high concentration of the parent drug. These side-effects disappear over a week or so, but it is nevertheless always advisable to start primidone at a low dose.

CLINICAL USE IN EPILEPSY

Primidone is available as 250 mg tablets, which have identical efficacy to 60 mg of phenobarbital.

Measurement of the derived phenobarbital—and not primidone—levels is usually carried out if plasma concentration monitoring is required. An average starting dose for an adult would be 125 mg at night, with increments every 2–4 weeks to an average maintenance total daily dose of 500–1500 mg per day in one or two divided doses.

Tiagabine

Primary indications	Adjunctive therapy in partial and secondarily generalized seizures
Usual preparations	Tablets: 5, 10, 15 mg
Usual dosages	Initial: 15 mg per day. Maintenance: 30–45 mg per day (combination with enzyme-inducing drugs), 15–30 mg per day (comedication with non-enzyme inducing drugs)
Dosage intervals	2–3 times per day
Significant drug interactions	Tiagabine levels are lowered by comedication with hepatic enzyme-inducing drugs
Serum level monitoring	Not useful
Target range	6–74 µmol/L
Common/important side-effects	Dizziness, tiredness, nervousness, tremor, diarrhoea, headache, confusion, psychosis, flu-like symptoms, ataxia, depression
Main advantages	Clinical experience is too limited to define the place of tiagabine in clinical practice, but initial experience is favourable
Main disadvantages	CNS side-effects
Mechanisms of action	Inhibits GABA reuptake
Oral bioavailability	96%
Time to peak levels	1 h
Metabolism and excretion	Hepatic oxidation then conjugation
Volume of distribution	1.0 L/kg
Elimination half-life	3.8–4.9 h
Plasma clearance	12.8 L/h
Protein binding	96%
Active metabolites	Nil
Comment	Newly licensed antiepileptic drug with promise for use in therapy of refractory partial seizures

Tiagabine was introduced into clinical practice in 1998, first in the UK. It has been the subject of a well-conducted preclinical programme of clinical trial, but postlicensing experience is very limited and the relative role of the drug in routine therapy is not yet established.

PHYSICAL AND CHEMICAL CHARACTERISTICS

It is a derivative of the GABA uptake inhibitor nipe-cotic acid, rendering the parent compound lipid-soluble by the attachment of a lipophilic side-chain. Tiagabine is thus able freely to cross the blood–brain barrier, unlike the parent compound.

Mode of action

Tiagabine greatly increases cerebral GABA concentrations, via the inhibition of the GABA transporter-1 (GAT-1) which is one of at least four specific GABA transporting compounds which carry GABA from the synaptic space into neurones and glial cells. Measurements in human and experimental models have confirmed that extracellular GABA concentrations are indeed raised after administration of tiagabine. The action of tiagabine on GAT-1 is reversible, unlike the action of vigabatrin on GABA-T, and its affinity is greater for glial than for neuronal uptake. Its effect seems remarkably specific, and studies have shown little or no effect at other receptor systems, including glutamate, benzodiazepine, 5-HT, dopamine 1 or 2, adenosine, serotonin, glycine, or β1 or β2 adrenoreceptor or muscarinic receptors. Tiagabine also appears not to affect the sodium or calcium channels.

PHARMACOKINETICS

Absorption and distribution

The oral bioavailability of the drug is about 96% in these studies, and almost complete absorption has been found at all ages. Drug concentrations are linear over the range of usual clinical dosages, and peak concentrations occur about 1 h after intake. A second peak of the plasma concentrations of tiagabine is seen 12 h after ingestion, and is presumably caused by enterohepatic recycling. Food slows down absorption by two- or threefold; however, the total amount absorbed (AUC, area under the serum level/time curve) is unchanged by food. The peak concentrations (C_{max}) is also reduced by food. The volume of distribution is 1 L/kg, and the drug is extensively bound (96%) to human plasma proteins.

Metabolism and excretion

Tiagabine is extensively metabolized in the liver. This is a relative disadvantage, although one shared by many other antiepileptics. *In vitro* studies suggest that the main enzymatic degradation is by the isoform CYP3A of the cytochrome P450 family. At least five major metabolites are found both in plasma and two additional metabolites in faeces. None of these known metabolites has any antiepileptic action. After oral ingestion of a single dose, less than 3% of the drug appeared in the urine unchanged. The plasma half-life of tiagabine has been found to be between 4.5 and 8.1 h in normal volunteers, and this is reduced to 3.8–4.9 h in patients with epilepsy comedicated with enzyme-inducing drugs. The shorter half-life in patients with epilepsy is presumably caused largely by the hepatic-inducing effects of other antiepileptics. The plasma clearance of tiagabine has been found to be 12.8 L/h in patients with epilepsy without concomitant therapy and is faster in patients receiving adjunctive therapy with enzyme-inducing

antiepileptic drugs. There are no differences in metabolism in the elderly. Kinetics in young children seem more variable and are less well studied but, generally speaking, the clearance of tiagabine is greater in children. Racial differences were not found to alter the pharmacokinetic parameters of tiagabine in a population analysis. The elimination of the drug is reduced in patients with mild to moderate liver impairment. In a study of four subjects with mild hepatic impairment, three with moderate impairment and six matched controls, tiagabine half-life was found to be 7, 12 and 16 h, respectively, and similar effects on C_{max} and AUC were found. Renal impairment has no effect on the kinetics of the drug.

Drug interactions

Tiagabine does not itself induce or inhibit hepatic metabolic enzymatic activity, and therefore should not alter the concentration of other adjunctive antiepileptic drugs. A small decrease in valproate concentrations has, however, been reported in patients taking concomitant tiagabine, but the mechanism of this effect is uncertain and the extent of the change is unlikely to be clinically significant. Interaction studies with theophylline, warfarin, digoxin, cimetidine, alcohol and also triazolam have not demonstrated any change in kinetics caused by tiagabine comedication. No significant change in plasma concentrations of progesterone, oestradiol follicular-stimulation hormone or luteinizing hormone were found in one small short-term study of comedication with the contraceptive pill.

Although tiagabine comedication does not affect the kinetics of other drugs, the metabolism of tiagabine itself is markedly changed by coadministration of hepatic-inducing drugs, such as carbamazepine, phenytoin and primidone. In one large-population kinetic analysis, the clearance of tiagabine was increased by two-thirds, and the AUC and C_{max} are similarly reduced in patients taking concomitant anticonvulsants. Higher tiagabine dosage is therefore necessary for those receiving concomitant enzyme-inducing antiepileptic drug therapy. Valproate, cimetidine and erythromycin has been found not to affect tiagabine plasma concentrations.

SIDE-EFFECTS

The frequency of side-effects on tiagabine therapy has been based on a pooled analysis of the five randomized double-blind placebo-controlled trials, in which a total of 675 patients (aged between 12 and

77 years) were treated with the drug at 64 mg per day or less, compared with 363 patients treated with placebo. In addition to this analysis, side-effect profiles are also available from the six non-blinded long-term studies which were either extensions of the short-term study (i.e. in which patients who did not tolerate the drug initially have been excluded) or newly initiated trials. At the time of writing, 1978 patients have been treated with tiagabine (at doses of 80 mg per day or less) and of these 814 received the drug for more than 1 year. Only 24 of the patients were over 65 years old, and 162 patients were between 12 and 17 years.

In the randomized placebo-controlled trials, 91% of the 675 patients taking tiagabine reported at least one side-effect compared with 79% of those taking placebo. The most common side-effects of tiagabine involved the central nervous system, with the following central nervous system symptoms significantly more frequent on tiagabine than on placebo (Table 4.12): dizziness, asthenia, nervousness, tremor, depressed mood and emotional lability. Diarrhoea was also significantly more frequent among tiagabine than placebo-treated patients. Other side-effects, which included somnolence, headaches, abnormal thinking, abdominal pain, pharyngitis, ataxia, confusion, psychosis and skin rash, occurred at a similar frequency in treated and placebo groups. Most of these side-effects were categorized as mild or moderate in severity, and only 15% of patients on tiagabine withdrew therapy because of side-effects.

In view of the potential for vigabatrin to result in psychosis or severe depression, these side-effects were particularly monitored, but neither occurred more frequently on tiagabine than on placebo. The side-effect profile from the database of 1978 patients in the long-term trials showed broadly similar results. On long-term therapy, the adverse events reported to occur with a frequency of 10% or more were: dizziness (34%), accidental injury (25%), somnolence (25%), asthenia (24%), headache (23%), infection (23%), tremor (20%), nervousness (15%), abnormal thinking (13%), confusion (13%), ataxia (12%), nausea (12%), flu-like symptoms (11%) and nystagmus (10%).

In the whole database by December 1994, serious adverse events (i.e. those requiring hospitalization or resulting in permanent disability or death) had occurred in 398 of 2600 patients (15.3%), although most were considered unrelated to the tiagabine therapy. The most common were accidental injury (3%), confusion (1%), somnolence (0.8%) and depression (0.8%). There were no changes in biochemical or haematological parameters. The adverse-event profile in the open and monotherapy studies was similar to that in the controlled studies. Serious idiosyncratic side-effects were rare, and recorded as commonly on placebo as on tiagabine.

Initial animal data suggested that tiagabine may induce status epilepticus, and there have been a few clinical reports reporting the occurrence of convulsive and non-convulsive status epilepticus, and tiagabine therapy should be used cautiously in patients with a history of status epilepticus (convulsive or non-convulsive).

A recently described side-effect of vigabatrin is a reduction of visual function in the peripheral visual fields. This is probably caused by elevation of retinal GABA concentrations, and tiagabine shares a similar biochemical potential. There have been a small number of open studies which have reassuringly failed to show any effect of tiagabine on visual fields. However, further studies are necessary before the safety of tiagabine in this regard can be assumed.

ANTIEPILEPTIC EFFECT

Tiagabine has been the subject of a series of clinical trials designed to demonstrate efficacy, including five double-blind placebo-controlled studies of the drug as adjunctive therapy, three trials (one open and two

Table 4.12 Side-effects of tiagabine in the randomized placebo controlled studies (side-effects occurring at a frequency of = <5%).

	Tiagabine (*n* = 675) Percentage of patients	Placebo (*n* = 276) Percentage of patients
Dizziness	30	13
Tiredness	24	12
Nervousness	12	3
Tremor	9	3
Diarrhoea	7	2
Depressed mood	5	1

double-blinded) in monotherapy and six open long-term studies. The randomized double-blind placebo-controlled studies in refractory partial epilepsy in adults form the core of the definitive efficacy studies. Pooling the results, 661 of the 951 enrolled patients entered into a double-blind phase, and 23% of patients showed a >50% reduction vs. 9% of patients on placebo. The overall seizure frequency was also reduced by 25% on tiagabine vs. 0.1% on placebo. Tiagabine was effective at doses of 32 and 56 mg per day. Although the magnitude of the effect seems relatively slight, in a meta-analysis comparing these results with placebo-controlled randomized trials of other drugs, no significant differences in efficacy were demonstrated between tiagabine, gabapentin, lamotrigine, topiramate, vigabatrin or zonisamide. In the long-term extension studies (i.e. of responders in the short-term clinical trials), a total of 772 patients were treated with tiagabine (at less than 80 mg per day), with 50% or greater reduction in seizure frequency in about 30–40% of patients treated for between 3 and 6 months. For partial seizures this effect was maintained during 12 months, but not for secondary generalized seizures.

Tiagabine has also been studied in monotherapy. In one multicentre, double-blind randomized parallel group design of 198 patients, with high-dose tiagabine (36 mg per day; 102 patients) and low-dose tiagabine (6 mg per day; 96 patients) arms. Concomitant antiepileptic drugs were withdrawn in the titration phase (6 weeks) and seizure frequencies were compared during a 12-week fixed dosage period. Fifty-seven (29%) completed the study, with no difference between the numbers withdrawing from each arm. The intent-to-treat analysis showed no major difference in the seizure frequencies in either arm when compared to baseline, but those on the lower dose seemed to do rather better than those on the higher dose. Open monotherapy studies have also been reported.

CLINICAL USE IN EPILEPSY

The drug is available for use as second-line add-on therapy in refractory patients with partial or secondary generalized seizures. It has been introduced too recently to allow a clear judgement to be made about its relative role in routine clinical practice, and concerns about any possible effect on visual function will need to be addressed before the drug is taken up widely.

In adults receiving concomitant medication with enzyme-inducing drugs, the European dosage recommendations are as follows. Tiagabine should be initiated at a doses of 15 mg per day followed by weekly increments of 5–15 mg. The recommended oral maintenance dose is between 30 and 45 mg per day for patients comedicated with enzyme-inducing drugs and 15–30 mg for those who are not. When total doses exceed 30 mg per day, tiagabine should be given three times a day with food. The dosage recommendations from the USA are slightly different: initial dose of 4 mg per day, titration of 4–8 mg per day each week, and usual maintenance doses of 32–56 mg per day.

In adolescents, the incremental increase initially should be slightly slower and the maintenance dose should be 32 mg per day. If there is a history of behavioural problems or depression, treatment should be initiated at a low initial dose under close supervision. No antiepileptic drug should be suddenly withdrawn. Although there are no clinical data, it seems sensible to withdraw tiagabine gradually, at a decremental rate of 5 mg every 2 weeks.

In monotherapy or in patients not taking concomitant enzyme-inducing drugs, experience is limited, but the European recommendations are that the maintenance dose of tiagabine should be reduced to between 15 and 30 mg per day.

Tiagabine is contraindicated in severe hepatic impairment. Dosage recommendations in children are not yet available. The drug should not be used in pregnant or lactating women.

Topiramate

Primary indications	Adjunctive therapy in partial and secondarily generalized seizures. Also for Lennox–Gastaut syndrome and primary generalized tonic–clonic seizures
Usual preparations	Tablets: 25, 50, 100, 200 mg; sprinkle: 15, 25 mg
Usual dosages	Initial: 25–50 mg per day (adults), 0.5–1 mg/kg per day (children). Maintenance: 200–600 mg per day (adults), 9–11 mg/kg per day (children)
Dosage intervals	2 times per day
Significant drug interactions	Topiramate levels are lowered by carbamazepine, phenobarbital and phenytoin
Serum level monitoring	Not generally useful
Target range	6–74 µmol/L
Common/important side-effects	Dizziness, ataxia, headache, paraesthesia, tremor, somnolence, cognitive dysfunction, confusion, agitation, amnesia, depression, emotional lability, nausea, diarrhoea, diplopia, weight loss
Main advantages	Highly effective, recently introduced antiepileptic drug
Main disadvantages	CNS side-effects
Mechanisms of action	Blockage of sodium channels, enhancement of GABA-mediated chloride influx and modulatory effects of the $GABA_A$ receptor and actions at the AMPA receptor
Oral bioavailability	<100%
Time to peak levels	2 h
Metabolism and excretion	Mainly renal excretion without metabolism
Volume of distribution	0.6–1.0 L/kg
Elimination half-life	18–23 h (but varies with comedication)
Plasma clearance	0.022–0.036 L/kg/h
Protein binding	15%
Active metabolites	Nil
Comment	Highly effective recently introduced antiepileptic drug

Topiramate is derived from D-fructose, a naturally occurring monosaccharide, and was initially developed as an antidiabetic drug. It is structurally quite distinct from other antiepileptic drugs. It was found to have striking antiepileptic action in animal models. It underwent a series of controlled trials in North America and in Europe and was licensed, first in the UK, in 1994. The strength of its antiepileptic action has differentiated topiramate from other newer antiepileptics, and it has gained a reputation as a powerful new antiepileptic drug, effective in some patients in whom all other medications have failed.

Physical and chemical characteristics
Topiramate is an insoluble compound with a complex sugar structure.

Mode of action
Topiramate appears to have multiple actions which may contribute to its antiepileptic potential. Possi-

bly the most important is its inhibitory effect on sodium conductance in neuronal membranes. In this sense its action is similar to that of phenytoin and carbamazepine. It reduces the duration of spontaneous antiepileptic bursts on neuronal firing and the number of action potentials generated within each burst. It also reduces the frequency of action potentials elicited by a depolarizing electrical current. Its second action is related to its enhancement of GABA action and, like diazepam, it increases GABA-mediated chloride influx into neurones. However, topiramate does not bind at the benzodiazepine binding site, and the exact mechanism of its GABA action is not known. Topiramate also inhibits glutamate receptors, particularly of the AMPA subtype. It is unique amongst the antiepileptic drugs in this regard. Finally, topiramate is also known to inhibit weakly carbonic anhydrase. This activity is several orders of magnitude less than acetazolamide, but nevertheless could contribute to its antiepileptic action. Recent evidence has suggested that acetazolamide may be particularly effective in patients whose epilepsy is related to genetically determined ion channel defects, and one can speculate that the same might apply to topiramate.

As a result of these actions, topiramate is effective in a wide range of experimental models of epilepsy. In experimental settings, no tolerance to topiramate has been recorded. The neuroprotective index of topiramate exceeds that of carbamazepine, phenytoin and phenobarbital.

PHARMACOKINETICS

Absorption and distribution
Topiramate is rapidly absorbed after oral dosage with a bioavailability approaching 100%. The time to peak blood levels is about 2 h. Food delays absorption but does not affect its extent. The volume of distribution is between 0.6 and 1.0 L/kg, although this falls at higher doses. In humans, approximately 15% of the topiramate is bound to plasma protein. Plasma concentrations increase linearly with dose within the normal dosage range.

Metabolism and elimination
Topiramate is metabolized in the liver, by the P450 microsomal enzymes. At least eight metabolites have been identified formed by hydroxylation, hydrolysis or cleavage of the sulphamate group. None of the metabolites have antiepileptic action. The plasma elimination half-life of topiramate is between 18 and 23 h, and is independent of dose over the normal clinical range. In monotherapy, metabolism is slight, plasma concentrations show little intraindividual variability, and the majority of the drug (85%) is excreted unchanged in the urine. In polytherapy, however, metabolism is much more extensive, presumably as a result of enzyme induction. The elimination of topiramate and its metabolites is via renal mechanisms. In patients in renal failure, topiramate drug doses may need to be reduced.

Drug interactions
Topiramate does not generally affect the steady-state concentrations of other drugs given in comedication (sodium valproate, phenytoin, carbamazepine or carbamazepine epoxide) although phenytoin levels do rise in occasional cases. However, enzyme-inducing drugs, such as phenytoin and carbamazepine, do decrease serum topiramate concentrations by approximately 50%. Sodium valproate administration has no effect on topiramate concentrations. The potential interactions of other non-antiepileptic drugs and topiramate has been inadequately studied. Topiramate reduces ethyl estradiol levels by 30% and will inactivate the low dose contraceptive pill in some cases. Comedication also results in a mild reduction in digoxin levels.

SIDE-EFFECTS

The side-effects of topiramate have been extensively studied in the controlled trials, and also during open experience of the drug in the past 5 years. Adverse effects include ataxia, impairment of concentration, confusion, dizziness, ataxia, fatigue, paraethesia in the extremities, somnolence, disturbance of memory, depression, agitation and slowness of speech. In monotherapy, side-effects, particularly CNS effects, are less common. These adverse events are prominent in about 15% of patients, and there is no doubt that topiramate is badly tolerated by a higher proportion of patients than with other less effective medication. However, many side-effects subside within a few weeks if the drug is continued, and it is worth emphasizing this point. Furthermore, the adverse events noted in the clinical trials largely occurred as the dose was being titrated upwards, often to high levels relatively rapidly. Indeed, three quarters of those who withdrew from the randomized clinical trials did so within the first two months of therapy, often during the rapid titration phase. In clinical practice, the frequency and severity of these side-effects seems to be greatly reduced by slow titration to lower doses (Table 4.13). The drug is well tolerated in children and the commonest side-effects are somnolence, anorexia, fatigue and nervousness.

Topiramate also causes weight loss in many patients. This effect is dose-related and also greatest in those who are overweight. The weight loss can in some cases be marked—a loss of over 10 kg has been reported—and patients need to be warned about this to prevent misinterpretation. Exactly how this effect is mediated is unclear, but it is probably via a suppressive effect on appetite. To some patients this is a welcome eventuality and can counter the tendency of other antiepileptic drugs (notably valproate, gabapentin and vigabatrin) to promote weight gain.

As the drug is a carbonic anhydrase inhibitor, topiramate also has a propensity to cause renal calculi. It has been estimated that symptomatic calculi occur in one patient per 1200 per year and topiramate should be used cautiously in those with a history of renal calculi or a family history. Patients should be encouraged to drink plenty of fluids.

Allergic rash due to topiramate has not been reported, and there is no evidence to date of any clinically significant haemotoxicity, hepatotoxicity, cardiotoxicity or serious gastrointestinal toxicity.

ANTIEPILEPTIC EFFECT

Topiramate has demonstrated marked antiepileptic effect in six double-blind parallel group placebo-controlled add-on trials and in a variety of open studies. In the six studies, topiramate was administered at doses between 200 and 1000 mg per day. Pooled results demonstrated that 44% of adult patients had a >50% reduction in seizures compared with 12% of placebo controls, 21% had a >75% reduction (4% of placebo controls) and 5% became seizure free (none of the placebo-controlled patients). The mean percentage reduction in simple partial seizures was 57% on topiramate (25% of controls), of complex partial seizures 43% (2% of controls) and of secondarily generalized tonic–clonic seizures 50% (vs. 3% of controls). These effects were seen regardless of age, gender, concomitant medication or the baseline seizure frequency. Meta-analysis of placebo-controlled parallel group studies of topiramate and the other new antiepileptic drugs has shown greater effects from topiramate than any of the other drugs compared to placebo, although the power of these studies was insufficient to demonstrate significant differences. Significantly smaller numbers of patients are required to find a responder to topiramate treatment than to gabapentin or lamotrigine. The trials studied the drug at var-

Table 4.13 Adverse events associated with topiramate as adjunctive or monotherapy, expressed as percentage of patients.

Adverse effects*	Adjunctive therapy		Monotherapy	
	Placebo (n = 291)	200–400 mg (n = 183)	25–50 mg (n = 125)	200–500 mg (n = 127)
Somnolence	12	29	14	17
Dizziness	15	25	19	12
Ataxia	7	16	1	4
Nervousness	6	16	6	6
Abnormal vision	2	13	3	3
Psychomotor slowing	2	13	0	7
Speech disorders	2	13	2	2
Memory difficulty	3	12	4	9
Confusion	5	11	5	6
Paraesthesia	4	11	13	35
Diplopia	5	10	0	2
Anorexia	4	10	8	10

*≥10% and/or ≥5% difference in incidence of adverse effects vs. placebo in controlled trials. 25 and 200 mg in children, 50 and 500 mg in adults.

Table 4.14 The results of five double-blind, placebo-controlled clinical trials of topiramate in adults with partial epilepsy.

Topiramate dosage (mg/day)	No. of subjects	Median percent reduction in monthly seizure rate	Percentage of patients with 50% decrease in seizures	Percentage of patients with 75–100% decrease in seizures
Placebo	24	1	8	4
400	23	41*	35†	22
Placebo	30	−12††	10	3
600	30	46‡	47§	23
Placebo	28	−18††	0	0
800	28	36§	43§	36
Placebo	45	13	18	9
200	45	30§	27	9
400	45	48**	47†	22
600	46	45§	46†	22
Placebo	47	1	9	0
600	48	41§	44§	23
800	48	41§	40§	13
1000	47	38§	38§	13

*, $P = 0.065$; †, $P \leq 0.05$; ‡, $P \leq 0.005$; §, $P \leq 0.001$; ¶, $P = 0.051$; **, $P \leq 0.01$, ††, negative number indicates an increase in seizure rate.

ious different dosages and, based on the mean responses, doses between 200–800 mg per day were found to produce optimal effect.

There have also been double-blind placebo-controlled add-on trials of topiramate in generalized tonic–clonic seizures. Again, a significant antiepileptic effect has been demonstrated, 56% of patients experiencing a 75% or more reduction in seizures and 13% seizure free. The power of the antiepileptic effect is confirmed in open clinical experience. A multicentre randomised placebo controlled trial in 86 children with partial epilepsy showed a median reduction in seizures of 33% compared with 10% on placebo, but no significant difference in the number of patients achieving a 50% seizure reduction. A similar trial in 98 patients with the Lennox–Gastaut syndrome showed a significant effect on drop attacks

(a 15% reduction vs. a 5% increase on placebo) and an improvement in seizure severity scales. Anecdotal evidence suggests good effect in typical absence seizures (petit mal) and in myoclonus. Finally, the drug has been shown to be effective as monotherapy in a blinded controlled study in partial epilepsy. The drug therefore appears to have a wide spectrum of antiepileptic action, although further clinical experience is needed to establish its relative role in therapy of these epilepsies in routine clinical practice. Controlled studies have shown that the drug is effective in monotherapy and also in children.

CLINICAL USE IN EPILEPSY

Topiramate is a powerful new antiepileptic drug, but

Table 4.15 Percentage reduction in seizures in adults with partial epilepsy in five double-blind, placebo-controlled clinical trials of topiramate.

Treatment*	Median per cent reduction by seizure type			Overall per cent reduction	
	Generalized seizures	Complex partial seizures	Simple partial seizures	75% reduction	100% reduction
Placebo	36	2	−15§	3	0
Topiramate	76†	41†	58†	19†	4‡

*, dosages of topiramate were 200–1000 mg/day; †, $P = 0.001$; ‡, $P < 0.01$; §, negative number indicates an increase in seizure rate.

with a relatively high rate of side-effects. It has already gained a place in the treatment of severe epilepsy and is sometimes strikingly effective where other drugs have completely failed. It will be interesting to see what its place will be in a wider context, for instance in children, in monotherapy, in the generalized epilepsies and in less severe cases. Preliminary trial work is promising in all these areas, but more routine clinical experience is needed. When first introduced, topiramate was found frequently to cause side-effects. It has since become evident that the incidence and severity of the side-effects can be reduced by starting the drug at low doses and titrating upwards slowly.

Topiramate is available in 25, 50, 100 and 200 mg tablets and as a sprinkle formulation. Parenteral administration is not possible. In adults, the author's practice is to initiate therapy at 25 mg per day and increase this fortnightly to 50 mg, then 100 mg, and then increase in 100 mg increments to an initial maintenance dose of 200–600 mg per day. The drug is given in two divided doses. Some patients have been usefully treated with much higher doses, up to, in exceptional cases, 1600 mg per day. In children, the usual starting dose is 0.5–1 mg/kg per day with incremental increases of 0.5–1 mg/kg per day each fortnight. Further experience is needed to define a range of paediatric dosing, but 9–11 mg/kg per day produced optimal seizure control in the clinical trials.

Valproate

COOH

Primary indications	First-line or adjunctive therapy in generalized seizures (including myoclonus and absence) and also partial seizures, Lennox–Gastaut syndrome and drug of first choice in the syndrome of primary generalized epilepsy. Also for childhood epilepsy syndromes and febrile convulsions
Usual preparations	Enteric-coated tablets: 200, 500 mg; crushable tablets: 100 mg; capsules: 150, 300, 500 mg; syrup: 200 mg/5 mL; liquid: 200 mg/5 mL; slow-release tablets: 200, 300, 500 mg; Divalproex tablets: 125, 300, 500 mg; sprinkle
Usual dosages	Initial: 400–500 mg per day (adults); 20 mg/kg per day (children under 20 kg); 40 mg/kg per day (children over 20 kg). Maintenance: 500–2500 mg per day (adults); 20–40 mg/kg per day (children under 20 kg); 20–30 mg/kg per day (children over 20 kg) (slow-release formulation not suitable for children)
Dosage intervals	2–3 times per day
Significant drug interactions	Valproate has a number of complex interactions with antiepileptic and other drugs
Serum level monitoring	Not generally useful
Target range	300–600 µmol/L
Common/important side-effects	Nausea, vomiting, metabolic effects, endocrine effects, severe hepatic toxicity, pancreatitis, drowsiness, cognitive disturbance, aggressiveness, tremor, weakness, encephalopathy, thrombocytopenia, neutropenia, aplastic anaemia, hair thinning and hair loss, weight gain
Main advantages	Drug of choice in primary generalized epilepsy and a wide spectrum of activity
Main disadvantages	Cognitive effects, weight gain, tremor and hair loss. Potential for severe hepatic and pancreatic disturbance in children
Mechanism of action	Uncertain but may affect GABA glutaminergic activity, calcium (T) conductance and potassium conductance
Oral bioavailability	<100%
Time to peak levels	1–8 h (dependent on formulation)
Metabolism and excretion	Hepatic oxidation and then conjugation
Volume of distribution	0.1–0.4 L/kg
Elimination half-life	4–12 h
Plasma clearance	0.010–0.115 L/kg/h
Protein binding	85–95%
Active metabolites	Nil
Comment	Drug of choice in primary generalized epilepsy and useful in a wide spectrum of other epilepsies

Valproate was first synthesized in 1882 and used as an organic solvent. Its antiepileptic properties were recognized, entirely by accident, while being used as a solvent for the experimental screening of new antiepileptic compounds. It was licensed in Europe in the early 1960s, where it became very widely used, and then in the USA in 1978. It has been marketed as a magnesium or calcium salt, an acid, and also as sodium hydrogen divalproate (Depakote). None of these derivatives show any real superiority. Sodium valproate is the usual form in the UK and Depakote in Europe. Valpromide (dipropylacetamide), a prodrug of valproate, is also marketed, as is a delayed-release formulation, and these have certain pharmacokinetic differences. Valproate is widely available throughout the world, and has become a drug of choice in primary generalized epilepsy and for treating a wide spectrum of seizure types.

PHYSICAL AND CHEMICAL CHARACTERISTICS

Valproic acid is a simple molecule, a branched-chain carboxylic acid, similar in clinical structure to endogenous fatty acids. It is slightly soluble in water and very soluble in organic solvents. Its pKa is 4.8. The sodium salt is very water-soluble, whereas the calcium and magnesium salts are insoluble.

Mode of action

The mechanism of action is uncertain. Valproate enhances GABA function, but this effect is only observed at high concentrations. There is a potentiation of GABA-mediated postsynaptic inhibition, but the significance of this is unclear. The drug also inhibits GABA degrading enzymes and succinate semialdehyde dehydrogenase, and may increase the synthesis of GABA by stimulating glutamic acid decarboxylase. Valproate also inhibits excitatory transmission by aspartate, glutamate and gamma-hydroxybutyrate, via mechanisms which are not fully understood. In hippocampal slices, valproate reduces the threshold for calcium and potassium conductance. The relative importance of these mechanisms in human epilepsy is unclear. In animal models, valproate is highly effective against pentylenetetrazol seizures but less effective in the maximal electric shock model. It suppresses the photically induced seizures in the photosensitive baboon. In kindling models it inhibits the spread of seizure activity but does not suppress focal discharges.

PHARMACOKINETICS

Absorption and distribution

Valproate is rapidly and nearly completely absorbed, with a bioavailability approaching 100%. The peak plasma concentration of sodium valproate, after oral administration, is reached within 13 min–2 h (usually by 1.5 h). The calcium salt has similar pharmacokinetic properties. Peak valproate concentrations are reached slightly more slowly with valproic acid (3–4 h), and slightly faster with sodium hydrogen divalproate. Valpromide is absorbed more slowly but has similar bioavailability. Administration with food slightly delays the absorption of most forms, but not their extent, although seems to speed up valpromide absorption. Sodium valproate is available in an enteric-coated formulation which results in peak plasma concentrations within 3–8 h, and this is a commonly used form. Slow-release formulations have also been developed to reduce fluctuation in plasma concentrations. The sprinkle formulation of sodium hydrogen divalproate has a slightly delayed absorption profile with peak concentrations reached in about 4 h. Rectal administration also results in complete absorption. The drug is 85–95% bound to plasma proteins. The free fraction is concentration-dependent and at higher plasma concentrations (above 100 µg/mL) protein binding decreases. Protein binding is reduced in renal and hepatic disease and during pregnancy and other drugs can displace valproate from its protein-binding sites (e.g. aspirin, phenylbutazone). The other antiepileptics, however, do not influence binding. Valproate distributes mainly in the extracellular space with an apparent volume of distribution of 0.1–0.4 L/kg. High concentrations are found in the liver, intestinal tract and gall bladder, kidney and urinary bladder. Valproate also enters the cerebrospinal fluid compartment and brain rapidly, although the exact mechanism of transport is unclear. It is an active process, and this transport mechanism is saturable at high doses with much less efficient brain absorption. The mean total plasma : cerebrospinal fluid ratio is about 0.15. The concentration of valproate obtained in the cerebral cortex is however low, and this indicates an active transport mechanism out as well as into the brain. This process is probably via the probenecid-sensitive monoamine transport systems of the blood–brain barrier. This has implications for the use of valproate in acute seizures or status epilepticus.

Metabolism and elimination

Valproate is rapidly eliminated from the body by

hepatic metabolism. There are a variety of pathways, the main one being beta-oxidation followed by glucuronidation. At least 30 metabolites have been identified, some of which may be responsible for adverse side-effects (notably the 4-ene metabolite and hepatic toxicity). Less than 4% of the drug is excreted unchanged. The plasma half-life is generally in the range of 4–12h, although the administration of other hepatic enzyme-inducing antiepileptic drugs increases clearance, often by 100%, and shortens the half-life. Young children (over 2 months of age) metabolize the drug faster than adults. The clearance of valproate and its metabolites is almost entirely by hepatic metabolism and follows linear kinetics at most dosage ranges, although at higher plasma concentrations reduced protein binding results in an increased clearance. Because of the relatively short half-life of the drug, there are marked diurnal variations in plasma levels (100% differences between peak and trough levels) on twice daily dosage. There is also marked intraindividual variation.

Drug interactions

Valproate is involved in a number of interactions with other antiepileptic drugs, the mechanism of which is often obscure. Valproate is extensively protein-bound, is metabolized in the liver but does not induce the metabolism of other drugs. Interactions are usually slight, and do not pose much of a clinical problem. The clinical effectiveness of the drug is also not as closely correlated to serum level as is the case with phenytoin or carbamazepine, for instance.

Effect of other drugs on valproate levels

Phenytoin, phenobarbital and carbamazepine can induce the hepatic metabolism of valproate, and levels can be reduced by comedication by as much as 50%. Antacids, Adriamycin and cisplatin have been shown to impair the absorption of valproate. Naproxen, phenylbutazone and salicylate displace valproate from its albumin-binding sites and occasionally result in valproate toxicity.

Effect of valproate on levels of other drugs

Valproate is a potent inhibitor of both oxidation and glucuronidation. Comedication elevates diazepam, phenobarbital, phenytoin, ethosuximide, carbamazepine and lamotrigine levels (Table 4.16). There is a particular interaction with nimodipine, levels of which can be almost doubled.

Table 4.16 Valproate interactions.

Drug	Effect
Valproate-induced changes	
Phenytoin	Decreased total concentration
	Increased free fraction
Phenobarbital	Increased
Carbamazepine	Increased epoxide concentration
Lamotrigine	Increased
Changes in valproate concentration	
Phenytoin	Decreased
Phenobarbital	Decreased
Carbamazepine	Decreased
Felbamate	Increased
Clobazam	Increased

SIDE-EFFECTS

As sodium valproate was introduced before the wide use of large controlled and blinded studies, the frequency of side-effects compared to placebo has not been established. Clinical experience has led to the view that the drug is well tolerated, and at least as well tolerated as carbamazepine, phenytoin or other of the newer antiepileptic drugs. The common dose-related side-effects include nausea, vomiting and gastrointestinal effects, common on initiation of therapy and avoided by the administration of enteric coated formulations. Weight gain is a frequent problem (30% of all patients), often troublesome and occasionally profound, especially in females. The mechanism is uncertain, but may be mediated by drug-induced decrease in beta-oxidation of fatty acids. Dose-related tremor is another common side-effect (10% of patients) although seldom severe enough to warrant treatment withdrawal. The typical sedative side-effects of antiepileptic drugs can also occur with valproate, severely so in about 2% of patients, and sometimes associated with other neurological symptoms, such as confusion and irritability. Rarely, severe sedation amounting to stupor or even coma has been reported (valproate encephalopathy). This has been inconsistently associated with hyperammonaemia, comedication with phenobarbital at high levels, or other drug interactions. In most instances, none of these factors are present, and the metabolic basis of the stupor is unclear. It is possible that carbamyl phosphate synthetase-1 deficiency is responsible. The EEG usually shows high-voltage slow activity and the encephalopathy rapidly reverses when valproate is withdrawn.

Another unusual side-effect of valproate is its propensity, rarely, to cause hair loss or more usually curling of hair. Again, this may be because of the formation of abnormal metabolites. The hair curling can sometimes be profound and striking changes of appearance—not always unwelcome—may result. It is said that the hair changes reverse if therapy is continued, but in the author's experience this is certainly not true in all cases.

Valproate also has a variety of metabolic effects resulting from the interference in mitochondrial-based intermediate metabolism. The common results are hypocarnitinaemia, hyperglycinaemia and hyperammonaemia. The metabolic effects may be exacerbated by genetically determined enzymic defects or by enzymic pathways already stressed because of acute illness or comedication. Ammonia levels are often slightly raised on valproate therapy and are usually asymptomatic. When hyperammonaemia is severe, stupor, coma or even death can result. Patients with existing urea cycle enzyme defects or those with hepatic disease are at particular risk. The most common defect is partial deficiency (heterozygosity) of ornithine transcarbamylase which can be asymptomatic and undiagnosed until valproate is prescribed or until valproate and metabolic stress combine to precipitate acute hyperammonaemia. This results in an encephalopathy which occasionally may be fatal.

Valproate also has endocrine effects. The importance of these is uncertain, and results somewhat conflicting. Insulin resistance can occur and drug-induced alterations in sex hormone levels possibly resulting in anovulatory cycles, amenorrhoea and polycystic ovary syndrome. The frequency of these effects is unclear, and assessment is complicated by inconsistent findings, the confounding effects of weight gain and other medications. Nevertheless, these effects should be considered when prescribing valproate to female patients in the reproductive age range.

Acute allergic rashes have been only rarely reported, as have severe bone marrow depression and neutropenia. The most common haematological effects of valproate are effects on clotting. These include thrombocytopenia, inhibition of platelet aggregation, reduction of factor VII complex and fibrinogen depletion. This can result in bruising and haematoma.

Usually mild, this is of little clinical significance except during surgical intervention; and it is sometimes advised that valproate is withdrawn, especially in children, prior to intracranial surgery, including epilepsy surgery.

Valproate-induced pancreatitis is a rare but serious complication. By 1993 there had been 24 cases reported. The mechanism of this effect is uncertain, but may be caused by valproate-induced reduction in free-radical scavenging enzyme activity. Pancreatitis should be suspected in any patient on valproate who develops acute abdominal pain. The pancreatitis usually reverses with withdrawal of valproate, but can be fatal.

The serious idiosyncratic side-effect which has caused most concern is acute hepatic failure (Table 4.17). This has been most frequently observed in children under the age of 2 years on polytherapy and with neurological handicaps. Initially, a rate of one case of hepatic failure per 500 children on polytherapy under the age of 2 years was reported. Some of these initial cases were in fact multifactorial with valproate precipitating an already existing diathesis (e.g. caused by underlying Alpers' disease) and, with more careful prescribing to avoid high-risk cases, the rate of valproate-induced hepatic failure has now fallen. Hepatic failure is rare above the age of 2 years, and in monotherapy. The pathological similarities to Reye's syndrome have also raised the possibility that the hepatic failure is caused by the 4-ene metabolite of valproate which inhibits beta-oxidation, although the administration of carnitine to correct coenzyme A depletion has not been found to reverse the hepatic failure. The routine analysis of valproate metabolites has not been useful as a general screening method. A useful set of recommendations have been made to diminish the risk of hepatotoxicity:
• to use the drug in monotherapy only, wherever possible, in children under 3 years;
• to administer the lowest possible dosage;
• to avoid comedication with salicylate;
• to avoid valproate in those with liver disease, or with metabolic disorders involving the urea cycle, organic acidaemias, mitochondrial disorders, free-radical scavenger deficiencies, carnitine or medium-chain acyl coenzyme A deficiency; and
• to advise parents to report nausea, vomiting, anorexia or jaundice immediately.

ANTIEPILEPTIC EFFECT

Valproate has activity against a wide range of sei-

Table 4.17 Rate of hepatic fatality by age-group in patients receiving valproate as monotherapy or polytherapy (1978–1984).

Age group	Monotherapy			Polytherapy		
	Total patients	Deaths	Rate per 10 million	Total patients	Deaths	Rate per 10 million
0–2	7 025	1	1.42	7 889	15	19.01
3–10	35 593	4	1.12	39 975	7	1.75
11–20	51 951	0	0	58 348	5	0.56
21–40	59 107	0	0	66 386	4	0.60
41+	34 125	0	0	38 351	1	0.26
Monotherapy total	187 821	5	0.27			
Polytherapy total				210 949	32	1.52
Combined total				398 770	37	0.93

Other anticonvulsants taken with valproate: phenytoin (17 patients); phenobarbital (16); clonazepam (10); carbamazepine (8); primidone (3), Diamox, diazepam and paraldehyde (2 each); ethosuximide and Mesantoin (1 each).

zure types and epilepsy syndromes. Indeed some authorities have recommended that valproate be used as first line therapy in *all* newly diagnosed epilepsies because of this.

There is little doubt that it is the drug of choice in the idiopathic (primary) generalized epilepsies, both for controlling generalized absence and generalized tonic–clonic seizures. A number of open and comparative studies have demonstrated control rates achieved in over 90% of new patients with typical absence seizures on valproate. In this, ethosuximide shows similar efficacy, but valproate is also highly effective in controlling the tonic–clonic seizures which often develop in idiopathic generalized epilepsy, for which ethosuximide is usually ineffective. Valproate is also the drug of choice for juvenile myoclonic epilepsy and approximately 80% of patients will become seizure-free on starting valproate. It can be used in other types of myoclonus, although with somewhat less effect, including postanoxic action myoclonus, benign myoclonic epilepsies of childhood and the more severe myoclonic epilepsies and progressive myoclonic epilepsy. In these latter severe myoclonic syndromes, valproate is a drug of first choice, but will seldom control these seizures altogether. Valproate is the drug of choice for photosensitive epilepsy—usually part of the syndrome of primary generalized epilepsy—and the EEG manifestations of photosensitivity will be abolished by valproate therapy.

The usefulness of valproate in partial seizures or in secondarily generalized seizures, however, is more contentious. Opinion is divided as to whether valproate is as effective as carbamazepine or phenytoin (the industry standards), and one certainly has a clinical impression that the more focal or more severe is the epilepsy, the less likely is valproate to be helpful. In mild focal epilepsy, however, valproate has been shown to be as effective as other first-line drugs. Overall, about 50% of new patients with tonic–clonic seizures, in all syndromic types, will become seizure-free when initiating therapy with valproate.

Valproate is also a drug of second choice in infantile spasms, controlling spasms in about 20–50% at normal doses and up to 90% at high doses. However, vigabatrin is now usually given as first-line therapy, and the risk of hepatic toxicity has rendered valproate use more circumspect. It is the first choice therapy in the Lennox–Gastaut syndrome, reportedly controlling seizures in up to 10% of cases and reducing attacks by 50% or more in one-third. The use of valproate in convulsive and non-convulsive status epilepticus and in the emergency treatment of epilepsy is considered in Chapter 5. It has been used in neonatal seizures and to prevent febrile seizures, although other drugs are preferable in children under 2 years in view of the potential hepatotoxic effects.

Serum level estimations can be made, but there is a poor relationship between level and effect. Moreover, the marked diurnal swings in blood levels on twice or three times daily dosage render measurements often rather meaningless. There is little point in a rigid adherence to the so-called therapeutic range (300–700 µmol/L).

CLINICAL USE IN EPILEPSY

Valproate is one of the most commonly used antiepileptics throughout the world. It is a drug of choice in primary generalized epilepsy, treating the generalized absence, myoclonus and tonic–clonic seizures in this syndrome. It is also useful in atypical absence and atonic seizures in the Lennox–Gastaut syndrome, where it is also still the drug of first choice. It is a drug of choice for myoclonic epilepsy and for photosensitivity. In partial and secondarily generalized epilepsy, carbamazepine is usually tried before valproate, although there is no conclusive evidence that valproate is less effective especially in new or mild cases.

Valproate is presented as the sodium, calcium, magnesium salt, as the acid, as sodium hydrogen divalproate or as valpromide. Enteric-coated, immediate and slow-release formulations also exist, as well as syrup, sprinkle, intravenous forms and a rectal suppository. There are no convincing therapeutic differences between any of these forms, although the enteric-coated form reduces gastrointestinal side-effects, and rates of absorption differ in different formulations. The pharmacokinetics of individual patients vary much more than any difference in formulation, and there is little logic in having so many different manufactured products.

The most popular form of sodium valproate is as 200 and 500 mg enteric-coated tablets. Divalproex tablets are another common preparation and are usually available as 125, 300 and 500 mg tablets. The usual starting dose for an adult is 200 mg at night increasing by 200 or 500 mg increments to a maintenance dose of between 600 and 1500 mg. Doses of up to 3000 mg per day are sometimes given. Twice daily dosage is usual. Patients on comedication often require higher doses than those on monotherapy. In children, the usual starting dose is 20 mg/kg per day and maintenance dose is 40 mg/kg per day, and on combination therapy doses may need to be higher. Although a target serum level range has been suggested by clinical studies, the levels fluctuate widely during a 24-h period, even on three times daily dosage, and the antiepileptic effectiveness is not influenced by these fluctuations. The controlled-release formulation lessens this fluctuation, but does not improve seizure control nor lessen side-effects and there seems little justification for its wide usage. Finally, because of the lack of correlation between serum level and effect, serum level monitoring is not generally clinically useful.

Vigabatrin

Primary indications	Adjunctive therapy in partial and secondarily generalized epilepsy. Also for infantile spasm and Lennox–Gastaut syndrome
Usual preparations	Tablets: 500 mg; powder sachet: 500 mg
Usual dosages	Initial: 1000 mg per day (adults). Maintenance: 1000–3000 mg per day (adults); 40 mg/kg per day (children) or 500–1000 mg per day (body weight 10–15 kg), 1000–1500 mg (body weight 15–30 kg), 1500–3000 mg (body weight over 30 kg)
Dosage intervals	2 times per day
Significant drug interactions	Vigabatrin may lower phenytoin levels
Serum level monitoring	Not useful
Target range	–
Common/important side-effects	Sedation, dizziness, headache, ataxia, paraesthesia, agitation, amnesia, mood change, depression, psychosis, aggression, confusion, weight gain, tremor, diplopia, severe visual field constriction, diarrhoea
Main advantages	Highly effective recently introduced antiepileptic drug
Main disadvantages	CNS side-effects and visual field constriction
Mechanisms of action	Inhibition of GABA transaminase activity
Oral bioavailability	<100%
Time to peak levels	2 h
Metabolism and excretion	Renal excretion without metabolism
Volume of distribution	0.8 L/kg
Elimination half-life	4–7 h
Plasma clearance	0.102–0.114 L/kg/h
Protein binding	Nil
Active metabolites	Nil
Comment	Highly effective recently introduced antiepileptic drug whose usage is limited by potential for neuropsychiatric side-effects and effects on visual field

Recognition in the 1970s that GABA was an important inhibitory neurotransmitter in the central nervous system raised the possibility that boosting GABA action may suppress seizures. This led the worldwide pharmaceutical industry to turn their attention to GABA analogues. The first developed and the most successful was vigabatrin, which was licensed in the UK in 1979 and subsequently in other European countries and worldwide. It is not licensed in the USA. It was the first of a new wave of antiepileptic drugs introduced in the 1980s. It has gained an important role in the treatment of epilepsy, although anxiety about its toxicity has been heightened by recently recognized side-effects and its future role seems in doubt.

PHYSICAL AND CHEMICAL CHARACTERISTICS

Vigabatrin (gamma-vinyl-GABA; 4-amino-hex-5-enoic acid) is a close structural analogue of GABA. The drug is a racemic mixture, but only the S-enantiomer is biologically active. It is a crystalline substance, highly water-soluble but only slightly soluble in ethanol.

Mode of action

Vigabatrin, being a close structural analogue of GABA, binds to GABA transaminase, the enzyme which metabolizes GABA in the synaptic cleft. Vigabatrin binds irreversibly to the active site on the enzyme, and enzymic activity therefore only recovers when new enzyme is synthesized. Vigabatrin greatly raises extracellular GABA concentrations in the brain and this has been demonstrated *in vitro*, in animal experimentation and in various ways *in vivo* in human subjects also. Enzyme activity returns to normal over 4–6 days, reflecting the rate of synthesis of new enzymes. Vigabatrin is effective in some but not all animal models of epilepsy. The time scale of the effect of local brain injections of vigabatrin mirrors that of the recovery of GABA-transaminase concentrations. In humans, elevations in cerebrospinal fluid and brain GABA levels have been measured after both single doses of vigabatrin and after long-term chronic therapy. Similar elevations in brain GABA have been recorded by magnetic resonance spectroscopy in animal and human studies. Vigabatrin has no other known action.

PHARMACOKINETICS

Vigabatrin has simple pharmacokinetics which pose few problems, unlike many other antiepileptic drugs. As vigabatrin acts by irreversibly inhibiting the cerebral enzyme GABA transaminase, its effect is dependent on the rate of production of new enzyme rather than on any pharmacokinetic parameters. The biological half-life of the drug (i.e. the time taken for the enzyme concentrations to recover to half their previous level) is several days, even after a single dose.

Absorption and distribution

Absorption is rapid following oral ingestion, with a peak concentration at about 2 h. The oral bioavailability is 100%. Food has little effect on the rate or extent of absorption. There is no appreciable protein binding in plasma, and the volume of distribution of the drug is 0.8 L/kg. The drug is distributed widely. The cerebrospinal fluid concentration of vigabatrin is about 10% that of the plasma. Only a small amount of the drug crosses the placenta. In children, bioavailability is somewhat lower.

Metabolism and excretion

Vigabatrin is only minimally metabolized in humans (<5%), and is eliminated primarily by renal excretion of the unchanged drug. Vigabatrin does not induce the activity of hepatic enzymes. Elimination is not dose-dependent, and the elimination half-life in subjects with normal renal function is between 4 and 7 h. The plasma clearance is 0.102–0.114 L/kg/h. Elimination is slower in the elderly and the half-life is doubled. A steady state is attained after stable dosage regimens within 2 days. In the elderly and in those with severe renal impairment, vigabatrin should be used at lower doses in view of the reduced clearance.

Drug interactions

Vigabatrin has virtually no pharmacokinetic or pharmacodynamic interactions with any other antiepileptic drug, except phenytoin. The addition of vigabatrin can result in a fall of plasma concentration of phenytoin by a mean of 25%, usually within a few weeks of polytherapy. The mechanism of this effect is uncertain, but presumably is caused by impairment of phenytoin absorption as phenytoin protein binding, metabolism and excretion are unchanged.

SIDE-EFFECTS

During the initial development of the drug, neuropathological studies in rats and dogs showed that vigabatrin caused widespread intramyelinic vacuolization throughout the brain. This could also be demonstrated *in vivo* by magnetic resonance spectroscopy (MRS). Primate studies, human surgical and postmortem pathology, human MRS and human evoked potential studies, however, failed to demonstrate any similar changes. On the basis of these reassuring data, the drug has been licensed, but vigilance still needs to be maintained to assess the possible development of neuropathological changes over more prolonged treatment periods. The drug also affected the retina in some rodent species but, until recently, problems in the human retina were not recognized clinically.

Acute hypersensitivity or idiosyncratic immunological adverse events (e.g. rash, hepatic disturbance, marrow dysplasia) are extremely rare, and vigabatrin has proved a safe drug in this regard. Minor side-effects were noted in about 40% of all patients taking vigabatrin in the clinical trials, and included fatigue, drowsiness, headache, dizziness, weight increase, tremor, double-vision and abnormal vision. Drowsiness is the most common effect. This occurs particularly at the initiation of treatment and often improves spontaneously over time (Table 4.18). In addition to these symptoms, vigabatrin can cause neuropsychiatric adverse events, notably depression (5%), agitation (7%), confusion and, in a few cases, psychosis. Although the frequency of the neuropsychiatric complications is relatively small (usually under 10%), they can be severe. If the drug is introduced slowly, and if it is stopped when such symptoms begin to appear, serious problems can generally be averted. The psychosis caused by vigabatrin has paranoid features and sometimes visual hallucinations. In the reported series, these psychotic reactions occur often when seizure control has been improved by the drug. Depression can be severe, and occasionally life-threatening. An increase in body weight of greater than 10% is seen in about 10–15% of adults taking long-term vigabatrin therapy, an effect which seems particularly to develop in the first 6 months of therapy, but the mechanism is unknown. Vigabatrin has little effect on cognitive function and indeed this can even improve. An encephalopathy has been recorded in patients with renal impairment in whom appropriate dose adjustments were not made.

Table 4.18 Incidence of the most frequent adverse events (>5%) reported in clinical trials of 2682 patients with epilepsy treated with vigabatrin.

Adverse event	Incidence (percentage of patients)
Drowsiness	18.6
Fatigue	15.1
Headache	12.7
Dizziness	10.3
Weight increase	7.9
Agitation	6.9
Abnormal vision	5.3
Diplopia	5.1
Tremor	5.1
Depression	5.1

A potentially very important side-effect of vigabatrin, recently reported, is the development of peripheral visual failure. Typically, this is asymptomatic, although there are now a number of patients (perhaps 10% of all those taking vigabatrin) who notice deterioration in vision and on occasions this deterioration has been severe. Visual fields show the pattern of nasal then concentric constriction (tunnel vision), with central vision preserved (Fig. 4.5). In one series, visual field disturbances were found in over 50% of cases. Field testing to confrontation in the clinic is usually normal, and the visual field disturbances are picked up by careful testing using either Goldmann perimetry or the computerized Humphries testing battery. The mechanism of this effect is unknown, although it does seem intuitively likely that the visual field failure is caused by GABA inhibition in the retina, which is a structure rich in $GABA_C$ receptors. It is unclear whether this effect is dose-related, or after what duration of therapy it develops, but alarmingly it seems to be irreversible, at least in some cases. The first reports of visual field failure were made only recently, and the full extent of this potentially serious adverse event has, at the time of writing, not been established (Fig. 4.5).

ANTIEPILEPTIC EFFECT

Nine well conducted double-blind controlled studies, four single-blind studies and one open label study have reported of a total of 479 patients. Evaluation periods range from 4 to 20 weeks, and the dose of vigabatrin has been between 1000 and 4000 mg (usually 3000 mg). Overall, these studies have shown 40–50% patients with refractory partial seizures to have a more than 50% reduction in seizure frequency, and up to 10% became seizure-free. These are excellent figures in this refractory group, and in this sense vigabatrin is superior to the other novel antiepileptic drugs, with the exception of topiramate. The value of vigabatrin can be further confirmed by the fact that a high proportion of responders from the clinical trials opted to stay on the drug in the long term. In paediatric studies too, vigabatrin had a good effect against complex partial seizures.

There are seizure types and syndromes which usually fail to respond to vigabatrin therapy. Secondarily generalized seizures are notably less well controlled than partial seizures, and less well than with other first-line antiepileptic drugs, even where the two seizure types coexist. Patients with Len-

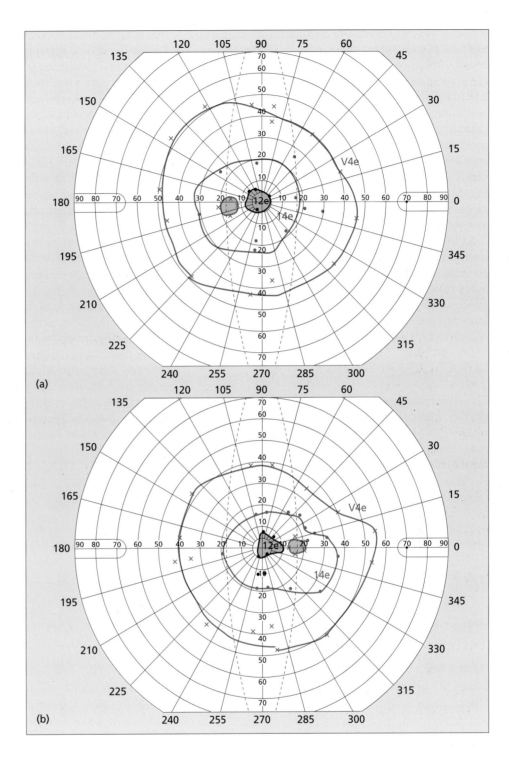

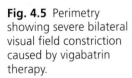

Fig. 4.5 Perimetry showing severe bilateral visual field constriction caused by vigabatrin therapy.

nox–Gastaut syndrome or myoclonic epilepsy also typically show little improvement. Vigabatrin is less effective against primarily generalized tonic–clonic seizures, and may also worsen myoclonic seizures or generalized absence seizures. Absence status can be precipitated by vigabatrin therapy. Monotherapy studies have also shown efficacy. How-ever, one comparative study of monotherapy with vigabatrin or carbamazepine in newly diagnosed pa-tients showed significantly fewer patients becom-ing seizure-free on vigabatrin (32%) than with carbamazepine (52%), perhaps because of the het-erogeneous patient population, which included gen-eralized epilepsy. A second blinded comparative study, however, showed no difference in effectiveness. In placebo-controlled trials in refractory epilepsy, 20% of children and 5% of adults showed an increase in seizures. Seizures may also flare-up during too rapid vigabatrin withdrawal.

Vigabatrin is particularly effective in controlling infantile spasms, with most patients experiencing a great reduction of spasms and many becoming seizure-free. Vigabatrin seems superior to corticosteroids or ACTH in this indication, and has become the drug of choice, especially it has been claimed in children whose infantile spasm is caused by tuberous sclerosis.

As the drug irreversibly inhibits a cerebral enzyme, therapeutic drug monitoring of the serum concentrations is unhelpful. It is possible to measure the activity of the same enzyme in platelets, and to use this as a guide to dosage, but these measurements have not proved useful in clinical practice.

CLINICAL USE IN EPILEPSY

The usual starting dose for an adult is 500 mg twice per day, increasing by 250–500 mg incremental steps every 1–2 weeks. The average daily maintenance dose is between 1000–2000 mg, although 25% of patients have better control on 3000 mg than on 2000 mg. The maximum dose is 4000 mg. In children 40 mg/kg per day is the usual starting dose, with maintenance doses of 80–100 mg/kg per day. Lower doses should be used in patients with renal impairment, especially when the creatinine clearance is <60 mL/min. When the drug is being withdrawn it is recommended that this be done slowly, with 250 or 500 mg decrements every 2–4 weeks.

Vigabatrin is currently indicated for second-line use in patients with refractory partial epilepsy. Unlike lamotrigine or topiramate, it does not appear to be useful in the generalized epilepsies, although its effect in partial epilepsy is better than that of lamotrigine or gabapentin. It would be much more widely used were it not for anxiety about its toxicity. Apart from its propensity to cause neuropsychiatric disturbance, there has been the recent observation that visual failure can also occur. Because of this, the use of the drug in the future is likely to be very much further restricted.

It is the drug of choice for infantile spasms, and it appears—on circumstantial evidence—to be particularly useful when the spasms are caused by tuberous sclerosis. Its effects are so beneficial in these children that it is likely to remain the drug of choice in this indication, even if its more widespread use becomes more limited.

Other drugs

ACETAZOLAMIDE

Acetazolamide is an interesting substance which was introduced as an antiepileptic drug in 1952. The drug inhibits the enzyme carbonic anhydrase (CA) with subsequent generation of carbon dioxide. How this results in an antiepileptic action is unclear. An intriguing possibility is that, by analogy with the periodic paralyses, it acts on the ion channels in epileptic patients who have genetic defects in channel structure (channelopathies).

Absorption, distribution and excretion
The drug is absorbed largely in the duodenum and upper jejunum. Peak levels in the plasma are reached 2–4 h after oral intake. Acetazolamide diffuses into tissue water as the free form, where is binds to CA. The highest concentrations are found in those tissues that contain the highest concentrations of CA, reflecting the high affinity of acetazolamide for this enzyme. Within the brain, glial cells are the main CA-containing cells and acetazolamide is localized to these cells. The subcellular distribution of the enzyme is predominantly in the cytoplasm and in mitochondria. Acetazolamide in humans is completely excreted in urine without metabolism.

Drug interactions
Reports of interactions between acetazolamide and other drugs are rare. As acetazolamide is not metabolized by the liver, its plasma concentration cannot be affected by drugs that induce or inhibit the metabolizing enzymes in the liver. In children with seizures resistant to carbamazepine, the administration of acetazolamide is reported occasionally to increase the plasma concentrations of carbamazepine.

Side-effects
Side-effects are mostly mild or transient, including lethargy, paraesthesias, anorexia, headache, nausea, diarrhoea and visual changes. Renal calculi can develop as a consequence of the carbonic anhydrase activity of acetazolamide, at an annual frequency of 235 per 10 000 patients.

Antiepileptic effect
In animal models, acetazolamide has been shown to prevent audiogenic seizures. It blocks the tonic extensor component in the maximal electroshock sei-zure pattern test and it is effective against seizures induced by pentylenetetrazol. Acetazolamide has not been subjected to rigorous clinical trials, and the assessment of its effectiveness in epilepsy is based on unblinded observations only.

Therapeutic use
Acetazolamide has been shown to be effective in the treatment of a variety of seizure types. The usual dose is 250 mg given once to three times a day. Frequently, tolerance develops over 3–6 months, and a period of drug withdrawal will restore its efficacy. It can be effective in monotherapy, in tonic–clonic seizures, in cases of juvenile myoclonic epilepsy, in absences and as an adjunctive antiepileptic drug in partial epilepsy. In a total of 48 patients with refractory partial epilepsy, 44% had a 50% decrease in seizure frequency when acetazolamide was given in addition to carbamazepine. Catamenial epilepsy is another indication for acetazolamide, which can be started 8–10 days before the expected onset of menses, and continued for up to 10 days.

ADRENOCORTICOTROPIC HORMONE

Adrenocorticotropic hormone (ACTH) is an endogenous hormone released by the anterior pituitary gland which regulates secretion of glucocorticoids and sex hormones. The anticonvulsant mechanism of action of ACTH is unclear. If it is assumed that there is no difference in efficacy between ACTH and oral steroids, the anticonvulsant effect may be mediated through cortisol. However, it has also been suggested that fragments of the ACTH molecule, independent of cortisol, have antiepileptic drug properties.

Absorption, distribution and excretion
As ACTH is inactivated in the gastrointestinal tract, it must be administered parenterally. Adrenocorticotropic hormone is rapidly metabolized and has a short half-life of only 15 min.

Side-effects
Treatment with ACTH may have a number of severe side-effects. Most children will develop Cushingoid features and exhibit irritability. Other side-effects include the risk of infection, heart failure caused by

steroid-induced cardiomyopathy and renal and pancreatic calcification, electrolyte abnormalities, hypertension and glucosuria.

Therapeutic use

It is an anticonvulsant of choice for infantile spasms and is also used in status epilepticus. There has been some discussion as to whether corticosteroids are more effective compared to ACTH and, although a double-blind study has shown no difference, most paediatricians seem to favour ACTH.

The recommended dosage for infantile spasms is $150\,IU/m^2$ per day in two divided doses for 1 week, followed by $75\,IU/m^2$ per day in a single dose for another week and then this same dose only on alternate days for 2 weeks. Four weeks after starting treatment the alternate-day dose of ACTH is gradually reduced over 8 or 9 weeks, until discontinued. Adrenocorticotropic hormone has an all or nothing effect in infantile spasms; monitoring is therefore relatively straightforward. In about 70–75% of children ACTH is effective in stopping the seizures.

KETOGENIC DIET

The ketogenic diet was introduced in 1921 as a treatment for intractable epilepsy. The diet is high in fat and low in carbohydrate and protein, and produces an increase in blood acetone concentration and a reduction in blood sugar concentration. The mechanisms by which the ketogenic diet works are still poorly understood. Several hypotheses have been suggested, including alterations in acid–base balance, in water and electrolyte distribution, in lipid and ketone bodies concentrations. Recently, detailed investigations of the metabolic effects of three ketogenic diets have been reported. The diets included the classical (4:1) ketogenic diet, the medium-chain triglycerides (MCT) diet and a modified MCT diet. Over a study period of 24 h, continuous measurements were carried out to assess concentrations of ketone bodies, glucose, pyruvate, lactate, glycerol and alanine. All three diets produced a significant increase in ketone body concentration. No significant increases in plasma cholesterol, high-density lipoproteins (HDL), low-density and very low-density lipoproteins (LDL, VLDL) were seen. Hypoglycaemia was not observed in any patient and no significant change in plasma sodium, potassium, chloride or bicarbonate levels were seen. All three regimens were associated with a marked improvement in seizure control, but this was not always related to ketone

levels. On the other hand, no correlation between blood lipid levels and seizure control was seen.

Side-effects

Reported side-effects include optic neuropathy, impaired neutrophil function, renal stones and hyperuricaemia. Acetazolamide combined with the ketogenic diet can lead to severe metabolic acidosis and acetazolamide therapy should be stopped 1–2 weeks before starting the diet. Valproate and the ketogenic diet elevate medium-chain fatty acids, which increases the risk of enhancing valproate-induced hepatotoxicity. The ketogenic diet can cause an elevation of very long-chain fatty acids (VLCFA) in plasma, similar to that in patients with adreno-leucodystrophy, adrenomyeloneuropathy and in Zellweger's syndrome. Diagnostic confusion can be caused, and plasma levels of VLCFA should be interpreted cautiously in this clinical setting.

Therapeutic use

The diet should be initiated in the hospital after 24–72 h of fasting. Once ketosis is established, caloric intake is increased until a 4:1 ketogenic diet is reached. The diet includes 1 g/kg body weight per day and 75 kcal/kg per day derived from four parts fat and one part protein/carbohydrate. Vitamins and minerals are supplemented, but sugar is not allowed. The diet requires strict supervision.

The ketogenic diet can be effective in most types of seizures. The main indications include medically refractory seizures of childhood and atonic, myoclonic and atypical absence seizures in patients with the Lennox–Gastaut syndrome. In 58 children with refractory seizures and severe neurological handicaps, 38% had a decrease in seizure frequency of at least 50%, and 29% had complete seizure control.

MEPHENYTOIN

Mephenytoin has a structure that clearly resembles phenytoin and ethotoin. Its mechanisms of action are presumed to be similar to phenytoin, but its efficacy against pentylenetetrazol-induced seizures is greater. It inhibits post-tetanic potentiation and prevents the tonic phase in tonic–clonic seizures. It also is effective against seizures induced by bicuculline and picrotoxin.

Side-effects

Side-effects include skin rashes, hepatotoxicity, periarteritis nodosa and lupus erythematosus. Other adverse effects are psychotic reactions and behavioural disturbances.

Therapeutic use

Mephenytoin has the same spectrum of indications as phenytoin but, because of its common side-effects, its use should be limited to those cases unable to tolerate other drugs. It is effective in complex partial seizures and tonic–clonic attacks, but it may exacerbate absence seizures. The usual daily dose is 300–600 mg in adults, given in divided doses.

MESUXIMIDE

Mesuximide is an N,2-dimethyl-2-phenyl-succinimide, chemically related to ethosuximide, but with a phenyl substituent similar to that of phenytoin.

Mesuximide is indicated for the treatment of absence seizures when conventional treatment has failed, and is, unlike ethosuximide, also indicated as adjunctive therapy for complex partial seizures. The mechanism of action of mesuximide is unknown. It has been shown to be effective against pentylenetetrazol-induced seizures and against maximal electroshock seizures, but less so than ethosuximide.

Pharmacokinetics

Mesuximide is rapidly absorbed after oral administration and thereafter undergoes rapid and complete demethylation to N-desmethylmesuximide (NDMSM). This compound is pharmacologically active and is assumed to be primarily responsible for the anticonvulsant effect of mesuximide. During chronic treatment, NDMSM plasma levels are about 700 times that of ethosuximide. N-desmethylmesuximide is slowly metabolized with an apparent half-life of 34–80h. The therapeutic plasma level of mesuximide has been proposed to be between 10–40 µg/mL. In one clinical trial, the optimal effect was obtained with plasma levels of 20–24 µg/mL.

The recommended starting dose of mesuximide is 150 mg per day with a gradual increase of the dose up to a maximal daily dose of 1200 mg. Studies have reported that the addition of mesuximide as concomitant therapy significantly increases the plasma level of phenytoin by 43.4%, and of phenobarbital derived from primidone by 17%, whereas carbamazepine levels are decreased by a mean of 23.2%. In a single study, plasma phenobarbital levels increased by 40% and those of phenytoin by 78%.

Side-effects

The incidence of side-effects is similar to that of ethosuximide, but the side-effects are more severe and persistent. The most commonly reported side-effects are drowsiness, lethargy, gastrointestinal disturbances, hiccups, irritability and headache. In one study, two of 26 patients experienced psychic changes including depression, weepiness and impulsive behaviour.

Indications and efficacy

The efficacy of mesuximide in the treatment of absence seizures has not been systematically studied and no studies seem to have compared the drug to ethosuximide. Ten of 16 patients with absences in one study became seizure-free and there was a reduction of 75% in seizures in another five. Of four patients with juvenile myoclonic epilepsy, two became seizure-free and in two there was a >75% reduction in attacks. Only 20% of patients with absence seizures had a 50% or greater reduction in seizure frequency when mesuximide was used in previously untreated patients, and no patients achieved complete seizure control. Unlike ethosuximide, mesuximide is also effective against complex partial and secondarily generalized seizures. In a study of previously untreated complex partial seizures, 27% of patients achieved a 50% or greater reduction and 18% became completely seizure-free. When mesuximide was used as an adjunctive drug for refractory complex partial seizures, 71% of the patients had 90–100% seizure control. More than 50% of the patients complained of adverse effects, particularly somnolence and lethargy. Only 30% of patients with refractory complex partial seizures had a 50% seizure reduction following addition of mesuximide, and only five of eight patients continued a 50% seizure reduction after 3–34 months of follow-up. This study controlled for alterations of plasma levels of concomitant drugs which were reduced when plasma concentrations increased by more than 10%. Mesuximide is rarely used today, as less toxic drugs are available. Nevertheless, it is a powerful antiepileptic with a wide spectrum of action, and still has a place as adjunctive therapy in the occasional patient.

NITRAZEPAM

Nitrazepam is the only benzodiazepine, apart from clobazam and clonazepam, which has a place (albeit small) in contemporary non-emergency therapy in epilepsy. Its use is largely confined to severe epilepsies in childhood.

Pharmacokinetics

The oral administration of 10 mg of nitrazepam will result in 78% absorption with peak plasma levels of 83–164 ng/mL appearing in just under 1 h. Protein binding is 86%, and the volume of distribution is 2.4 L/kg. The elimination half-life of 24–31 h is the same following acute and chronic administration. The volume of distribution is greater in elderly subjects with prolongation of the elimination half-life by 40–46%. Hepatic metabolism results in reduction of the nitro group to yield 7-aminonitrazepam; this is then acetylated. Excretion occurs via both urine and faeces (45–65% and 14–20%, respectively) with prolonged tissue binding of the remainder. In a group of 44 children under satisfactory control, the mean plasma concentration was 114 ng/mL at a dose of 0.27 mg/kg per day.

Clinical use in epilepsy

The seizure type for which nitrazepam had been found most effective is infantile spasm, with a reported positive response of between 52 and 68%. This compared favourably with ACTH, with fewer side-effects from nitrazepam. The drug is also used as adjunctive therapy in the severe generalized and secondary generalized epilepsies of childhood, in Lennox–Gastaut syndrome and in myoclonic epilepsy. Maintenance doses range from up to 1 mg/kg per day in children to less than 0.5 mg/kg per day in elderly adults. Intoxication is likely at levels above 200 ng/mL. Dose-related side-effects include drowsiness, which may be minimized by a gradual upward taper, ataxia, hypersecretion and hypersalivation, which can be severe and occasionally has resulted in aspiration pneumonia. Idiosyncratic side-effects include leucopenia and urticaria. Delirium tremens can follow sudden withdrawal of nitrazepam.

The usual dose is between 1.25 and 10 mg per day, with some children taking the drug on an alternate-day regimen—a fashion which seems to have no published evidential support.

FURTHER READING

Adkins, J.C., Noble, S. (1998) Tiagabine: A review of its pharmacodynamic and pharmacokinetic properties and therapeutic potential in the management of epilepsy. *Drugs*, **55**, 437–60.

Aicardi, J., Mumford, J.P., Dumas, C., Wood, S. (1996) Vigabatrin as initial therapy for infantile spasms: a European retrospective survey. Sabril IS Investigator and Peer Review Groups. *Epilepsia*, **37**, 638–42.

Anon (1998) Vigabatrin and visual defects. WHO Drug information. 2.6; 12/3 147.

Barron, T.F. & Hunt, S.L. (1997) Review of the newer antiepileptic drugs and the ketogenic diet. *Clin Pediatr Phila*, **36**, 513–21.

Baruzzi, A., Michelucci, R. & Tassinari, C.A. (1989) Benzodiazepines: nitrazepam. In: *Antiepileptic Drugs*, 3rd edn (eds R.H. Levy, F.E. Dreifuss, R.H. Mattson, B.S. Meldrum & J.K. Penry), pp. 785–804. Raven Press, New York.

Ben-Menachem, E. & Abrahamsson, H. (1994) Gastroscopic evaluation of patients with complex partial seizures treated with topiramate. *Epilepsia*, **35S8**, 116 (abstract).

Booth, F., Buckley, D., Camfield, C. *et al.* (1998) Clobazam has equivalent efficacy to carbamazepine and phenytoin as monotherapy for childhood epilepsy. *Epilepsia*, **39**, 952–9.

Brodie, M.J. (1992) Lamotrigine. *Lancet*, **339**, 1397–400.

Browne, T.R., Dreifuss, F.E., Dyken, P.R. *et al.* (1975) Ethosuximide in the treatment of absence (petit mal) seizures. *Neurology*, **25**, 515–24.

Bruni, J. & Albright, P. (1983) Valproic acid therapy for complex partial seizures. Its efficacy and toxic effects. *Arch Neurol*, **40**, 135–7.

Bruni, J. (1998) Efficacy of topiramate. *Can J Neurol Sci*, **25**: S6–7.

Callaghan, N., O'Hare, J., O'Driscoll, D., O'Neill, B. & Daly, M. (1982) Comparative study of ethosuximide and sodium valproate in the treatment of typical absence seizures (petit mal). *Develop Med Child Neurol*, **24**, 830–6.

Canadian Study Group for Childhood Epilepsy. Clobazam has equivalent efficacy to carbamazepine and phenytoin as monotherapy for childhood epilepsy. *Epilepsia*, **39**, 952–9.

Chadwick, D. (1994) Gabapentin. *Lancet*, **343**, 89–91.

Chadwick, D.W., Anhut, H., Greiner, M.J. *et al.* (1998) A double-blind trial of gabapentin monotherapy for newly diagnosed partial seizures. International Gabapentin Monotherapy Study Group 945–77. *Neurology* **51**, 1282–8.

Convanis, A., Gupta, A.K. & Jeavons, P.M. (1982) Sodium valproate: monotherapy and polytherapy. *Epilepsia*, **23**, 693–700.

Crawford, P., Ghadiali, E., Lane, E., Blumhardt, L. & Chadwick, D. (1986) Gabapentin as an antiepileptic drug in man. *J Neurol Neurosurg Psychiat*, **50**, 682–6.

Croiset, G. & de Wied, D. (1992) ACTH: a structure–activity study on pilocarpine-induced epilepsy. *Eur J Pharmacol*, **229**, 211–16.

de Silva, M., MacArdle, B. & McGowan, M. (1996) Randomised comparative monotherapy trial of phenobarbitone, phenytoin, carbamazepine, or sodium valproate for newly diagnosed childhood epilepsy. *Lancet*, **347**, 709–13.

Duncan, J.S., Shorvon, S.D. & Fish, D.R. (1995) *Clinical Epilepsy*. Churchill Livingstone, London.

Engel, J., Pedley, T.A. (1997) *Epilepsy: a comprehensive textbook*. Lippincott Raven, Philadelphia.

Faught, R.E. (1993) *Topiramate: US clinical trial experience in partial epilepsy* (abstract). Presented at the 20th International Epilepsy Congress, Oslo, Norway, July 1993.

Felbamate Study Group in Lennox–Gastaut Syndrome (1993) Efficacy of felbamate in childhood epileptic encephalopathy (Lennox–Gastaut syndrome). *N Engl J Med*, **328**, 29–33.

Glauser, T.A. (1998) Topiramate use in pediatric patients. *Can J Neurol Sci*, **25** S8–S12.

Goa, K.L., Ross, S.R. & Chrisp, P. (1993) Lamotrigine: a review of its pharmacological properties and clinical efficacy in epilepsy. *Drugs* **46**, 152–76.

Graves, N.M., Brundage, R.C., Wen, Y. (1998) Population pharmacokinetics of carbamazepine in adults with epilepsy. *Pharmacotherapy*, **18**, 273–81.

Hopkins, A., Shorvon, S. & Cascino, G. (1995) *Epilepsy*, 2nd edn. Chapman & Hall, London.

Jeavons, P.M., Bishop, A. & Harding, G.F.A. (1986) The prognosis of photosensitivity. *Epilepsia*, **27**, 569–75.

Kasteleijn Nolst Trenite, D.G., Marescaux, C., Stodieck, S., Edelbroek, P.M. & Oosting, J. (1996) Photosensitive epilepsy: a model to study the effects of antiepileptic drugs. Evaluation of the piracetam analogue, levetiracetam. *Epilepsy Res*, **25**(3): 225–30.

Kaufman, D.W., Kelly, J.P., Anderson, T., Harmon, D.C. & Shapiro, S. (1997) Evaluation of case reports of aplastic anemia among patients treated with felbamate [see comments]. *Epilepsia*, **38**, 1265–9.

Kinsman St, L., Vining, E.P.G., Quaskey, S.A., Mellits, D. & Freeman, J.M. (1992) Efficacy of the ketogenic diet for intractable seizure disorders: review of 58 cases. *Epilepsia*, **33**(6), 1132–6.

Koskiniemi, M., Van Vleymen, B., Hakamies, L., Lamusuo, S. & Taalas, J. (1998) Piracetam relieves symptoms in progressive myoclonus epilepsy: a multicentre, randomised, double blind, crossover study comparing the efficacy and safety of three dosages of oral piracetam with placebo. *J Neurol Neurosurg Psychiatry*, **64**(3), 344–8.

Krauss, G.L., Johnson, M.A. & Miller, N.R. (1998) Vigabatrin-associated retinal cone system dysfunction: electroretinogram and ophthalmologic findings. *Neurology*, **50**, 614–18.

Langtry, H.D., Gillis, J.C. & Davis, R. (1997) Topiramate. A review of its pharmacodynamic and pharmacokinetic properties and clinical efficacy in the management of epilepsy. *Drugs*, **54**, 752–73.

Leppilk, I.E., Dreifuss, F.E., Pledger, G.W. *et al.* (1991) Felbamate for partial seizures: results of a controlled clinical trial. *Neurology*, **41**(11), 1785–9.

Levy, R.H., Mattson, R. & Medrum, B.S. (1998) *Antiepilepsy Drugs* (4th edn). Raven Press, New York.

Marson, A.G., Kadir, Z.A., Hutton, J.L. & Chadwick, D.W. (1997) The new antiepileptic drugs: a systematic review of their efficacy and tolerability [see comments] *Epilepsia*, **38**, 859–80.

Meador, K.J. & Baker, G.A. (1997) Behavioral and cognitive effects of lamotrigine. *J Child Neurol*, **12** Suppl 1: S44–7.

Mullens, E.L. (1998) Clinical experience with lamotrigine monotherapy in adults with newly diagnosed epilepsy: A review of published randomised clinical trials. *Clin Drug Invest*, **16**, 125–33.

Obeso, J.A., Artieda, J., Rothwell, J.C. *et al.* (1989) The treatment of severe action myoclonus. *Brain*, **112**, 756–77.

Oles, K.S., Penry, J.K., Cole, D.L. & Howard, G. (1989) Use of acetazolamide as an adjunct to carbamazepine in refractory partial seizures. *Epilepsia*, **30**(1), 74–8.

Pellock, J.M. & Brodie, M.J. (1997) Felbamate: 1997 update [editorial; comment]. *Epilepsia*, **38**, 1261–4.

Perucca, E. (1996) The new generation of antiepileptic drugs: advantages and disadvantages. *Br J Clin Pharmacol*, **42**, 531–43.

Resor, S.R. & Resor, L.D. (1990) Chronic acetazolamide monotherapy in the treatment of juvenile myoclonic epilepsy. *Neurology*, **40**, 1677–81.

Rosenfeld, W.E. (1997) Topiramate: a review of preclinical, pharmacokinetic, and clinical data. *Clin Ther* **19**, 1294–308; discussion 1523–4.

Sachdeo, R.C., Sachdeo, S.K., Walker, S.A. *et al.* (1996) Steady-state pharmacokinetics of topiramate and carbamazepine in patients with epilepsy during monotherapy and concomitant therapy. *Epilepsia*, **37**, 774–80.

Sato, S., White, B.G., Penry, J.K. *et al.* (1982) Valproic acid versus ethosuximide in the treatment of absence seizures. *Neurology*, **32**, 157–63.

Sherwin, A.L., Robb, J.P. & Lechter, M. (1973) Improved control of epilepsy by monitoring plasma ethosuximide. *Arch Neurol*, **28**, 178–81.

Shorvon, S.D. (1998) The use of clobazam, midazolam, and nitrazepam in epilepsy. *Epilepsia*, **39**/Suppl. 1, 15–23.

Shorvon, S.D., Dreifuss, F., Fish, D. & Thomas, D. (eds) (1996) *The Treatment of Epilepsy*. Blackwell Science, Oxford.

Snead, O.C. (1989a) Adrenocorticotropic hormone (ACTH). In: *Antiepileptic Drugs* (eds R.H. Levy, F.E. Dreifuss, R.H. Mattson, B.S. Meldrum & J.K. Penry), pp. 905–12. Raven Press, New York.

Suzuki, M., Maruyama, H., Ishibashi, Y. *et al.* (1972) A double-blind comparative trial of sodium dipropylacetate and ethosuximide in children with special emphasis on pure petit mal seizures. *Med Prog (Jap)*, **82**, 470–88.

Tanganelli, P. & Regesta, G. (1996) Vigabatrin vs. carbamazepine monotherapy in newly diagnosed focal epilepsy: a randomized response conditional cross-over study. *Epilepsy Res*, **25**, 257–62.

Tassinari, C.A., Michelucci, R., Riguzzi, P. *et al.*

(1998) The use of diazepam and clonazepam in epilepsy. *Epilepsia*, **39** (Suppl. 1) S7–S14.

UK Gabapentin Study Group (1990) Gabapentin in partial epilepsy. *Lancet*, **i**, 1114–17.

US Gabapentin Study Group (1993) Gabapentin therapy in refractory epilepsy: a double-blind placebo-controlled parallel group study. *Neurology*, **43**, 2292–8.

Wallace, S.J. Myoclonus and epilepsy in childhood: a review of treatment with valproate, ethosuximide, lamotrigine and zonisamide (1998) *Epilepsy Res*, **29**, 147–54.

Drug	Primary indications
Carbamazepine	First-line or adjunctive therapy in partial and generalized seizures (excluding absence and myoclonus). Also in Lennox–Gastaut syndrome and childhood epilepsy syndromes
Clobazam	Adjunctive therapy for partial and generalized seizures. Also for intermittent therapy, one-off prophylactic therapy, and non-convulsive status epilepticus
Clonazepam	Adjunctive therapy in partial and generalized seizures (including absence and myoclonus). Also, Lennox–Gastaut syndrome, status epilepticus
Ethosuximide	First-line or adjunctive therapy in generalized absence seizures
Felbamate	Adjunctive therapy in refractory partial and secondarily generalized epilepsy. Also in Lennox–Gastaut syndrome
Gabapentin	Adjunctive therapy in adults with partial or secondarily generalized epilepsy
Lamotrigine	Adjunctive or monotherapy in partial and generalized epilepsy. Also in Lennox–Gastaut syndrome
Levetiracetam	Adjunctive therapy in partial seizures with or without secondarily generalized seizures
Oxcarbazepine	Adjunctive or monotherapy in partial and secondarily generalized seizures
Phenobarbital	Adjunctive or first-line therapy for partial or generalized seizures (including absence and myoclonus). Also for status epilepticus, Lennox–Gastaut syndrome, childhood epilepsy syndromes, febrile convulsions and neonatal seizures
Phenytoin	First-line or adjunctive therapy for partial and generalized seizures (excluding myoclonus and absence). Also for status epilepticus, Lennox–Gastaut syndrome and childhood epilepsy syndromes
Piracetam	Adjunctive therapy for myoclonus
Primidone	Adjunctive therapy in partial and secondarily generalized seizures (including absence and myoclonus). Also Lennox–Gastaut syndrome
Tiagabine	Adjunctive therapy in partial and secondarily generalized seizures
Topiramate	Adjunctive therapy in partial and secondarily generalized seizures. Also for Lennox–Gastaut syndrome and primary generalized tonic–clonic seizures
Valproate	First-line or adjunctive therapy in generalized seizures (including myoclonus and absence) and also partial seizures, Lennox–Gastaut syndrome and drug of first choice in the syndrome of primary generalized epilepsy. Also for childhood epilepsy syndromes and febrile convulsions
Vigabatrin	Adjunctive therapy in partial and secondarily generalized epilepsy. Also for infantile spasm and Lennox–Gastaut syndrome

Drug	Usual preparations
Carbamazepine	Tablets: 100, 200, 400 mg; chewtabs: 100, 200 mg; slow-release formulations; 200, 400 mg; liquid: 100 mg/5 mL; suppositories: 125, 250 mg
Clobazam	Tablet, capsule: 10 mg
Clonazepam	Tablets: 0.5, 2 mg; liquid: 1 mg in 1 mL diluent
Ethosuximide	Capsules: 250 mg; syrup: 250 mg/5 mL
Felbamate	Tablets: 400, 600 mg; syrup: 600 mg/5 mL
Gabapentin	Capsules: 100, 300, 400 mg
Lamotrigine	Tablets: 25, 50, 100, 200 mg; chewtabs: 5, 25, 100 mg
Levetiracetam	Tablets: 250, 500, 750, 1000 mg
Oxcarbazepine	Tablets: 150, 300, 600 mg
Phenobarbital	Tablets: 15, 30, 50, 60, 100 mg: elixir: 15 mg/5 mL; injection: 200 mg/mL
Phenytoin	Capsules: 25, 50, 100, 200 mg; chewtabs: 50 mg; liquid suspension: 30 mg/5 mL, 125 mg/50 mL; injection: 250 mg/5 mL.
Piracetam	Tablets: 800, 1200 mg; sachets: 1.2, 2.4 g; ampoules: 1, 3 g; baxter: 12 g; solution: 20, 33%
Primidone	Tablets: 250 mg; oral suspension: 250 mg/5 mL
Tiagabine	Tablets: 5, 10, 15 mg
Topiramate	Tablets: 25, 50, 100, 200 mg; sprinkle: 15, 25 mg
Valproate	Enteric-coated tablets: 200, 500 mg; crushable tablets: 100 mg; capsules: 150, 300, 500 mg; syrup: 200 mg/5 mL; liquid: 200 mg/5 mL; slow-release tablets: 200, 300, 500 mg; Divalproex tablets: 125, 300, 500 mg; sprinkle
Vigabatrin	Tablets: 500 mg; powder sachet: 500 mg

Drug	Usual dosages
Carbamazepine	Initial: 100 mg at night. Maintenance: 400–1600 mg per day (maximum 2400 mg). (Slow-release formulation, higher dosage.) Children: <1 year, 100–200 mg; 1–5 years, 200–400 mg; 5–10 years, 400–600 mg; 10–15 years, 600–1000 mg
Clobazam	10–30 mg per day (adults); higher doses can be used. Children aged 3–12 years, up to half adult dose
Clonazepam	Initial: 0.25 mg. Maintenance: 0.5–4 mg (adults); 1 mg (children under 1 year), 1–2 mg (children 1–5 years), 1–3 mg (children 5–12 years). Higher doses can be used
Ethosuximide	Initial: 250 mg (adults); 10–15 mg/kg per day (children). Maintenance: 750–2000 mg per day (adults); 20–40 mg/kg per day (children)
Felbamate	Initial: 1200 mg per day (adults); 15 mg/kg per day (children). Maintenance: 1200–3600 mg per day (adults); 45–80 mg/kg per day (children)
Gabapentin	Initial: 300 mg per day. Maintenance: 900–3600 mg per day
Lamotrigine	Initial: 12.5–25 mg per day. Maintenance: 100–200 mg (monotherapy or comedication with valproate); 200–400 mg (comedication with enzyme inducing drugs)
Levetiracetam	Initial: 1000 mg per day. Maintenance dose: 1000–3000 mg per day
Oxcarbazepine	Initial starting dose: 600 mg per day. Titration rate of 600 mg per week. The usual maintenance dose is 900–2400 mg per day
Phenobarbital	Initial: 30 mg per day. Maintenance: 30–180 mg per day (adults); 3–8 mg/kg per day (children); 3–4 mg/kg per day (neonates)
Phenytoin	Initial: 100–200 mg per day (adults); 5 mg/kg (children). Maintenance: 100–300 mg per day (adults), higher doses can be used guided by serum level monitoring: 4–8 mg/kg (children)
Piracetam	Initial: 7.2 g per day. Maintenance: up to 24 g per day
Primidone	Initial: 125 mg per day. Maintenance: 500–1500 mg per day (adults), 250–500 mg (children under 2 years), 500–750 mg (children 2–5 years), 750–1000 mg (children 6–9 years)
Tiagabine	Initial: 15 mg per day. Maintenance: 30–45 mg per day (combination with enzyme-inducing drugs), 15–30 mg per day (comedication with non-enzyme inducing drugs)
Topiramate	Initial: 25–50 mg per day (adults), 0.5–1 mg/kg per day (children). Maintenance: 200–600 mg per day (adults), 9–11 mg/kg per day (children)
Valproate	Initial: 400–500 mg per day (adults); 20 mg/kg per day (children under 20 kg); 40 mg/kg per day (children over 20 kg). Maintenance: 500–2500 mg per day (adults); 20–40 mg/kg per day (children under 20 kg); 20–30 mg/kg per day (children over 20 kg). (Slow-release formulation not suitable for children)
Vigabatrin	Initial: 1000 mg per day (adults). Maintenance: 1000–3000 mg per day (adults), 40 mg/kg per day (children) or 500–1000 mg per day (body weight 10–15 kg), 1000–1500 mg (body weight 15–30 kg), 1500–3000 mg (body weight over 30 kg)

Drug	Dosage intervals
Carbamazepine	2–3 times per day (2–4 times per day at higher doses or in children)
Clobazam	1–2 times per day
Clonazepam	1–2 times per day
Ethosuximide	2–3 times per day
Felbamate	3–4 times per day
Gabapentin	2–3 times per day
Lamotrigine	2 times per day
Levetiracetam	2 times per day
Oxcarbazepine	2 times per day
Phenobarbital	1–2 times per day
Phenytoin	1–2 times per day
Piracetam	2–3 times per day
Primidone	1–2 times per day
Tiagabine	2–3 times per day
Topiramate	2 times per day
Valproate	2–3 times per day
Vigabatrin	2 times per day

Drug	Significant drug interactions
Carbamazepine	Carbamazepine has a large number of interactions with antiepileptic and other drugs
Clobazam	Minor interactions are common, but usually not clinically significant
Clonazepam	Minor interactions are common, but usually not clinically significant
Ethosuximide	Ethosuximide levels are increased by valproate. Levels may be reduced by carbamazepine, phenytoin and phenobarbital
Felbamate	Felbamate increases the concentration of phenobarbital, phenytoin, carbamazepine epoxide and valproate. Felbamate lowers the concentration of carbamazepine. Phenytoin, phenobarbital and carbamazepine lower felbamate levels; valproate increases felbamate levels
Gabapentin	None
Lamotrigine	Autoinduction. Lamotrigine levels are lowered by phenytoin, carbamazepine, phenobarbital and other enzyme-inducing drugs. Lamotrigine levels increased by sodium valproate
Levetiracetam	None
Oxcarbazepine	Fewer than with carbamazepine
Phenobarbital	Phenobarbital has a number of interactions with antiepileptic and other drugs
Phenytoin	Phenytoin has a large number of interactions with antiepileptic and other drugs
Piracetam	None
Primidone	Primidone has a large number of interactions with antiepileptic and other drugs
Tiagabine	Tiagabine levels are lowered by comedication with hepatic enzyme-inducing drugs
Topiramate	Topiramate levels are lowered by carbamazepine, phenobarbital and phenytoin
Valproate	Valproate has a number of complex interactions with antiepileptic and other drugs
Vigabatrin	Vigabatrin may lower phenytoin levels

Drug	Serum level monitoring
Carbamazepine	Useful
Clobazam	Not useful
Clonazepam	Not useful
Ethosuximide	Useful
Felbamate	Value not established
Gabapentin	Not useful
Lamotrigine	Value not established
Levetiracetam	Value not established
Oxcarbazepine	Value not established
Phenobarbital	Useful
Phenytoin	Useful
Piracetam	Not useful
Primidone	Primidone, not generally useful. Derived phenobarbital, useful
Tiagabine	Not useful
Topiramate	Not generally useful
Valproate	Not generally useful
Vigabatrin	Not useful

Drug	Target range (µmol/L)
Carbamazepine	20–50
Clobazam	–
Clonazepam	–
Ethosuximide	300–700
Felbamate	200–460
Gabapentin	–
Lamotrigine	4–60
Levetiracetam	–
Oxcarbazepine	50–125
Phenobarbital	40–170
Phenytoin	40–80
Piracetam	–
Primidone	<60 primidone; 40–170 derived phenobarbital
Tiagabine	–
Topiramate	6–74
Valproate	300–600
Vigabatrin	–

Drug	Common/important side-effects
Carbamazepine	Drowsiness, fatigue, dizziness, ataxia, diplopia, blurring of vision, sedation, headache, insomnia, gastrointestinal disturbance, tremor, weight gain, impotence, effects on behaviour and mood, hepatic disturbance, rash and other skin reactions, bone marrow dyscrasias, hyponatraemia, water retention, nephritis
Clobazam	Sedation, dizziness, weakness, blurring of vision, restlessness, ataxia, aggressiveness, behavioural disturbance, withdrawal symptoms
Clonazepam	Sedation (common and may be severe), cognitive effects, drowsiness, ataxia, personality and behavioural changes, hyperactivity, restlessness, aggressiveness, psychotic reaction, seizure exacerbations, hypersalivation, leucopenia, withdrawal symptoms
Ethosuximide	Gastrointestinal symptoms, drowsiness, ataxia, diplopia, headache, sedation, behavioural disturbances, acute psychotic reactions, extra-pyramidal symptoms, blood dyscrasia, rash, systemic lupus erythematosus
Felbamate	Severe hepatic disturbance and aplastic anaemia are rare but serious side-effects. Insomnia, weight loss, gastrointestinal symptoms, fatigue, dizziness, lethargy, behavioural change, ataxia, visual disturbance, mood change, psychotic reaction, rash, neurological symptoms
Gabapentin	Drowsiness, dizziness, seizure exacerbation, ataxia, headache, tremor, diplopia, nausea, vomiting, rhinitis
Lamotrigine	Rash (sometimes severe), headache, blood dyscrasia, ataxia, asthenia, diplopia, nausea, vomiting, dizziness, somnolence, insomnia, depression, psychosis, tremor, hypersensitivity reactions
Levetiracetam	Somnolence, asthenia, infection, dizziness, headache
Oxcarbazepine	Somnolence, headache, dizziness, rash, hyponatraemia, weight gain, alopecia, nausea, gastrointestinal disturbance
Phenobarbital	Sedation, ataxia, dizziness, insomnia, hyperkinesis (children), mood changes (especially depression), aggressiveness, cognitive dysfunction, impotence, reduced libido, folate deficiency, vitamin K and vitamin D deficiency, osteomalacia, Dupuytren's contracture, frozen shoulder, connective-tissue abnormalities, rash
Phenytoin	Ataxia, dizziness, lethargy, sedation, headaches, dyskinesia, acute encephalopathy, hypersensitivity rash, fever, blood dyscrasia, gingival hyperplasia, folate deficiency, megaloblastic anaemia, vitamin K deficiency, thyroid dysfunction, decreased immunoglobulins, mood changes, depression, coarsened facies, hirsutism, peripheral neuropathy, osteomalacia, hypocalcaemia, hormonal dysfunction, loss of libido, connective-tissue alterations, pseudolymphoma, hepatitis, vasculitis, myopathy, coagulation defects, bone marrow hypoplasia
Piracetam	Dizziness, insomnia, nausea, gastrointestinal discomfort, hyperkinesis, weight gain, tremulousness, agitation, drowsiness, rash
Primidone	Acute dizziness and nausea on initiation of therapy. Other side-effects as for phenobarbital
Tiagabine	Dizziness, tiredness, nervousness, tremor, diarrhoea, headaches, confusion, psychosis, flu-like symptoms, ataxia, depression
Topiramate	Dizziness, ataxia, headache, paraesthesia, tremor, somnolence, cognitive dysfunction, confusion, agitation, amnesia, depression, emotional lability, nausea, diarrhoea, diplopia, weight loss
Valproate	Nausea, vomiting, metabolic effects, endocrine effects, severe hepatic toxicity, pancreatitis, drowsiness, cognitive disturbance, aggressiveness, tremor, weakness, encephalopathy, thrombocytopenia, neutropenia, aplastic anaemia, hair thinning and hair loss, weight gain
Vigabatrin	Sedation, dizziness, headache, ataxia, paraesthesia, agitation, amnesia, mood change, depression, psychosis, aggression, confusion, weight gain, tremor, diplopia, severe visual field constriction, diarrhoea

Drug	Main advantages
Carbamazepine	Highly effective and usually well-tolerated therapy
Clobazam	Highly effective in some patients with epilepsy resistant to first-line therapy. Better tolerated than other benzodiazepines
Clonazepam	Useful add-on action, especially in children
Ethosuximide	Well-established treatment for absence epilepsy without the risk of hepatic toxicity carried by valproate
Felbamate	Highly effective novel antiepileptic drug for refractory patients
Gabapentin	Lack of side-effects (especially at low doses) and good pharmacokinetic profile
Lamotrigine	Effective and well tolerated
Levetiracetam	A recently licensed drug which, on the basis of clinical trial evidence, is well-tolerated and highly effective
Oxcarbazepine	Better tolerated and fewer interactions than with carbamazepine
Phenobarbital	Highly effective and cheap antiepileptic drug
Phenytoin	Highly effective and cheap antiepileptic drug
Piracetam	Well tolerated and very effective in some resistant cases
Primidone	Highly effective and cheap antiepileptic drug
Tiagabine	Clinical experience is too limited to define the place of tiagabine in clinical practice, but initial experience is favourable
Topiramate	Highly effective, recently introduced antiepileptic drug
Valproate	Drug of choice in primary generalized epilepsy and a wide spectrum of activity
Vigabatrin	Highly effective recently introduced antiepileptic drug

Drug	Main disadvantages
Carbamazepine	Transient adverse effects on initiating therapy. Occasional severe toxicity
Clobazam	Development of tolerance in as many as 50% of subjects within weeks or months
Clonazepam	Side-effects are sometimes prominent, particularly sedation, tolerance and a withdrawal syndrome
Ethosuximide	Side-effects common
Felbamate	Severe hepatic and aplastic anaemia in occasional patients. Other side-effects also frequent on initial therapy, and in patients on polytherapy
Gabapentin	Lack of therapeutic effect in severe cases. Seizure exacerbation
Lamotrigine	High instance of rash (occasionally severe), and other side-effects
Levetiracetam	Limited experience in routine clinical practice, as it is recently licensed
Oxcarbazepine	25% cross-sensitivity with carbamazepine. Higher incidence of hyponatraemia than with carbamazepine
Phenobarbital	CNS side-effects
Phenytoin	CNS and systemic side-effects
Piracetam	Not effective in many cases
Primidone	CNS side-effects. Also acute reaction on initiation of therapy
Tiagabine	CNS side-effects
Topiramate	CNS side-effects
Valproate	Cognitive effects, weight gain, tremor and hair loss. Potential for severe hepatic and pancreatic disturbance in children
Vigabatrin	CNS side-effects and visual field constriction

Drug	Mechanisms of action
Carbamazepine	Action on neuronal sodium-channel conductance. Also action on monoamine, acetylcholine and NMDA receptors
Clobazam	GABA$_A$ receptor agonist. Also action on ion-channel conductance
Clonazepam	GABA$_A$ receptor agonist. Also action on sodium channel conductance
Ethosuximide	Effects on calcium T-channel conductance
Felbamate	Probably by effect on NMDA receptor (glycine recognition site) and sodium-channel conductance
Gabapentin	Not known. Possible action on calcium channels
Lamotrigine	Blockage of voltage-dependent sodium conductance
Levetiracetam	Not known
Oxcarbazepine	Sodium-channel blockade. Also affects potassium conductance and modulates high-voltage activated calcium-channel activity
Phenobarbital	Enhances activity of GABA$_A$ receptor, depresses glutamate excitability and affects sodium, potassium and calcium conductance
Phenytoin	Blockade of sodium channels and action on calcium and chloride conductance and voltage-dependent neurotransmission
Piracetam	Unclear
Primidone	Enhances activity of GABA$_A$ receptor, depresses glutamate excitability and affects sodium, potassium and calcium conductance
Tiagabine	Inhibits GABA reuptake
Topiramate	Blockade of sodium channels, enhancement of GABA-mediated chloride influx and modulatory effects of the GABA$_A$ receptor and actions at the AMPA receptor
Valproate	Uncertain but may affect GABA glutaminergic activity, calcium (T) conductance and potassium conductance
Vigabatrin	Inhibition of GABA transaminase activity

Drug	Oral bioavailability
Carbamazepine	75–85%
Clobazam	90%
Clonazepam	>80%
Ethosuximide	<100%
Felbamate	90%
Gabapentin	<60%
Lamotrigine	<100%
Levetiracetam	<100%
Oxcarbazepine	<100%
Phenobarbital	80–100%
Phenytoin	95%
Piracetam	<100%
Primidone	<100%
Tiagabine	96%
Topiramate	<100%
Valproate	<100%
Vigabatrin	<100%

Drug	Time to peak levels
Carbamazepine	4–8 h
Clobazam	1–4 h
Clonazepam	1–4 h
Ethosuximide	<4 h
Felbamate	1–4 h
Gabapentin	2–4 h
Lamotrigine	1–3 h
Levetiracetam	0.6–1.3 h
Oxcarbazepine	4–5 h
Phenobarbital	1–3 h (but variable)
Phenytoin	4–12 h
Piracetam	30–40 min
Primidone	3 h
Tiagabine	1 h
Topiramate	2 h
Valproate	1–8 h (dependent on formulation)
Vigabatrin	2 h

Drug	Metabolism and excretion
Carbamazepine	Hepatic epoxidation and then conjugation
Clobazam	Hepatic oxidation and then conjugation
Clonazepam	Hepatic reduction and then acetylation
Ethosuximide	Hepatic oxidation then conjugation
Felbamate	Hepatic hydroxylation and then conjugation (60%); renal excretion as unchanged drug (40%)
Gabapentin	Renal excretion without metabolism
Lamotrigine	Hepatic glucuronidation (without phase I reaction)
Levetiracetam	Partially hydrolysed in the blood to inactive compound
Oxcarbazepine	Hepatic hydroxylation then conjugation
Phenobarbital	Hepatic oxidation, glucosidation and hydroxylation, then conjugation
Phenytoin	Hepatic oxidation and hydroxylation, then conjugation
Piracetam	Renal excretion without metabolism
Primidone	Metabolized to phenobarbital and phenylmethylmalonamide
Tiagabine	Hepatic oxidation then conjugation
Topiramate	Mainly renal excretion without metabolism
Valproate	Hepatic oxidation and then conjugation
Vigabatrin	Renal excretion without metabolism

Drug	Volume of distribution (L/kg)
Carbamazepine	0.8–1.2
Clobazam	–
Clonazepam	2.0
Ethosuximide	0.65
Felbamate	0.75
Gabapentin	0.9
Lamotrigine	0.9–1.3
Levetiracetam	0.5–0.7
Oxcarbazepine	0.3–0.8
Phenobarbital	0.42–0.75
Phenytoin	0.5–0.8
Piracetam	0.6
Primidone	0.6–1.0 (derived phenobarbital)
Tiagabine	1.0
Topiramate	0.6–1.0
Valproate	0.1–0.4
Vigabatrin	0.8

Drug	Elimination half-life
Carbamazepine	5–26 h (but very variable)
Clobazam	10–50 h (clobazam); 50 h (*N*-desmethylclobazam)
Clonazepam	20–80 h
Ethosuximide	30–60 h
Felbamate	20 h (13–30 h; lowest in patients comedicated with enzyme inducers)
Gabapentin	5–9 h
Lamotrigine	30 h (monotherapy approx.); 15 h (enzyme-inducing comedication); 60 h (valproate comedication)
Levetiracetam	6–8 h
Oxcarbazepine	8–10 h (10-monohydroxy metabolite (MHD)
Phenobarbital	75–120 h
Phenytoin	7–42 h (mean, 20 h: dependent on plasma level)
Piracetam	5–6 h
Primidone	5–18 h primidone; 75–120 h derived phenobarbital
Tiagabine	3.8–4.9 h
Topiramate	18–23 h (varies with comedication)
Valproate	4–12 h
Vigabatrin	4–7 h

Drug	Plasma clearance
Carbamazepine	0.133 L/kg/h (but very variable)
Clobazam	–
Clonazepam	0.09 L/kg/h
Ethosuximide	0.010–0.015 L/kg/h
Felbamate	0.027–0.032 L/kg/h (but variable)
Gabapentin	0.120–0.130 L/kg/h
Lamotrigine	0.044–0.084 L/kg/h (but variable)
Levetiracetam	0.6 mL/min/kg
Oxcarbazepine	–
Phenobarbital	0.006–0.009 L/kg/h
Phenytoin	0.003–0.02 L/kg/h (dependent on plasma level)
Piracetam	–
Primidone	0.006–0.009 L/kg/h (derived phenobarbital)
Tiagabine	12.8 L/kg/h
Topiramate	0.022–0.036 L/kg/h
Valproate	0.010–0.115 L/kg/h
Vigabatrin	0.102–0.114 L/kg/h

Drug	Active metabolites
Carbamazepine	Carbamazepine epoxide
Clobazam	*N*-desmethylclobazam
Clonazepam	Nil
Ethosuximide	Nil
Felbamate	Nil
Gabapentin	Nil
Lamotrigine	Nil
Levetiracetam	Nil
Oxcarbazepine	MHD
Phenobarbital	Nil
Phenytoin	Nil
Piracetam	Nil
Primidone	Phenobarbital
Tiagabine	Nil
Topiramate	Nil
Valproate	Nil
Vigabatrin	Nil

Drug	Protein binding
Carbamazepine	75%
Clobazam	83%
Clonazepam	86%
Ethosuximide	Nil
Felbamate	20–25%
Gabapentin	Nil
Lamotrigine	55%
Levetiracetam	Nil
Oxcarbazepine	38% (MHD)
Phenobarbital	45–60%
Phenytoin	70–95%
Piracetam	Nil
Primidone	25% primidone; 45–60% derived phenobarbital
Tiagabine	96%
Topiramate	15%
Valproate	85–95%
Vigabatrin	Nil

Emergency Treatment of Epilepsy: Acute Seizures, Serial Seizures, Seizure Clusters and Status Epilepticus

ACUTE SEIZURES

General measures

Convulsive seizures which are short-lived do not require emergency drug treatment. Nothing can be done to influence the course of the seizure. The sufferer should be made as comfortable as possible, lying down, or eased to the floor if seated, the head should be protected and tight clothing or neckwear released. During the attack, measures should be taken to avoid injury (e.g. from hot radiators, top of stairs, hot water, road traffic). No attempt should be made to open the mouth or force anything between the teeth. After the convulsive movements have subsided, the onlooker should put the person into the recovery position, check that the airway is not obstructed and that there are no injuries. When fully recovered, the patient should be comforted and reassured. An ambulance or emergency treatment is required only if:

• injury has occurred;
• the convulsive movements continue for longer than 10 min, or longer than is customary for the individual patient;
• the patient does not recover consciousness rapidly; or
• the seizures rapidly recur.

Non-convulsive seizures are less dramatic but can still be disturbing to onlookers and embarrassing to the victim. Again, drug treatment is not indicated in short attacks. If consciousness is not lost, the patient should be treated sympathetically and with the minimum of fuss. If consciousness is impaired or in the presence of confusion, it is necessary to prevent injury or danger (for instance, from wandering about), at the same time minimizing restraint which often exacerbates the confusion and causes agitation or occasionally violence.

If a person with epilepsy is likely to have a seizure in any particular situation (for instance, at school or at work) it is usually best to inform those who might be present (e.g. fellow students, colleagues, supervisors, etc.), and to provide simple advice about first-aid measures. This lessens the impact of a sudden epileptic seizure which can be particularly frightening and disturbing if unexpected.

Emergency antiepileptic drug therapy

This is needed in convulsive attacks if the convulsions persist for more than 10 min or longer than is customary for the individual patient. It is usual to give a fast-acting benzodiazepine. The traditional choice is diazepam, administered either intravenously or rectally. Intravenous diazepam is given in its undiluted form at a rate not exceeding 2–5 mg/min, using the Diazemuls formulation. Rectal administration is either as the intravenous preparation infused from a syringe via a plastic catheter, or as the ready-made proprietary rectal tube preparation such as Stesolid which is convenient and easy. Diazepam suppositories should not be used, as absorption is too slow. The adult bolus intravenous or rectal dose is 10–20 mg, and in children the equivalent bolus dose is 0.2–0.3 mg/kg. More recent work has shown that midazolam or lorazepam are alternatives with some advantages over diazepam, although the long experience enjoyed by diazepam is not shared by these other drugs. Lorazepam can be given by an intravenous bolus of 4 mg in adults or 0.1 mg/kg in children, its antiepileptic effect is longer lasting than that of diazepam and the rate of injection is not critical. Midazolam has the advantage that it can be given by intramuscular injection, intranasally or by buccal instillation. A published randomized trial has shown that buccal midazolam has equal efficacy and as rapid an action as rectal diazepam and is more convenient, potentially faster to administer and less stigmatizing. The dose used is 10 mg drawn up into a syringe and instilled into the mouth or between the cheeks and gums.

SERIAL SEIZURES

Serial seizures are defined as seizures recurring at

frequent intervals, with full recovery between attacks—and in the latter sense differ from status epilepticus. The premonitory stage of status epilepticus, however, often takes the form of serial seizures, and drug therapy is advisable if status threatens, even if the individual seizures are short. The emergency antiepileptic drug treatment is as outlined above for acute seizures.

SEIZURES OCCURRING IN CLUSTERS

In some patients, clusters of seizures regularly occur at certain times (for instance, around menstruation). Acute therapy after the first seizure can be given in an attempt to prevent subsequent attacks. Clobazam (10–20 mg) or acetazolamide (250–500 mg per day) are common choices. Both are given orally, and will take effect within 1 h.

A cluster of seizures is sometimes the result of the withdrawal or dose reduction of an antiepileptic drug. The reintroduction of the drug will usually terminate the seizure cluster.

STATUS EPILEPTICUS

Status epilepticus is defined as a condition in which epileptic activity persists for 30 min or more. The seizures can take the form of prolonged seizures or repetitive attacks without recovery in between. There are various types of status epilepticus and classification is controversial. As the clinical forms of status epilepticus are dependent on age, seizure type, underlying aetiology and underlying pathophysiology, a composite classification has been proposed and this is outlined in Table 5.1.

Tonic–clonic status epilepticus
Tonic–clonic status epilepticus is defined as a condition in which prolonged or recurrent tonic–clonic seizures persist for 30 min or more. The annual incidence of tonic–clonic status has been estimated to be approximately 18–28 cases per 100 000 persons. It occurs most commonly in children, people with learning difficulties and in those with structural cerebral pathology, especially in the frontal lobes. Most episodes of status epilepticus develop *de novo*, without a prior history of epilepsy, and in such cases are almost always caused by acute cerebral events; common causes are cerebral infection, trauma, cerebrovascular disease, cerebral tumour, acute toxic or metabolic disturbances, or childhood febrile illness.

Table 5.1 Revised classification of status epilepticus.

Status epilepticus confined to early childhood
Neonatal status epilepticus
Status epilepticus in specific neonatal epilepsy
   syndromes
Infantile spasms

Status epilepticus confined to later childhood
Febrile status epilepticus
Status in childhood partial epilepsy syndromes
Status epilepticus in myoclonic–astatic epilepsy
Electrical status epilepticus during slow wave sleep
Landau–Kleffner syndrome

Status epilepticus occurring in childhood and adult life
Tonic–clonic status epilepticus
Absence status epilepticus
Epilepsia partialis continua
Status epilepticus in coma
Specific forms of status epilepticus in learning
   difficulty
Syndromes of myoclonic status epilepticus
Simple partial status epilepticus
Complex partial status epilpeticus

Status epilepticus confined to adult life
De novo absence status and late onset

In patients with pre-existing epilepsy, status epilepticus can be precipitated by drug withdrawal, intercurrent illness or metabolic disturbance, or the progression of the underlying disease, and is more common in symptomatic than in idiopathic epilepsy (Table 5.2). About 5% of all adult patients attending an epilepsy clinic will have at least one episode of status in the course of their epilepsy, and in children the proportion is higher (10–25%).

There is often a premonitory stage of several hours, during which epileptic activity increases in frequency or severity from its habitual level. This clinical deterioration is a warning of impending status, and urgent therapy at this stage can prevent full-blown status. At the onset of status, the attacks typically take the form of discrete tonic–clonic seizures, the motor activity becomes continuous, the jerking becomes less pronounced and finally ceases altogether. This is the stage of 'subtle status epilepticus' by which time the patient will be deeply unconscious. There is also sometimes a progressive change in the electroencephalogram (EEG). This state can persist for days if left untreated (or partially treated) and will eventually result in death.

The physiological changes in status can be divided into two phases, the transition from phase 1 to 2

Table 5.2 Aetiology of status epilepticus in 554 patients from 5 case series.

Underlying aetiology	No previous history of epilepsy (%)	Previous history of epilepsy (%)	All patients (%)
Cerebral trauma	12	17	14
Cerebral tumour	16	10	13
Cerebrovascular disease	20	19	20
Intracranial infection	15	6	11
Acute metabolic disturbance	12	5	9
Other acute event	14	3	10
No cause found	11	41	23

occurring after about 30–60 min of continuous seizures (see Table 5.3 and Fig. 5.1).

Phase 1 (Phase of compensation). As the status develops, cerebral metabolism is markedly increased. Homeostatic physiological mechanisms are initially sufficient to compensate for these changes. There is a massive increase in cerebral blood flow, and the delivery of glucose to the active cerebral tissue is maintained. Systemic and cerebral lactate levels rise, and a profound lactic acidosis may develop. Endocrine changes result in initial hyperglycaemia. Blood pressure rises, as does cardiac output and rate. Massive autonomic activity results in sweating, hyperpyrexia, bronchial secretion, salivation and vomiting, and epinephrine (adrenaline) and norepinephrine (noradrenaline) release.

Phase 2 (Phase of decompensation). Compensatory physiological mechanisms begin to fail as seizure activity continues. Cerebral autoregulation breaks down progressively, and thus cerebral blood flow becomes increasingly dependent on systemic blood pressure. Hypotension develops because of seizure-related autonomic and cardiorespiratory changes and drug treatment, and in terminal stages may be severe. The falling blood pressure results in falling cerebral blood flow and cerebral metabolism. The high metabolic demands of the epileptic cerebral tissue cannot be met and this results in ischaemic or metabolic damage. The hypotension can be greatly exacerbated by intravenous antiepileptic drug therapy, especially if infusion rates are too fast.

Other common problems in status epilepticus are hypoxia and cardiac dyrhythmias, both of which may require urgent therapy. Intracranial pressure can rise dramatically in late status, and the combined effects of systemic hypotension and intracranial hypertension can result in a compromised cerebral circulation and cerebral oedema, particularly in children. Pulmonary hypertension and pulmonary oedema occur, and pulmonary artery pressures can exceed the osmotic pressure of blood, causing oedema and stretch injuries to lung capillaries. Cardiac output can fall because of decreasing left ventricular contractility and stroke volume, and cardiac failure. Profound hyperpyrexia is also a risk in tonic–clonic status.

At the onset of status autonomic changes are prominent and sometimes profound. There are also many metabolic and endocrine disturbances in status, the most common and most important are: acidosis (including lactic acidosis), hypoglycaemia, hypo- and hyperkalaemia and hyponatraemia. Lactic acidosis is almost invariable in tonic–clonic status epilepticus from its onset. Other potentially fatal metabolic complications include acute tubular necrosis, renal failure, hepatic failure and disseminated intravascular coagulation. Rhabdomyolysis, resulting from persistent convulsive movements, can precipitate renal failure if severe. This can be prevented by artificial ventilation and muscle paralysis.

The mortality of tonic–clonic status is about 5–10%, most patients dying of the underlying condition, rather than the status itself or its treatment. In the phase of decompensation (but not of compensation), tonic–clonic status epilepticus also carries a significant risk of causing cerebral damage and morbidity. Permanent epilepsy follows in over 75% of children who develop staus without a history of epilepsy, and in a smaller proportion of adults. In patients with a prior history of epilepsy, the epilepsy is often worse after an episode of status. Neurological deterioration and also focal neurological deficit (e.g. hemiparesis) can follow status, as can mental and intellectual determination. The risks are greatest in young children, and are greatly increased the longer the duration of the status episode.

Phase I: compensation

During this phase, cerebral metabolism is greatly increased because of seizure activity, but physiological mechanisms are sufficient to meet the metabolic demands, and cerebral tissue is protected from hypoxia or metabolic damage. The major physiological changes are related to the greatly increased cerebral blood flow and metabolism, massive autonomic activity and cardiovascular changes.

Cerebral changes	Systemic and metabolic changes	Autonomic and cardiovascular changes
Increased blood flow	Hyperglycaemia	Hypertension (initial)
Increased metabolism	Lactic acidosis	Increased cardiac output
Energy requirements matched by supply of oxygen and glucose (increased glucose and oxygen utilization)		Increased central venous pressure
		Massive catecholamine release
Increased lactate concentration		Tachycardia
		Cardiac dysrhythmia
Increased glucose concentration		Salivation
		Hyperpyrexia
		Vomiting
		Incontinence

Phase II: decompensation

During this phase, the greatly increased cerebral metabolic demands cannot be fully met, resulting in hypoxia and altered cerebral and systemic metabolic patterns. Autonomic changes persist and cardiorespiratory functions may progressively fail to maintain homeostasis.

Cerebral changes	Systemic and metabolic changes	Autonomic and cardiovascular changes
Failure of cerebral autoregulation; thus cerebral blood flow becomes dependent on systemic blood pressure	Hypoglycaemia	Systemic hypoxia
	Hyponatraemia	Falling blood pressure
	Hypokalaemia/ hyperkalaemia	Falling cardiac output
Hypoxia	Metabolic and respiratory acidosis	Respiratory and cardiac impairment (pulmonary oedema, pulmonary embolism, respiratory collapse, cardiac failure, dysrrhythmia)
Hypoglycaemia		
Falling lactate concentrations	Hepatic and renal dysfunction	
Falling energy state	Consumptive coagulopathy, DIC, multiorgan failure	Hyperpyrexia
Rise in intracranial pressure and cerebral oedema	Rhabdomyolysis, myoglobulinuria	
	Leucocytosis	

DIC, disseminated intravascular coagulopathy.

Note: the physiological changes listed above do not necessarily occur in all cases. The type and extent of the changes depend on aetiology, clinical circumstances and the methods of therapy employed.

Table 5.3 Physiological changes in tonic–clonic status epilepticus.

Fig. 5.1 Temporal changes which occur as tonic–clonic status epilepticus progresses. Motor activity lessens, the electroencephalogram (EEG) evolves and profound physiological changes occur, both systemically and cerebrally. In the first 30 min or so, physiological changes are largely compensatory, but as the seizures continue these compensatory mechanisms break down. The biphasic evolution is emphasized. PED, periodic epileptic discharge; 1, loss of reactivity of brain oxygen tension; 2, mismatch between the sustained increase in oxygen and glucose utilization and a fall in cerebral blood flow; 3, a depletion of cerebral glucose and glycogen concentrations; 4, a decline in cerebral energy state.

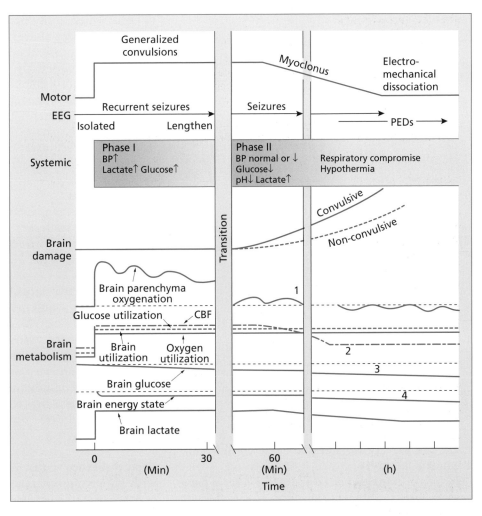

Epilepsia partialis continua

This form of status epilepticus can be defined as spontaneous regular or irregular clonic muscle jerking of cerebral cortical origin, sometimes aggravated by action or sensory stimuli, confined to one part of the body, and continuing for hours, days or weeks. There are many potential causes (Table 5.4).

The clonic jerks in epilepsia partialis continua can affect any muscle group. In some individuals, they are confined to a single muscle or muscle group, but in others the distribution is more widespread, and the distribution of the jerks can vary over time. Agonists and antagonists are affected together, and distal muscles are more commonly involved than proximal musculature. The jerks are spontaneous and often exacerbated on action, startle or sensory stimuli. They can be single or cluster, may have a rhythmic quality and a wide range of frequencies and amplitudes. Some jerks recur only every few minutes and others are more frequent. In chronic cases the jerks can have continued relentlessly for months or years.

Complex partial status epilepticus

This form of non-convulsive status can be defined as a prolonged epileptic episode in which fluctuating or frequently recurring focal electrographic epileptic discharges result in a confusional state. There are highly variable clinical symptoms, and the focal epileptic discharges may arise in temporal or extratemporal cortical regions.

Confusion is the leading clinical feature of complex partial status. This can fluctuate or be fairly continuous. The severity of the confusion can vary from profound stupor with little response to external stimuli in some cases, to others in whom subtle abnormalities on cognitive testing are the only sign. Amnesia is usual but not invariable. Associated with the confusion are behavioural changes, speech and language disturbance, motor and autonomic features.

Table 5.4 Causes of epilepsia partialis continua.

Cerebral tumour	Metastasis
	Primary tumour
Cerebral infection	Abscess
	Tuberculoma
	Parasitic mass (e.g. cysticercosis)
	Viral encephalitis
	Meningo-encephalitis
Cerebral inflammatory disease	Rasmussen's chronic encephalitis
	Granuloma
Cerebrovascular disease	Cerebral infarction
	Cerebral haemorrhage/ haematoma
	Arterio-venous malformation
	Venous thrombosis
	Cavernous haemangioma
Other cerebral disorders	Cerebral tumour
	Cortical dysgenesis
	Mitochondrial disease
Drug-induced	Penicillin
	Cefotaxime
	Metrizamide

These can be very variable and cause considerable diagnostic difficulty.

Periods of complex partial status can last for days or even weeks, although typically an episode will persist for several hours. It is most common in adults, usually with long histories of complex partial epilepsy. Precipitating factors include menstruation, alcohol and drug withdrawal; but not usually photic stimulation or overbreathing as in typical absence status. The onset and offset are usually less well defined than in absence status, and the response to intravenous therapy more gradual. Complex partial status may follow in the aftermath of a secondarily generalized tonic–clonic seizure (or cluster of seizures), but is rarely terminated by a generalized convulsion, in contrast to typical absence status. Episodes of complex partial status are usually recurrent, and occasionally there is a remarkable periodicity. Complex partial status can arise in focal epilepsies of widely varying aetiologies.

The abnormalities on scalp EEG may be slight although the EEG is seldom normal. A whole range of EEG patterns are seen including continuous or frequent spike or spikes/slow wave, or spike/wave par-oxysms which are sometimes widespread or focal, and also episodes of desynchronization. The longer the status proceeds, the less likely is discrete ictal activity to be noticeable.

The prognosis of complex partial status is good. It is not usually life-threatening, and resolves with oral or intravenous therapy. There is, however, a strong tendency for recurrence. Permanent neurological or psychological sequelae are rare, in contrast to the poor prognosis of tonic–clonic status.

Absence status

Absence status can be best subdivided into at least two separate syndromes, with overlapping clinical and EEG features. Both should be distinguished from complex partial status which can take a similar clinical form.

• Typical absence status: non-convulsive status, occurring in the syndrome of idiopathic generalized epilepsy.
• Atypical absence status: status that occurs largely in secondarily generalized epilepsy of the Lennox–Gastaut type, and also in other patients with compromised cerebral function.

Whilst this is a tidy classification scheme, there are transitional cases which do not fit happily into either category.

Typical absence status. This occurs only in patients with idiopathic generalized epilepsy, and a history of absence status occurs in about 3–9% of patients with a history of typical absences. The attacks can recur, and can last for hours or occasionally days. Precipitating features are common and include menstruation, withdrawal of medication, hypoglycaemia, hyperventilation, flashing or bright lights, sleep deprivation, fatigue and stress. The principal clinical feature is clouding of consciousness. This can vary from slight clouding to profound stupor. At one extreme, patients have nothing more than slowed ideation and expression, and deficits in activities requiring sustained attention, sequential organization or spatial structuring. Amnesia may be slight or even absent. At the other extreme, there may be immobility, mutism, simple voluntary actions performed only after repeated requests, long delays in verbal responses, monosyllabic and hesitant speech. Typically, the patient is in an expressionless, trance-like state with slow responses and a stumbling gait. Motor features occur in about 50% of cases, including myoclonus, atonia, rhythmic eyelid blinking, quivering of the lips and face. Facial, especially eyelid, myoclonus is common in absence status, but rare in complex partial status. Episodes of absence status are often terminated by a tonic–clonic seizure. The diagnostic electrographic pattern is continuous or almost continuous bilaterally synchronous and symmetrical spike/wave activity.

Atypical absence status. This form of status is common in patients with diffuse cerebral damage and is typically seen as part of the Lennox–Gastaut syndrome. Although the clinical phenomenology of typical and atypical absence status overlap greatly, there are important differences. The clinical context is very different; typical absence status occurs in patients without intellectual deterioration, very unlike the clinical picture of the Lennox–Gastaut syndrome. The episodes of atypical absence status are usually longer and more frequent, with a gradual onset and offset. Atypical absence status is often preceded by changes in motor activity, mood or intellectual ability, for hours or days before the overt seizures develop. This prodromal stage might be caused by subclinical status. Atypical absence status tends to fluctuate and minor motor, myoclonic or, more typically, tonic seizures interrupt, but do not terminate an episode. In some patients, the mental state fluctuates gradually in and out of this ill-defined epileptic state over long periods of time—some attacks last weeks or even months—with little distinction possible between ictal and interictal phases. Unlike typical absence status, tonic–clonic seizures seldom occur at the beginning or end of the status episode, and atypical absence status often responds poorly to injection of a benzodiazepine. Indeed antiepileptic drug therapy has little effect, and the condition fluctuates apparently uninfluenced by external factors. Atypical absence status is more likely to occur if the patient is drowsy or understimulated, and it is thus important not to overmedicate these patients. The EEG during atypical absence status may show continuous irregular slow (2 Hz) spike/wave, hypsarrhythmia or more discrete ictal patterns.

DRUG PHARMACOKINETICS

Acute drug pharmacokinetics

Fast drug absorption is essential in the treatment of status epilepticus, and thus almost all drugs need to be administered parenterally. Paraldehyde and midazolam can be given intramuscularly, and diazepam and paraldehyde rectally. All the others must be given by intravenous injection.

In order to act rapidly, the drugs need to cross the blood–brain barrier readily. Drugs achieve this either by being lipid-soluble or by having an active transport mechanism. Thus most drugs that are effective in status epilepticus have a high lipid solubility. This lipid solubility has one drawback, a tendency to redistribution.

During parenteral administration, a drug directly enters the central compartment (blood and extracellular fluid of highly perfused organs) and from here it is distributed to peripheral compartments, in particular fat and muscle. As most of these drugs are highly lipid-soluble, they are rapidly redistributed into the peripheral compartment from the central compartment. This leads to an initial drop in plasma concentrations, which can be quantified as a distribution half-life. In addition, the drug may be eliminated from the central compartment either through renal excretion, hepatic metabolism (the major route of elimination for most antiepileptic drugs) or exhalation, at a rate that can be quantified as the elimination half-life. The antiepileptic drugs used in status epilepticus have a much shorter distribution half-life than elimination half-life (Fig. 5.2). Thus, following acute administration, the initial fall in plasma levels and brain levels, and hence loss of activity, as measured by the distribution half-life can be relatively rapid. This has led to the practice of repeat boluses or infusions in order to maintain adequate plasma levels. However, persistent administration leads to accumulation of the drug within the peripheral compartment, and this has two important effects.
• The peripheral compartment becomes saturated, the drug no longer redistributes, and thus its clearance from the central compartment becomes solely dependent on the elimination half-life (Fig. 5.3).
• The drug accumulated in the peripheral compartment can act as a reservoir, such that following prolonged administration the plasma levels may be maintained by diffusion from the peripheral compartment back into the central compartment, even if drug administration has ceased (Fig. 5.3).

These two effects are commonly seen. For example, following intravenous administration of a diazepam bolus, there is a transient peak level and then a rapid fall in plasma levels due to redistribution, resulting in recurrence of the seizures. If repeat bo-

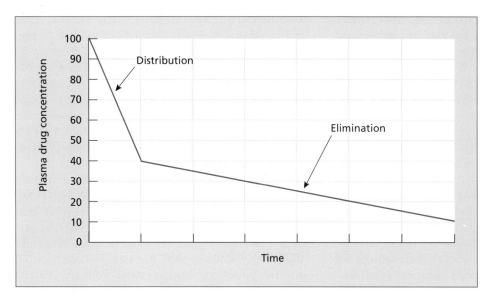

Fig. 5.2 Lipid soluble drugs: the two phases of fall in plasma drug concentration.

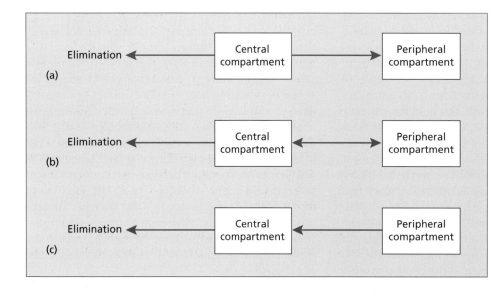

Fig. 5.3 (a) Following initial injection into the central (blood) compartment, drug distributes into the peripheral compartment, and the plasma half-life is mainly determined by this distribution. (b) During an infusion, the peripheral compartment and central compartment eventually reach equilibrium. The plasma half-life is then determined by elimination. (c) When the infusion is stopped, drug diffuses from the peripheral compartment into the central compartment, thus prolonging the half-life.

luses are given, the peripheral compartment becomes saturated, and the rapid redistribution from the central compartment to the peripheral compartment does not readily occur. Plasma half-life increases as it becomes solely dependent on elimination. This leads to a prolongation of the action, and further boluses lead to persistently very high brain levels, which may result in cardiorespiratory collapse. With prolonged infusion, the saturated peripheral compartment acts as a reservoir for the drug and, even after stopping an infusion, plasma and brain levels are maintained by diffusion from this compartment. The patient may thus remain obtunded for a much longer period than would necessarily be predicted from the elimination half-life. These effects are potentially very dangerous, and some of the mortality and morbidity of status epilepticus are caused by injudicious use of repeated boluses or continuous infusions of lipid-soluble drugs.

Kinetics of drugs during seizures

Seizures—especially convulsive seizures—may affect both the peripheral and the central pharmacokinetics of drugs. During convulsive seizures, there is a fall in the pH of the blood, resulting in a change in the degree of ionization, and thus lipid solubility, of drugs in plasma. This will affect their distribution half-lives, their ability to cross the blood–brain barrier and their protein binding. In addition, the pH in blood decreases to a greater degree than in the brain; this pH gradient facilitates the movement of a weakly acid drug from blood to brain. This effect occurs, for instance, with phenobarbital. Other, peripheral pharmacokinetic effects are also apparent during status epilepticus. These may result from increased blood flow to muscle and from hepatic and renal compromise. Status epilepticus can result in a breakdown in the blood–brain barrier during convulsive seizures, which again results in more effective brain penetration of anticonvulsant drugs. During seizures there is increased blood flow to the seizing brain; thus drugs in which the cortical blood flow determines the rate at which the drug crosses the blood–brain barrier (e.g. phenobarbital) will concentrate preferentially in active seizure foci.

Brain pharmacokinetics

It is an obvious, but often forgotten point, that the critical drug concentration is the concentration at the point of action (e.g. synapses, receptors, etc.). Plasma concentrations may be a poor indication of this concentration and this is especially so with acute administration. Additionally, it is not enough to picture the brain as a single compartment. The brain consists of extracellular, intracellular, lipid and cerebrospinal fluid compartments. The presence of these compartments may lead to complex kinetic effects which can be predicted from a knowledge of plasma kinetics. This is certainly seen in the case of phenytoin, where there may be increasing extracellular brain levels despite falling plasma levels. Unfortunately, the acute pharmacokinetic properties of antiepileptic drugs in compartments of interest are not well described. This contrasts with the situation after chronic administration (i.e. when a steady state is achieved), when the plasma kinetics give a useful index of the brain kinetics.

THE MANAGEMENT OF TONIC–CLONIC STATUS EPILEPTICUS

General measures

Cardiorespiratory function

In all patients presenting in status, the protection of cardiorespiratory function takes first priority. Cardiorespiratory function should be assessed, the airway secured and resuscitation carried out if necessary. Hypoxia is usually much worse than appreciated, and oxygen should always be administered.

Emergency investigations

Blood should be taken for measurement of arterial blood gases, glucose, renal and liver function, calcium and magnesium, full blood count, clotting screen and anticonvulsant levels. Serum should be saved for possible future analysis. An electrocardiogram (ECG) should be performed.

Monitoring

Regular neurological observations, pulse, blood pressure and temperature need to be taken. Continuous ECG monitoring and oximetry are necessary, and regular measurements of glucose, electrolytes, arterial blood gases and pH should be performed.

Emergency drug treatment

Emergency drug treatment should be started (see below).

Intravenous glucose and thiamine

If there is any suspicion of hypoglycaemia, 50 mL of 50% glucose should be given intravenously. In anyone with a history of poor nutrition or alcoholism, 250 mg of thiamine should be administered intravenously. This is especially important if intravenous glucose is going to be given, as glucose infusions can precipitate Wernicke's encephalopathy in susceptible individuals. There is some evidence that glucose, given to a normoglycaemic person, will worsen or intensify the status. For this reason, sugar should only be given if there are good grounds for suspecting hypoglycaemia.

Correction of metabolic abnormalities

Correction of severe metabolic abnormalities is best managed on the intensive care unit (ICU). Acidosis is a common complication of status epilepticus, and is usually corrected through the rapid control of respiration and the abolition of motor seizure activity. In severe acidosis, however, bicarbonate infusion should be given. Hyperthermia may be treated by successful abolition of the motor seizure activity.

Hypotension and cardiac dysrhythmias

Hypotension results from the status epilepticus itself, and most of the drugs used in the treatment of status epilepticus exacerbate this problem. As the cerebral blood flow becomes dependent on systemic blood pressure, maintenance of the blood pressure is of paramount importance and pressor agents are indicated; this is especially so if barbiturate anaesthesia is used. Continuous ECG monitoring is mandatory as dysrhythmias and other ECG abnormalities are commonplace in prolonged status, and are associated with a high mortality. Electrocardiogram monitoring should be continued for at least 24 h after the status epilepticus has stopped.

Respiratory compromise

This can result not only from the continued seizure activity and from pulmonary oedema, but also from the drugs used. There should be a low threshold for intubation and initiating ventilatory support. The use of subanaesthetic doses of anaesthetic agents without the rapid availability of ventilatory support is not to be recommended. Aspiration pneumonia is not an uncommon problem and, if suspected, broad-spectrum antibiotics should be started.

Hypoglycaemia

This is common in the later stages of status epilepticus. It should not, however, be routinely corrected with glucose, unless severe. Hyperglycaemia in the later stages of status epilepticus may result in an increase in cerebral damage and mild hypoglycaemia can be neuroprotective.

Hyperthermia and lactic acidosis

These are usually controlled by halting the motor seizure activity, but, if these persist despite adequate treatment, paralysing agents may be indicated. Sodium bicarbonate can be used in severe cases of acidosis, but is a large sodium load and can compound the problems of cerebral and pulmonary oedema. Cooling is indicated if the temperature rises above 40 °C.

Rhabdomyolysis

This can be prevented by halting motor seizure activity and maintaining serum electrolyte concentrations. If it occurs, it may lead to myoglobinuria, acute renal failure and life-threatening hyperkalaemia. Provided that the acute electrolyte disturbances are adequately dealt with, the prognosis for the renal failure in this circumstance is usually good.

Renal and hepatic failure

A number of factors in status epilepticus may be involved in the aetiology of acute renal failure, including myoglobinuria, disseminated intravascular coagulation, hypoxia and hypotension. In the early stages of renal failure there may be benefit in giving mannitol and a dopamine infusion. Electrolytes and renal function should always be closely monitored. Acute hepatic failure too can have various causes, including hypersensitivity reactions to administered drugs. Care should be taken to avoid these drugs in cases with a prior history of drug hypersensitivity.

Cerebral oedema

This may be a complication in the later stages, and continuous intracranial pressure monitoring is advisable in certain situations, especially in children. Depending on the underlying cause, active therapy with dexamethasone or mannitol may be necessary, and occasionally neurosurgical decompression is required.

Establish aetiology

The outcome of status to a great extent depends on the aetiology, and the urgent treatment of causative factors is vital. Computed tomography (CT) scanning and cerebrospinal fluid examination are often necessary, but the choice of investigations depends on the clinical circumstances.

Other complications

Some of the complications encountered in tonic–clonic status are listed in Table 5.5 and these often need emergency treatment in their own right. Failure to treat can perpetuate the status and worsen the outcome.

Intensive care and seizure monitoring

If seizures are continuing in spite of the measures taken above, the patient must be transferred to an intensive care setting, where intensive monitoring can be performed, including intra-arterial blood pressure, capnography, oximetry, central venous pressure and Swan–Ganz monitoring.

Motor activity in status diminishes over time, and may cease in spite of ongoing epileptic electrographic activity. Neurophysiological monitoring can thus be the only way of detecting electrographic activity. The electrographic activity is potentially damaging to the cortical neurones and anaesthetic therapy is targeted to suppress it by the attainment of the anaesthetic level of burst suppression (see below). Both ongoing epileptic activity and also burst suppression require neurophysiological monitoring and this can be provided by either a full EEG or a cerebral function monitor (CFM). The CFM has to be calibrated for each individual patient, but then has the advantage over EEG of simplicity of use. Burst suppression provides an arbitrary physiological target for the titration of barbiturate or anaesthetic therapy, with drug dosage set at a level to produce interburst intervals of between 2 and 30 s.

If there is evidence of persisting, severe or progressively elevated intracranial pressure (ICP), ICP mon-

Table 5.5 Medical complications in tonic–clonic status epilepticus.

Cerebral
Hypoxic/metabolic cerebral damage
Seizure-induced cerebral damage
Cerebral oedema and raised intercranial pressure
Cerebral venous thrombosis
Cerebral haemorrhage and infarction

Cardiorespiratory and autonomic
Hypotension
Hypertension
Cardiac failure, tachy- and bradydysrhythmia, cardiac arrest, cardiogenic shock
Respiratory failure
Disturbances of respiratory rate and rhythm, apnoea
Pulmonary oedema, hypertension, embolism, pneumonia, aspiration
Hyperpyrexia
Sweating, hypersecretion tracheobronchial obstruction
Peripheral ischaemia

Metabolic and systemic
Dehydration
Electrolyte disturbance (especially hyponatraemia, hyperkalaemia, hypoglycaemia)
Acute renal failure (especially acute tubular necrosis)
Acute hepatic failure
Acute pancreatitis

Other
Disseminated intravascular coagulopathy/multi-organ failure
Rhabdomyolysis
Fractures
Infections (especially pulmonary, skin, urinary)
Thrombophlebitis, dermal injury

---

itoring is advisable in some patients. The need for this is usually determined by the underlying cause rather than the status, and its use is more common in children. If ICP is critically raised, intermittent positive pressure ventilation, high-dose corticosteroid therapy (4 mg dexamethasone every 6 h), or mannitol infusion can be used to lower the pressure, and neurosurgical decompression is occasionally required.

Drug treatment

Convulsive status epilepticus can be temporally divided, both clinically and electrographically, into four stages, each requiring a distinctive therapeutic approach. The risk of status-induced brain damage is greatest after several hours of continuous seizure activity, and increases the longer the status persists. For this reason, stage 4 therapy (general anaesthesia) should be administered within 1–2 h after the onset of status if prior treatment has been unsuccessful.

Choosing the best drug treatment for each stage of status epilepticus is difficult, because of the lack of good comparative trials, the contradictory anecdotal reports of the use of various agents and the diversity of advice in the numerous reviews on the subject.

Nevertheless, it is mandatory to have a protocol for the treatment of status epilepticus as this simple measure has itself been shown to reduce mortality and morbidity, regardless of the treatment options chosen. Figure 5.4 outlines the protocol favoured by the author.

Premonitory stage of status epilepticus

Both in animal models and in human convulsive status epilepticus, there is often a prodromal period. During this period there is a gradual increase in the frequency of tonic–clonic seizures or of myoclonic jerking (Table 5.6). Parenteral drug treatment in this phase will often prevent the development of full-blown status, and the earlier treatment is given the more successful it is. If the patient is at home, antiepileptic drugs should be administered before transfer to hospital, or in the casualty department before transfer to the ward. Carers can be trained in the administration of emergency therapy to persons who have frequent or prolonged attacks. However, acute parenteral therapy will cause drowsiness or sleep, and occasionally cardiorespiratory collapse, and should therefore be carefully supervised.

The drugs used include rectal or intravenous diazepam, buccal, intranasal or intramuscular midazolam, intravenous lorazepam or rectal paraldehyde. All are highly effective and the choice will depend on local circumstances. Carers or non-medical personnel can sometimes be trained in the use of rectal diazepam, paraldehyde or buccal midazolam. Rectal diazepam is available in a very convenient formulation with a ready-prepared syringe and catheter. Similarly, buccal or intranasal midazolam is easy and quick to administer, and is especially useful for children.

Stage of early status epilepticus

This is defined as the first 30 min of status. It is usual to initiate treatment with a fast-acting benzodiazepine drug. Intravenous lorazepam is the drug of choice, at least in older children and adults. It is longer acting than other benzodiazepines, safer to admin-

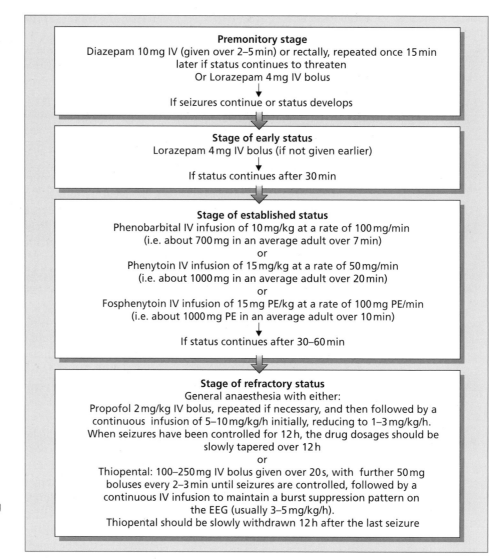

Fig. 5.4 Emergency drug treatment of status in adults. PE, phenytoin equivalent.

Within the figure:

Premonitory stage
Diazepam 10 mg IV (given over 2–5 min) or rectally, repeated once 15 min later if status continues to threaten
Or Lorazepam 4 mg IV bolus

If seizures continue or status develops

Stage of early status
Lorazepam 4 mg IV bolus (if not given earlier)

If status continues after 30 min

Stage of established status
Phenobarbital IV infusion of 10 mg/kg at a rate of 100 mg/min
(i.e. about 700 mg in an average adult over 7 min)
or
Phenytoin IV infusion of 15 mg/kg at a rate of 50 mg/min
(i.e. about 1000 mg in an average adult over 20 min)
or
Fosphenytoin IV infusion of 15 mg PE/kg at a rate of 100 mg PE/min
(i.e. about 1000 mg PE in an average adult over 10 min)

If status continues after 30–60 min

Stage of refractory status
General anaesthesia with either:
Propofol 2 mg/kg IV bolus, repeated if necessary, and then followed by a continuous infusion of 5–10 mg/kg/h initially, reducing to 1–3 mg/kg/h. When seizures have been controlled for 12 h, the drug dosages should be slowly tapered over 12 h
or
Thiopental: 100–250 mg IV bolus given over 20 s, with further 50 mg boluses every 2–3 min until seizures are controlled, followed by a continuous IV infusion to maintain a burst suppression pattern on the EEG (usually 3–5 mg/kg/h).
Thiopental should be slowly withdrawn 12 h after the last seizure

ister intravenously, and carries less risk of cardiorespiratory depression. Alternatives include other intravenous benzodiazepines or intravenous lidocaine, the latter drug may be preferable in patients with respiratory disease. Subanaesthetic doses of propofol have recently been shown to be effective and safe in terminating early status, but experience is limited. In most episodes of status, initial therapy treatment will be highly effective. Even if seizures cease, 24-h inpatient observation should follow. In persons without a previous history of epilepsy, chronic antiepileptic drug treatment should be introduced, and in those already on maintenance antiepileptic therapy, this should be reviewed.

Stage of established status epilepticus
Once the seizures have continued for 30 min, the stage of established status epilepticus is entered. It is practical also to define this period as that which occurs where early stage treatment has failed, or when no accurate estimate of the duration of seizures can be made.

There are three alternative first-line treatment options, but each has drawbacks and status at this stage carries an appreciable morbidity. These are subanaesthetic doses of phenobarbital, or phenytoin or fosphenytoin. All three are given by intravenous loading, and followed by repeated oral (phenytoin or phenobarbital) or intravenous supplementation.

Subanaesthetic infusions of benzodiazepine drugs were once fashionable in the stage of established status. The infusions can result in dangerous respiratory depression and hypotension, or sudden collapse. For all these reasons, benzodiazepine infusions should not be given. Clomethiazole infusion has been frequently used in the treatment of status, but carries

Table 5.6 Drug dosages for convulsive status epilepticus.

Drug	Route	Adult dose	Paediatric dose
Clomethiazole	IV infusion of 0.8% solution	40–100 mL (320–800 mg) at 5–15 mL/min, then 0.5–20 mL/min	0.1 mL/kg/min increasing every 2–4 h as required
Clonazepam	IV bolus	1 mg at <2 mg/min*	250–500 µg at <2 mg/min
	IV infusion	Maintenance dose: 10 mg/24 h	
Diazepam	IV bolus	10–20 mg at <5 mg/min*	0.25–0.5 mg/kg at <2–5 mg/min
	Rectal administration	10–30 mg*	0.5.–0.75 mg/kg
	IV infusion	3 mg/kg/day	200–300 µg/kg/day
Fosphenytoin	IV bolus	15 mg PE/kg at a rate of <100–150 mg PE/min Maintenance dose: 4–5 mg/kg/day IV or IM	
Isoflurane	Inhalation	End tidal concentrations of 0.8–2% to maintain burst suppression	
Lidocaine	IV bolus	1.5–2.0 mg/kg at <50 mg/min*	
	IV infusion	Maintenance dose: 3–4 mg/kg/h	
Lorazepam	IV bolus	4 mg*	0.1 mg/kg
Midazolam	IM or rectally	5–10 mg*	0.15–0.3 mg/kg*
	IV bolus	0.1–0.3 mg/kg at <4 mg/min*	
	IV infusion	0.05–0.4 mg/kg/h	
	Buccal	10 mg	10 mg
Paraldehyde	Rectally or IM	5–10 mL (approx. 1 g/mL) in equal vol. of water*	0.07–0.35 mL/kg*
Pentobarbital	IV infusion	5–20 mg/kg at a rate of <25 mg/min, then 0.5–1.0 mg/kg/h increasing to 1–3 mg/kg/h	
Phenobarbital	IV bolus	10 mg/kg at a rate of <100 mg/min	15–20 mg/kg at a rate of <100 mg/min
		Maintenance: 1–4 mg/kg/day	3–4 mg/kg/day
Phenytoin	IV bolus/infusion	15–18 mg/kg at a rate of <50 mg/kg	20 mg/kg at a rate of <25 mg/min
Propofol	IV infusion	2 mg/kg, then 5–10 mg/kg/h initially, reducing to 1–3 mg/kg/h to maintain burst suppression	
Thiopental	IV infusion	100–250 mg bolus given over 20 s, then further 50 mg boluses every 2–3 min until seizures are controlled. Then infusion to maintain burst suppression (3–5 mg/kg/h)	

* may be repeated.

IV, intravenous; IM, intramuscular.

similar risks. Intravenous valproate has been proposed as a suitable treatment, but experience is limited. Lorazepam and lidocaine are essentially short-term therapies, and so should not be employed at this stage.

Stage of refractory status epilepticus

In most patients, if seizures continue for 60–90 min in spite of the therapy outlined above, full anaesthesia is required. In some emergency situations (e.g.

postoperative status, severe or complicated convulsive status, patients already in ICU), anaesthesia can and should be introduced earlier. The prognosis is now much poorer, and there is a high risk of mortality and morbidity. The principles of therapy are similar for all anaesthetics, and a wide range of barbiturate and non-barbiturate anaesthetic agents could be used.

Barbiturate anaesthetics have the advantage of long experience in the treatment of status epilepticus and potent antiepileptic activity. Their main disadvantages, however, are due to their poor pharmacological and pharmacokinetic properties. Thiopental has saturable kinetics, with a resultant long half-life at high concentrations. It has a tendency to accumulate, and thus recovery times can be protracted with prolonged therapy. It can result in profound hypotension and concomitant inotropes are often required. Pentobarbital, which is one of the major metabolites of thiopental, has a shorter half-life, but is subject to many of the same problems as thiopental, and there is little to choose between them.

Non-barbiturate anaesthetics have more suitable kinetics, but less is known about their antiepileptic activity and there has been less experience of their use in status epilepticus. Propofol is easy to use and fast-acting and recovery is quick. There have been a number of favourable reports of its use in status epilepticus. It has, however, been reported to precipitate seizures and status epilepticus, although the status in these reports may, in fact, have been rebound seizures due to too rapid propofol withdrawal. In intracortical recordings during epilepsy surgery, propofol has activated epileptiform discharges on the electrocorticogram.

Other general anaesthetics which have been used include isoflurane, etomidate and ketamine. Experience with these agents in status is, however, meagre, and furthermore although all are powerful anaesthetics, they do not generally have antiepileptic properties and some exhibit proconvulsant properties at subanaesthetic doses. Whether such non-anticonvulsant anaesthesia is as effective in status as anticonvulsant anaesthesia is quite unclear.

Benzodiazepine infusions can be given at anaesthetic doses in an ICU setting. Drug-induced hypotension is a common side-effect and the risks of drug accumulation complicate their use. Midazolam is probably the drug of choice because of its short half-life and large volume of distribution, and encouraging early reports of its use in status have been published.

All the anaesthetic drugs are given in doses sufficient to induce deep unconsciousness; therefore assisted respiration, intensive cardiovascular monitoring and the full panoply of intensive care are essential. The depth of anaesthesia should be that which abolishes all clinical and EEG epileptic activity (often requiring sedation to the point of burst suppression on the EEG), and therefore cerebral electrical activity must be visualized, either with a formal EEG or a cerebral function monitor.

Failure to respond to treatment

In the great majority of cases, the above measures will control the seizures and the status will resolve. If drug treatment fails, there are often complicating factors. Common reasons for the failure to control seizures in status epilepticus are the following.

1 Inadequate drug treatment.
 • Insufficient emergency antiepileptic drug therapy. A particular problem is the administration of intravenous drugs at too low a dosage (a common mistake in A&E departments, for instance, with phenobarbital or phenytoin).
 • Failure to initiate or continue maintenance antiepileptic drug therapy in parallel with the acute emergency therapy. This will result in recrudescence of seizures once the effects of the emergency drug treatment have worn off.
2 Additional medical factors.
 • Medical complications can exacerbate seizures (see Table 5.5).
 • A failure to treat, or identify, the underlying cause. This is particularly the case in acute progressive cerebral disorders and cerebral infections.
3 Misdiagnosis.
 • A common problem is to fail to diagnose pseudostatus which, in specialist practice, is more common than true epileptic status.

Convulsive status epilepticus in special circumstances

Status epilepticus due to antiepileptic drug withdrawal. Although drug withdrawal is an important cause of status epilepticus in patients with epilepsy, it is easy, in attributing status to drug withdrawal, mistakenly to overlook other causes. Nevertheless, reintroduction of a withdrawn antiepileptic drug often effectively terminates status epilepticus, and for this reason alone antiepileptic withdrawal must be considered in all patients with prior epilepsy who develop status epilepticus.

Adverse drug reactions. Although rare, there may be adverse drug reactions (including acute anaphylaxis) to many of the agents used for the treatment of status epilepticus, which may necessitate the use of alternative agents. In the case of acute intermittent porphyria, the seizures can be controlled with a benzodiazepine, although this in itself can sometimes worsen the porphyria. Paraldehyde is probably the drug of choice in this instance, and, if anaesthesia is required, isoflurane may be safely used.

Status epilepticus following alcohol withdrawal. Both paraldehyde and clomethiazole have been traditionally used in this situation. Benzodiazepines are probably equally effective, and there is usually a good response to phenytoin.

Status epilepticus following drug overdose. These should be treated, on the whole, as above. There are, however, some exceptions. There is evidence from animal models to suggest that lidocaine potentiates the convulsant effects of cocaine and thus should be avoided in this circumstance. Opiates will potentiate the respiratory and circulatory compromise seen with many of the drugs used in status epilepticus, and immediate transfer to the ICU is recommended.

EMERGENCY TREATMENT OF OTHER FORMS OF STATUS EPILEPTICUS

Status epilepticus in coma (subtle generalized tonic–clonic status epilepticus)

If convulsive status epilepticus is allowed to progress, electromechanical dissociation may occur and the patient may enter a stage of subtle generalized convulsive status epilepticus, characterized by profound coma, bilateral EEG ictal discharges and only subtle motor activity. A similar syndrome can occur following a cerebral insult resulting in coma, especially postanoxia. In any classification of status epilepticus, it is difficult to know where to place these patients. It is not clear if presence of epileptiform activity on the EEG of patients in coma represents true seizure activity. It is, however, associated with a poor prognosis. In view of the poor prognosis of these patients and the animal evidence of status-

induced neuronal damage, however, aggressive treatment is recommended, as outlined above, for those with electrographic features of status epilepticus.

Epilepsia partialis continua

In acute cases, the seizures sometimes remit spontaneously. In a well-established case, however, epilepsia partialis continua can be particularly resistant to therapy, and intravenous therapy even to the point of anaesthesia can produce only temporary respite. It is usual to prescribe oral antiepileptic drugs, to prevent secondarily generalization, even if the epilepsia partialis continua itself is not controlled. Phenytoin, carbamazepine or phenobarbital are probably the drugs of first choice, and oral corticosteroids are sometimes helpful. There is one report of the use of intravenous nimodipine (2 mg/h for 1–2 days) in two patients with epilepsia partialis continua in the setting of an acute cerebral event. The long-term outcome depends on the underlying cause, but in many cases the clonic movements continue in spite of medical therapy. Resective neurosurgical treatment can be considered in refractory cases. Steroids, plasma exchange, intravenous immunoglobulin and zidovudine have been tried in uncontrolled settings in Rasmussen's chronic encephalitis, but definitive evidence of long-term efficacy is lacking.

Other forms of myoclonic status epilepticus

In myoclonic status in primary generalized epilepsy or the progressive myoclonic epilepsies, intravenous therapy is only occasionally required, and benzodiazepine infusion or valproate can be used. For oral therapy, valproate, benzodiazepines (e.g. diazepam, clobazam or clonazepam) or piracetam are the drugs of choice.

Non-convulsive simple partial status epilepticus

This form of status seldom requires intravenous therapy, and the principles of medical and surgical treatment are similar to that of ordinary partial epilepsy. In many patients, the seizures are refractory to conventional treatment.

Complex partial status epilepticus

How aggressively complex partial status epilepticus should be treated is uncertain. Therapy should be aimed at preventing neuronal damage developing consequent upon the status. Although animal models of limbic status show neuronal damage similar to that seen in convulsive status epilepticus, human data are far less convincing.

The relative merits of oral as compared with intravenous therapy are debatable. If it were undoubtedly true that complex partial status epilepticus causes neuronal damage similar to that seen with convulsive status epilepticus, there would be little difficulty in recommending a treatment regimen equivalent to that for convulsive status epilepticus. This has been advocated by a number of authors; however, because of the not insignificant morbidity of aggressive treatment and the uncertainty of the prognosis of complex partial status epilepticus, a different treatment regimen seems more appropriate.

An intravenous benzodiazepine in the acute stages may abort the attack, and if given during EEG recording may also help confirm the diagnosis; the acute response to benzodiazepines, however, may be disappointing. This should then be followed with a short course of an oral benzodiazepine as maintenance therapy. Concomitant antiepileptic drug treatment should be optimized. In a number of cases, intravenous phenytoin or phenobarbital may be necessary.

In recurrent cases, rectal and oral diazepam and oral clobazam given at home may abort the attacks. This is especially likely to be helpful if precipitating factors can be identified, such as a secondarily generalized seizure or menstruation, when an oral benzodiazepine can be given during the period of risk. In recurrent cases, which are self limiting, drug treatment is sometimes not necessary at all.

Treatment of complex partial status epilepticus may be disappointing, and even patients on optimal antiepileptic drug treatment may continue to have recurrent complex partial status epilepticus, although in most cases the episodes are self-terminating.

Absence status epilepticus

There is no evidence that absence status epilepticus induces neuronal damage, and thus aggressive treatment is not warranted. Typical absence status (petit mal status) can usually be terminated by intravenous benzodiazepine therapy; diazepam of 0.2–0.3 mg/kg, clonazepam 1 mg (0.25–0.5 mg in children) or lorazepam 0.07 mg/kg (0.1 mg/kg in children), repeated if required. If this is ineffective, intravenous clomethiazole, phenytoin or valproate can be used. In childhood absence epilepsy, maintenance therapy with valproate or ethosuximide is required once the status is controlled.

De novo absence status of late onset

This is a condition which presents in later life, usually without a history of recent epilepsy. It is commonly caused by drug withdrawal (especially psychotropic drugs or benzodiazepines), and can be safely treated by intravenous diazepam, lorazepam or clomethiazole. Long-term maintenance therapy is not usually required.

Atypical absence status epilepticus

This is usually poorly responsive to intravenous benzodiazepines, which should in any case be given cautiously as they can induce tonic status epilepticus in occasional cases. Oral rather than intravenous treatment is usually more appropriate, and the drugs of choice are valproate, lamotrigine, clonazepam and clobazam. Sedating medication, carbamazepine and vigabatrin have been reported to worsen these seizures. Conversely, arousal or stimulation can terminate the status. Often the episodes are self-limiting and therapy is not required.

Tonic status epilepticus

This is again poorly responsive to conventional treatment. It can be worsened with benzodiazepines, which should be used with care. Sedating medication may worsen all seizure types in the Lennox–Gastaut syndrome, and thus should be avoided. Conversely, stimulants, such as methylphenidate, may be helpful. Tonic status epilepticus has been terminated with oral lamotrigine.

DRUGS USED IN STATUS EPILEPTICUS

Clomethiazole

Clomethiazole has been widely used in established status epilepticus, in spite of the meagre published evidence of its value, and also the well-known risks of accumulation. It nevertheless has a loyal following. It is given by intravenous bolus followed by a continuous infusion. The drug is rapidly redistributed and has a very rapid and short-lived initial action. Dosage can be initially titrated against response, on a moment by moment basis—a unique property amongst the drugs used in status. The danger of clomethiazole is that it accumulates on prolonged use, with the risk of sudden cardiorespiratory collapse, hypotension and sedation. There is also a danger of respiratory arrest and hypotension if the maximum rate of injection is exceeded. Other side-effects include cardiac rhythm disturbances, vomiting, thrombophlebitis, and there is a tendency for seizure recurrence on discontinuing therapy. Prolonged therapy carries the risk of fluid overload and electrolyte disturbance. There is very limited published experience in status, particularly in children, and insufficient published data for neonatal use. Hepatic disease reduces the metabolism and elimination of the drug, and prolonged contact with plastic results in substantial resorption.

Usual preparation. 0.8% solution of clomethiazole edisylate in 500 mL in 4% dextrose (8 mg/mL).

Usual dosage. Intravenous infusion of 40–100 mL (320–800 mg), at rate of 5–15 mL/min, followed by a continuous infusion, with dosage titrated according to response (usually 1–4 mL/min, range 0.5–20 mL/min) (adults). Initially 0.1 mL/kg/min (0.08 mg/kg/min) increasing progressively every 2–4 h as required (children).

Clonazepam

Clonazepam is an alternative to diazepam in early status, and there is little to choose between the two drugs. It has a similar onset of action and a longer duration of action and a lower incidence of late relapse. There is wide experience with the drug in adults and children, although not in neonates, and the drug has proven efficacy in tonic–clonic, partial and absence status. Clonazepam accumulates on prolonged infusion, with the resulting risk of respiratory arrest, hypotension, and sedation; a side-effect profile similar to that of diazepam. There is also a danger of sudden collapse if the recommended rate of injection is exceeded. A continuous infusion of clonazepam is not now recommended.

Usual preparation. 1 mL ampoule containing 1 mg of clonazepam.

Usual dosage. 1 mg bolus injection over 30 s (adults), 250–500 µg (children), which can be repeated up to four times. The 1 mL ampoule of clonazepam is mixed with 1 mL of water for injection (provided as diluent) *immediately* before administration. The rate of injection should not exceed 1 mg in 30 s. The drug can also be given more slowly in a dextrose (5%) or 0.9% sodium chloride solution (1–2 mg in 250 mL).

Diazepam

Diazepam is useful in the premonitory or early stages of status. There is extensive clinical experience in adults, children and the newborn, the drug has well-proved efficacy in many types of status, a rapid onset of action, and well-studied pharmacology and pharmacokinetics. It can be given by rectal administration, and the rectal tubule is a convenient rectal preparation. Diazepam has two important disadvantages, however, which limit its usefulness in status. First, although it has a rapid onset of action, it is highly lipid-soluble and thus has a short duration of action after a single injection. This means that there is a strong tendency for seizure relapse after initial control. Secondly, diazepam accumulates on repeated injections or after continuous infusion, and this accumulation carries a high risk of sudden respiratory depression, sedation and hypotension. Other disadvantages are its dependency on hepatic metabolism and its metabolism to an active metabolite, which can complicate prolonged therapy. Diazepam has a tendency to precipitate from concentrated solutions and to interact with other drugs, and is absorbed onto plastic on prolonged contact.

Usual preparations. Intravenous formulation—diazepam emulsion (Diazemuls), 2 mL ampoule containing 5 mg/mL *or* intravenous solution 2 mL ampoules containing 5 mg/mL.
Rectal formulation—rectal tube containing 2.5, 5, 10 or 20 mg *or* using the intravenous solution, 2 mL ampoule containing 5 mg/mL.

Usual dosage. Intravenous bolus (undiluted) 10–20 mg (adults); 0.25–0.5 mg/kg (children), at a rate not exceeding <5 mg/min. The bolus dosing can be repeated. Rectal administration 10–30 mg (adults); 0.5–0.75 mg/kg (children), and this can be repeated.

Fosphenytoin

Fosphenytoin is a prodrug of phenytoin. It is converted in the plasma into phenytoin by widely distributed phosphatase enzymes. The half-life of conversion is about 15 min, and conversion is not affected by age, hepatic status or by the presence of other drugs. Fosphenytoin is water-soluble and prepared in a Tris buffer; it thus causes less thrombophlebitis than phenytoin when given intravenously. It can also be administered intramuscularly. Fosphenytoin itself is inert, and its action in status is due entirely to the derived phenytoin. The dosage of the drug is expressed in phenytoin equivalents (PE, thus 15 mg PE of fosphenytoin is the same as 15 mg of phenytoin). When fosphenytoin is infused at 150 mg PE/min, the rate at which free phenytoin levels are reached in the serum is similar to that achieved by a phenytoin infusion of 50 mg/min. Fosphenytoin can therefore be administered three times faster than phenytoin, with equivalent risks of hypotension, cardiac dysrhythmias and respiratory depression. Its rate of antiepileptic action is also similar and is no faster than phenytoin despite the fact that it can be administered more quickly. The faster rate of injection and the lower incidence of local side-effects are advantages over phenytoin, but in other ways the two drugs are equivalent and fosphenytoin is more expensive.

Usual preparation. Fosphenytoin is formulated in a Tris buffer at physiological pH. Vials of 50 mg PE are available for mixture with dextrose or saline. The solution must be diluted before IV infusion.

Usual dosage. Fosphenytoin is given at a dose of between 15 mg PE/kg at a rate of between 100 and 150 mg PE/min (an average adult dose of 1000 mg PE in 10 min). The drug is not recommended for children under the age of 5 years. For older children, the mg PE/kg dose is the same as for adults. A maintenance dose of 4–5 mg PE/kg can be given by IV infusion or IM injection.

Isoflurane

Where inhalational anaesthesia is used to treat status (a rare option), isoflurane is the drug of choice. It has advantages over other inhalational anaesthetics, such as halothane or enflurane: lower solubility, less hepatotoxicity or nephrotoxicity, less effect on cardiac output, fewer cardiac dysrhythmias, less hypotension, less effect on cerebral blood flow and autoregulation, less increase in intracranial pressure, less convulsant effect and linear kinetics. It has a very rapid onset of action and recovery, and no tendency to accumulate. Although hypotension is common it is generally mild. There is no hepatic metabolism, and the drug is unaffected by hepatic or renal disease. There is, however, little published experience in status or of long-term use, and the major disadvantage is logistical, as isoflurane requires the use of an anaesthetic system with a scavenging apparatus which is inconvenient in most ICU situations. The other facilities required are the usual ones of assisted ventilation, intensive care and cardiorespiratory monitoring.

Usual preparation. Nearly pure (99.9%) liquid, for use in a correctly calibrated vaporizer via an anaesthetic system.

Usual dosage. Inhalation of isoflurane at dosages producing end tidal concentrations of 0.8–2%, with the dose titrated to maintain a burst suppression pattern on the EEG.

Lidocaine

Lidocaine is a second-line drug for use in early status only. It is given as a bolus injection or short intravenous infusion. The clinical effects and pharmacokinetics have been extensively studied in patients of all ages, and the drug is highly effective. The main disadvantage of lidocaine is that its antiepileptic effects are short-lived and seizures are controlled for a matter of hours only. Lidocaine is thus useful only while more definitive antiepileptic drug treatment is administered. The risk of drug accumulation is low, and the incidence of respiratory or cerebral depression and hypotension is lower than with other antiepileptics. The drug may be particularly valuable in patients with respiratory disease. Other disadvantages include a possible proconvulsant effect at high levels, an active metabolite which may accumulate on prolonged therapy, the need for cardiac monitoring as cardiac rhythm disturbances are common, and the dependency of the clearance of lidocaine on hepatic blood flow.

Usual preparations. 5 mL ready-prepared syringe containing lidocaine 20 mg/mL (2%) *or* 10 mL ready-prepared syringe containing lidocaine 10 mg/mL (1%) (i.e. both syringes containing 100 mg). Lidocaine is also available as a 5-mL vial containing 20 mg/mL (i.e. 100 mg) of lidocaine (2%) or a 5-mL vial containing 200 mg/mL (i.e. 1000 mg) of lidocaine (20%), and as ready-made 0.1% (1 mg/mL) and 0.2% (2 mg/mL) infusions (in 500 mL containers in 5% dextrose).

Usual dosage. Intravenous bolus injections 1.5–2.0 mg/kg (usually 100 mg in adults), at a rate of injection not exceeding 50 mg/min. The bolus injection can be repeated once if necessary. A continuous infusion can be given at a rate of 3–4 mg/kg/h (usually of 0.2% solution in 5% dextrose, for no more than 12 h); 3–6 mg/kg/h (neonates).

Lorazepam

Lorazepam is the drug of choice in the early stage of status, given by intravenous bolus injection. A single injection is highly effective, and the drug has a longer initial duration of action and a smaller risk of cardiorespiratory depression than diazepam. There is little risk of drug accumulation, and also a lower risk of hypotension. The main disadvantage of lorazepam is a stronger tendency for tolerance to develop, the drug being usually effective for about 12 h only. It is thus usable only as initial therapy, and longer-term maintenance antiepileptic drugs must be given in addition. There is a large clinical experience in adults, children and the newborn, with well-proven efficacy in tonic–clonic and partial status, and the pharmacology and pharmacokinetics of the drug are well characterized. Preliminary experience of buccal installation is encouraging and it seems safe and effective by this route of administration. Lorazepam is a stable compound which is not likely to precipitate in solution, and is relatively unaffected by hepatic or renal disease.

Usual preparation. 1 mL ampoule containing 4 mg/mL for intravenous injection.

Usual dosage. Intravenous bolus of 0.07 mg/kg (usually 4 mg), repeated after 10 min if necessary (adults); bolus of 0.1 mg/kg (children). The rate of injection is not crucial.

Midazolam

Midazolam is another benzodiazepine which can be used in the premonitory or early stages of status. It is a water-soluble compound whose ring structure closes when in contact with serum to convert it into a highly lipophilic structure. Its water solubility provides one major advantage over diazepam, and that is that it can be rapidly absorbed by intramuscular injection or by intranasal or buccal administration. It is therefore useful in situations in which intravenous administration is difficult or ill-advised. Blinded comparisons with rectal diazepam, after intramuscular and buccal administration show midazolam to be equivalent in efficacy and speed of action. Although there is a danger of accumulation on prolonged or repeated therapy, this tendency is less than with diazepam. There is, however, only limited published experience in adults or children with status. Occasionally, severe cardiorespiratory depression occurs after intramuscular administration, and other adverse effects include hypotension, apnoea, sedation and thrombophlebitis. Like diazepam, the drug is short-acting, and there is a strong tendency for seizures to relapse after initial control and, as with diazepam, its metabolism is altered by hepatic disease. Its half-life is prolonged in hepatic disease or in the elderly. There are also encouraging reports of the use of intravenous infusions of midazolam as

an anaesthetic in the refractory stage of status, and midazolam is probably the only benzodiazepine which should be used as a continuous infusion.

Usual preparation. 2 or 5 mL ampoule containing 10 mg midazolam hydrochloride.

Usual dosage. Intramuscularly or rectally 5–10 mg (adults); 0.15–0.3 mg/kg (children). This can be repeated once after 15 min. Intravenous bolus of 0.1–0.3 mg/kg, at a rate not to exceed 4 mg/min, which can be repeated once after 15 min. Buccal instillation of 10 mg can be given by a syringe and catheter in children or adults. An intravenous infusion can be given at a rate of 0.05–0.4 mg/kg/h.

Paraldehyde

Paraldehyde still has a small role in premonitory and early status, as an alternative to the benzodiazepines in situations where facilities for resuscitation are not available. Paraldehyde is rapidly and completely absorbed after intramuscular injection or rectally. The risks of drug accumulation, hypotension or cardiorespiratory arrest are small, and seizures do not often recur after control has been obtained. Paraldehyde has been used for many years in status, and although there is wide experience in patients at all ages, no modern pharmacokinetic or clinical studies have been carried out. Toxicity is unusual provided the solution is freshly made, used immediately and correctly diluted. The use of decomposed or inadequately diluted intravenous solutions are dangerous, causing precipitation, microembolism, thrombosis or cardiorespiratory collapse. The intramuscular injection of paraldehyde is painful, can cause sterile abscess and sciatic nerve damage if wrongly placed. Other side-effects include cardiorespiratory depression, sedation and metabolic or lactic acidosis. The drug rapidly binds to plastic, and glass tubing and syringes are advisable unless injected immediately upon drawing the solution up. The drug should not be exposed unduly to light. The half-life of paraldehyde is markedly increased by hepatic disease.

Usual preparation. Ampoule containing 5 mL paraldehyde (equivalent to approximately 5 g; in darkened glass).

Usual dosage. Paraldehyde can be given rectally or intramuscularly 5–10 mL diluted by the same volume of water for injection (adults) or 0.07–0.35 mL/kg (children). This dose can be repeated after 15–30 min.

Pentobarbital

Pentobarbital is an alternative to thiopental, and it shares many of the characteristics of thiopental. It has certain advantages which include a shorter elimination half-life than thiopental, non-saturable kinetics, no active metabolites and a longer duration of action. It is a stable compound and does not react with plastic. There is, however, limited clinical experience, and published trials have shown a uniformly poor outcome. Respiratory depression and sedation are invariable, and hypotension and cardiorespiratory dysfunction are common. Decerebrate posturing and flaccid paralysis occur during induction of anaesthesia, and a flaccid weakness can persist for weeks in survivors. There is a tendency for seizures to recur when the drug is withdrawn. It requires intensive care, artificial ventilatory support, EEG and cardiovascular monitoring. Blood level monitoring is usually advised although there is only an inconsistent relationship between serum level and seizure control.

Usual preparation. 100 mg in a 2-mL injection vial, formulated in propylene glycol 40% and ethyl alcohol 10%.

Usual dosage. Intravenous loading dose of 10–20 mg/kg, at a rate not exceeding 25 mg/min, followed by a continuous infusion of 0.5–1.0 mg/kg/h, increasing if necessary to 1–3 mg/kg/h. Additional 5–20 mg/kg boluses can be given if breakthrough seizure occurs. The dose should be tapered 12 h after the last seizure by 0.5–1 mg/kg/h every 4–6 h (depending on blood level).

Phenobarbital

Phenobarbital is the drug of choice in established status. It is a reliable antiepileptic drug, with well-proven effectiveness in tonic–clonic and partial status and there is extensive clinical experience in adults, children and in neonates. Phenobarbital has a stronger anticonvulsant action than other barbiturates and an additional potential cerebral protective action. It has a rapid onset and long-lasting action, and can be administered much faster than can phenytoin. Its safety at high doses has been established, and the drug can be continued as chronic therapy. The disadvantages of the drug relate to prolonged use where, because of the long elimination half-life, there is a risk of drug accumulation and inevitable sedation, respiratory depression and hypotension. Marked autoinduction may also occur.

Usual preparation. 1 mL ampoule containing phenobarbital sodium 200 mg/mL in propylene glycol 90% and water for injection 10%.

Usual dosage. Intravenous loading dose of 10 mg/kg at rate of 100 mg/min (usual adult dose 600–800 mg), followed by maintenance dose of 1–4 mg/kg per day (adults). Intravenous loading dose of 15–20 mg/kg, followed by maintenance dose of 3–4 mg/kg per day (children and neonates). Higher doses can be given, with monitoring of blood concentrations.

Phenytoin

Phenytoin is a drug of choice and a highly effective medication for the stage of established status. Extensive clinical experience has been gained in adults, children and neonates, and phenytoin has proven efficacy in tonic–clonic and partial status. The drug has a prolonged action, with a relatively small risk of respiratory or cerebral depression and no tendency for tachyphylaxis. Its main disadvantage is the time necessary to infuse the drug and its delayed onset of action. Fosphenytoin is a prodrug of phenytoin which can be administered more quickly. The pharmacokinetics of phenytoin are problematic, with zero-order kinetics at conventional dosages and wide variation between individuals. Toxic side-effects include cardiac rhythm disturbances, thrombophlebitis and hypotension. The risk of cardiac side-effects is greatly increased if the recommended rate of injection is exceeded, and cardiac monitoring is advisable during phenytoin infusion. There is a risk of precipitation if phenytoin is diluted in other solutions than 0.9% saline or if mixed with other drugs.

Usual preparations. 5 mL ampoule containing 250 mg stabilized in propylene glycol, ethanol and water. Alternatives exist; e.g. phenytoin in Tris buffer or in infusion bottles of 750 mg in 500 mL of osmotic saline.

Usual dosage. In adults, an 15–18 mg/kg intravenous infusion. This can be given via the side arm of a drip or preferably directly via an infusion pump. The rate of infusion should not exceed 50 mg/min (20 mg/min in the elderly). In children, a 10–20-mg/kg intravenous infusion is usually given, at a rate not exceeding 1–3 mg/kg per min. The drug should never be given by intramuscular injection. The subsequent maintenance dose should be guided by blood levels.

Propofol

Propofol is the anaesthetic agent of choice for non-barbiturate infusional anaesthesia in status. It is an excellent anaesthetic with very good pharmacokinetic properties. In status, it has a very rapid onset of action and rapid recovery. There are few haemodynamic side-effects, and the drug has been used at all ages. There is, however, only limited published experience of its use in status, or indeed of prolonged infusions. Preliminary experience of the use of subanaesthetic bolus doses of propofol in acute seizures or the early stage of status is also encouraging. Unlike isoflurane, it is metabolized in the liver and affected by severe hepatic disease. As with all anaesthetics, its use requires assisted ventilation, intensive care and intensive care monitoring. It causes lipaemia and acidosis which may complicate its use, especially in long-term therapy and in infants. Involuntary movements (without EEG change) can occur, and should not be confused with seizure activity. Rebound seizures are a problem when it is discontinued too rapidly, and a decremental rate of 1 mg/kg or less every 2 h is recommended when the drug is to be withdrawn.

Usual preparation. 20 mL ampoule containing 10 mg/mL (i.e. 200 mg) as an emulsion.

Usual dosage. 2 mg/kg bolus, repeated if necessary, and then followed by a continuous infusion of 5–10 mg/kg/h initially, reducing to 1–3 mg/kg/h. When seizures have been controlled for 12 h, the drug doses should be slowly tapered over 12 h.

Thiopental

Thiopental is in most countries the usual choice for barbiturate anaesthesia. It is a highly effective antiepileptic drug, with additional potential cerebral protective action. It reduces intracranial pressure and cerebral blood flow, and has a very rapid onset of action, and there is wide experience of its use. The drug has a number of pharmacokinetic disadvantages including saturable kinetics, a strong tendency to accumulate and a prolonged recovery time after anaesthesia is withdrawn. Blood level monitoring of the parent drug and its active metabolite (pentobarbital) is advisable on prolonged therapy. There is often some tachyphylaxis to its sedative and to a lesser extent its anticonvulsant properties. Respiratory depression and sedation is inevitable, and hypotension is common. Other less common side-effects include pancreatitis, hepatic dysfunction and spasm at the injection site. Full intensive care facilities with artificial ventilatory support and intensive EEG and cardiovascular monitoring are needed. It can react with comedication, and with plastic-giving sets, and

is unstable when exposed to air. Autoinduction occurs and hepatic disease prolongs the elimination of thiopental.

Usual preparations. Injection of thiopental sodium 2.5 g with 100 mL, and 5 g with 200 mL diluent (to make 100 and 200 mL of a 2.5% solution). It is also available as 500 mg and 1 g vials to make 2.5% solutions.

Usual dosage. 100–250 mg intravenous bolus given over 20 s, with further 50 mg boluses every 2–3 min until seizures are controlled, followed by a continuous intravenous infusion to maintain a burst suppression pattern on the EEG (usually 3–5 mg/kg/h). The dose should be lowered if systolic blood pressure falls below 90 mmHg despite cardiovascular support. Thiopental should be slowly withdrawn 12 h after the last seizure.

FURTHER READING

Browne, T.R. (1983) Paraldehyde, chlormethiazole, and lidocaine for treatment of status epilepticus. *Adv Neurol*, **34**, 509–17.

Burstein, C.L. (1943) The hazard of paraldehyde administration: clinical and laboratory studies. *JAMA*, **121**, 187–90.

Kofke, W.A., Young, R.S., Davis, P. *et al.* (1989) Isoflurance for refractory status epilepticus: a clinical series. *Anesthesiology*, **71**, 653–9.

Kumar, A. & Bleck, T.P. (1992) Intravenous midazolam for the treatment of refractory status epilepticus. *Crit Care Med*, **20**, 483–8.

Leppik, I.E., Derivan, A.T., Homan, R.W. *et al.* (1983) Double-blind study of lorazepam and diazepam in status epilepticus. *JAMA*, **249**, 1452–4.

Leppik, I.E., Patrick, B.K. & Cranford, R.E. (1983) Treatment of acute seizures and status epilepticus with intravenous phenytoin. *Adv Neurol*, **34**, 447–51.

Lowenstein, D.H. & Aminoff, M.J. & Simon, R.P. (1988) Barbiturate anesthesia in the treatment of status epilepticus: clinical experience with 14 patients. *Neurology*, **38**, 395–400.

Mackenzie, S.J., Kapadia, F. & Grant, I.S. (1990) Propofol infusion for control of status epilepticus. *Anaesthesia*, **45**, 1043–5.

Pascual, J., Ciudad, J. & Berciano, J. (1992) Role of lidocaine (lignocaine) in managing status epilepticus. *J Neurol Neurosurg Psychiatry*, **55**, 49–51.

Pentikainen, P.J., Valtonen, V.V. & Miettien, T.A. (1976) Deaths in connection with chlormethiazole (Hemineurin) therapy. *Int J Clin Pharmacol Biopharm*, **14**, 225–30.

Rashkin, M.C., Youngs, C. & Penovich, P. (1987)

Pentobarbital treatment of refractory status epilepticus. *Neurology*, **37**, 500–3.

Remy, C., Jourdil, N., Villemain, D., Favel, P. & Genton, P. (1992) Intrarectal diazepam in epileptic adults. *Epilepsia*, **33**, 353–8.

Robson, D.J., Blow, C., Gaines, P., Flanagan, R.J. & Henry, J.A. (1984) Accumulation of chlormethiazole during intravenous infusion. *Intensive Care Med*, **10**, 315–16.

Scott, R.C., Besag, F.M., Boyd, S.G., Berry, D. & Neville, B.G. (1998) Buccal absorption of midazolam: pharmacokinetics and EEG pharmacodynamics. *Epilepsia*, **39**, 290–4.

Shorvon, S.D. (1994) *Status Epilepticus: Its Clinical Features and Treatment in Children and Adults*. Cambridge University Press, Cambridge.

Shorvon, S.D., Dreifuss, F., Fish, D. & Thomas, D. (eds) (1996) *The Treatment of Epilepsy*. Blackwell Science, Oxford.

Simon, R.P. (1985) Physiologic consequences of status epilepticus. *Epilepsia*, **26**, S58–S66.

Stecker, M.M., Kramer, T.H., Raps, E.C. *et al.* (1998) Treatment of refractory status epilepticus with propofol: clinical and pharmacokinetic findings. *Epilepsia*, **39**, 18–26.

Thomas, J.E., Reagan, T.J. & Klass, D.W. (1977) Epilepsia partialis continua: a review of 32 cases. *Arch Neurol*, **34**, 266–75.

Treiman, D.M. (1990) The role of benzodiazepines in the management of status epilepticus. *Neurology*, **40**, 32–42.

Treiman, D.M., Meyers, P.D., Walton, N.Y. *et al.* (1998) A comparison of four treatments for generalized convulsive status epilepticus. Veterans Affairs Status Epilepticus Cooperative Study Group. *N Engl J Med*, **339**, 792–8.

Treiman, D.M., Tyrrell, E., Lee, J. *et al.* (1983) Lorazepam versus phenytoin in the treatment of major motor status epilepticus: a preliminary report. *Epilepsia*, **24**, 520.

Turcant, A., Delhumeau, A., Premel Cabic, A. *et al.* (1985) Thiopentol pharmacokinetics under conditions of long-term infusion. *Anesthesiology*, **63**, 50–4.

Van Ness, P.C. (1990) Pentobarbital and EEG burst suppression in treatment of status epilepticus refractory to benzodiazepines and phenytoin. *Epilepsia*, **31**, 61–7.

Walker, M.C., Alavijeh, M.S., Patsalos, P.N. & Shorvon, S.D. (1994) The neuropharmacokinetics of acutely administered phenytoin in the rat. *J Neurol Neurosurg Psychiatry*, **57**, 1299.

Walker, M.C., Smith, S.J.M. & Shorvon, S.D. (1995) The intensive care treatment of convulsive status epilepticus in the UK: results of a national survey and recommendations. *Anaesthesia*, **50**, 130–5.

Surgical Treatment of Epilepsy

The evolution of surgical treatment for epilepsy in the past century has been critically dependent on technical developments. The first resective surgery was performed in 1880, following improvements in anaesthetics and surgical instrumentation. It remained a therapeutic curiosity until the late 1930s when the introduction of electroencephalography (EEG) ushered in a period of intensive development. The first temporal lobectomy was carried out in the 1940s and the standard operation with removal of the hippocampus was introduced in 1951. In the late 1980s, the advent of magnetic resonance imaging (MRI) opened a new era of epilepsy surgery. Magnetic resonance imaging has simplified presurgical investigation, rendered the identification of underlying aetiology far more sensitive and improved patient selection. As a result, there has been a considerable increase in the proportion of patients for whom resective surgery has become a realistic option. Figures have varied but, at a conservative estimate, between 2 and 5% of individuals with medically refractory partial epilepsy would benefit from epilepsy surgery.

DEFINITIONS

Epilepsy surgery is the form of surgery that is carried out specifically to control epileptic seizures. This will include operations on tumours and vascular lesions where epilepsy is the primary indication for surgery. There is clearly an overlap with lesional surgery carried out for other primary reasons if the lesion is causing epilepsy, and even if the operation influences the epilepsy. There are five main types of surgical approach.

• Focal resections for hippocampal sclerosis, which include temporal lobectomy for hippocampal sclerosis and more selective operations.
• Focal resections for other lesions (lesionectomies), which include lesions in temporal and non-temporal areas.
• Non-lesional focal resections.

• Multilobar resections, which include hemispherectomy.
• Functional procedures, which include multiple subpial transection, vagal nerve stimulation and corpus callosectomy.

Practice has changed substantially since the introduction of MRI, with a trend towards lesional surgery and away from non-lesional resections based on EEG. There is also a renewed interest in functional procedures, although to date much of this is still largely in the research phase. An approximate frequency of these operations in a modern surgical practice is shown in Table 6.1.

Epileptogenic zone

The conceptual basis of resective surgery is that there is an 'epileptogenic zone' underlying focal epilepsy,

Table 6.1 The approximate frequency of different forms of epilepsy surgery in modern surgical practice.

Focal resections for hippocampal sclerosis	>50%
Temporal lobectomy	
Amygdalohippocampectomy	
Focal resections for other lesions	20%
Lesionectomy in the temporal lobe	
Lesionectomy in other locations	
Non-lesional focal resections	<5%
Frontal lobectomy	
Other restricted neocortical resections	
Multilobar resections	<5%
Hemispherectomy	
Other multilobar resections	
Functional procedures	20%
Corpus callosectomy	
Multiple subpial transection	
Vagal nerve stimulation	
Stereotactic ablation/stimulation	

and that its resection will abolish the seizures. The aim of presurgical evaluation of a patient is to define the anatomical boundaries of the epileptogenic zone. The feasibility of complete or partial resection and its potential risks can then be estimated. Whilst the concept of the epileptogenic zone has the attractions of simplicity and apparent logicality, in practice often it can not be defined with accuracy and the boundaries of surgical resection are often chosen on a rather more empirical basis. In mesial temporal lobe epilepsy, for instance, there is good experimental and clinical evidence that the seizures are underpinned by a network which extends well beyond the mesial temporal lobe and that resection of the hippocampus will remove only part of this network, yet such a resection is often successful in controlling seizures. Similarly, resection of large areas of frontal cortex in apparently well-localized frontal lesional epilepsy will stop seizures in a relatively small proportion of patients. Nevertheless, provided its limitations are recognized, the concept of the epileptogenic zone provides a simple and convenient basis for the presurgical investigation of most patients with epilepsy.

Two important components of the epileptogenic zone are the pathological lesion and the EEG disturbance. These almost always overlap, but are not necessarily contiguous. Thus, epilepsy may be generated from part of the lesion only, and independent EEG disturbances can occur well away from the pathological abnormality.

Concordance of investigations

The investigation of patients prior to resective surgery has four main components: radiological, neurophysiological, psychological and clinical. If investigations in each area point to a similar epileptogenic zone (i.e. are concordant), then the outcome of surgery is likely to be good. Conversely, if results are discordant, resective surgery is likely to be less successful. It follows from this that all patients require multimodal investigation aimed at defining the epileptogenic zone, and this is best carried out in a designated centre with multidisciplinary experience in presurgical evaluation. Incomplete or unfocused investigation is fraught with danger and is negligent practice.

Importance of aetiology

The advent of MRI has greatly changed the focus of presurgical investigation. It has become apparent that the underlying aetiology (i.e. the nature of the structural abnormality) of the epilepsy is the primary de-

terminant of outcome in competently evaluated and operated patients. The starting point of any surgical evaluation should therefore be to determine the aetiology and its extent. If the MRI shows no abnormality and thus no structural cause for the epilepsy can be determined, the chances of resective surgery being possible even after intensive investigation are greatly reduced. In one study, for instance, of 40 patients with normal MRI, investigation even with intensive intracranial EEG revealed a well-localized epileptogenic zone concordant with other tests in only five cases and only three could proceed to surgery. In routine practice, the MRI has become in effect the first screening test for considering surgical intervention, and has now displaced EEG from this role.

SURGERY FOR HIPPOCAMPAL SCLEROSIS

The most commonly performed epilepsy surgery is the resection of hippocampal sclerosis in patients with refractory mesial temporal lobe seizures.

Which patients should be evaluated?

Intractable epilepsy

Because of its risks, surgery should in most situations be offered only to patients in whom there is no hope of seizure control by medical means (refractory epilepsy) without unacceptable side-effects. To define such intractability is obviously difficult, and the nature and severity of the seizure disorder are also important factors to consider. However, in practice, it would be rare to proceed to surgery without attempting a trial of adequate treatment with at least four of the major antiepileptic drugs.

Duration of epilepsy

It is usual to require that the epilepsy has been present for at least 5 years before considering surgical therapy, as spontaneous (or medically induced) remission is frequent in early epilepsy. Exceptions can be made, but only after careful counselling and consideration.

Quality of life

Surgical therapy should (in view of its risks) be offered only to those patients whose quality of life is being seriously compromised by the epilepsy and also in whom seizure freedom will result in major quality of life improvements. While this might seem obvious to the point of banality, it is often by no means easy to decide and there are many patients successfully rendered seizure-free who regret the operation and whose life has shown little improvement. Preoperative counselling on this point is essential.

The gains in quality of life are greatest before life patterns are fixed, and epilepsy surgery should be carried out as soon as possible in the life of the young patient. Conversely, surgery after the age of 40 years would be unusual as quality of life gains have proved generally disappointing.

Preoperative evaluation

The evaluation needs to decide the following questions.

• Do the seizures arise from the sclerotic hippocampus?

• What are the likely functional consequences of temporal lobe (or hippocampal) resection, both in terms of controlling seizures and of neuropsychological, neurological and psychiatric sequelae?

• Are the chances of quality of life gain, and its extent, sufficient to warrant the risks of deleterious consequences of surgery?

In addition to the normal medical and neurological investigations, the presurgical evaluation should be concentrated particularly on the following aspects.

Clinical history and examination

It is imperative to obtain a detailed history of the seizure disorder, its prior treatment and its causation. Hippocampal sclerosis usually causes complex partial seizures of mesial temporal lobe type. Additional secondarily generalized tonic–clonic seizures are typically absent or infrequent, and indeed a history of secondarily generalized seizures reduces the chances of a good outcome following temporal lobe surgery. Other seizure types are not to be expected in hippocampal epilepsy, and their presence indicates an epileptogenic zone which extends beyond the mesial temporal lobe structures. A history of childhood febrile convulsions, especially if prolonged or focal, is very strongly associated with hippocampal sclerosis, and the outcome of hippocampal surgery is better if such a history is present.

The patient's general medical status should be assessed, and the suitability for an anaesthetic of long duration and for intracranial surgery.

Magnetic resonance imaging

Computed tomography (CT) cannot demonstrate hippocampal sclerosis because of the middle fossa bony artefact close to the hippocampus and the inherently poor grey–white contrast of CT. Conversely, with modern techniques, MRI can demonstrate hippocampal sclerosis with high specificity and sensitivity. High-quality imaging is now an absolute requirement in the presurgical work-up of all patients with hippocampal sclerosis (Fig. 6.1). The changes of hippocampal sclerosis are quite subtle, and their detection requires experience and appropriate scanning protocols. If the MRI sequence is not tailored to identify hippocampal atrophy, many cases of hippocampal sclerosis will be missed. It follows therefore that a negative routine MRI study in a patient with temporal lobe epilepsy should not be taken as evidence of normality.

Hippocampal sclerosis, on MRI, causes loss of volume, and increased T_2 signal on views through the structure. Additional changes, seen inconsistently, are atrophy of the ipsilateral fornix, mammillary body, amygdala and temporal lobe. The temporal horn of the lateral ventricle may be dilated but this is an unreliable sign and should never be interpreted as isolated evidence of ipsilateral hippocampal atrophy. Some workers have emphasized other changes such as decreased T_1 signal intensity and loss of internal mesial temporal structure. As this latter feature is not noted on fine T_1-weighted cuts, it may be an artefact related to slice thickness.

Volume loss. Hippocampal volume measurement has proved to be the most consistently reliable method of detecting hippocampal sclerosis (Fig. 6.1). Visual analysis of T_1-weighted coronal image will be sufficient to identify atrophy in most severe cases of hippocampal sclerosis. Formal quantitation of the hippocampal volume will be needed to detect milder cases. Formal quantitation should be employed in all potential surgical cases. An asymmetry of over 10% is unequivocal evidence of hippocampal sclerosis.

To estimate volume accurately, the scanning sequence should produce high-anatomical-resolution coronal T_1-weighted images, with fine contiguous slices of less than 2 mm thickness. A volumetric sequence is generally used to acquire these, using a 1.5 Tesla system. Thicker slices cause unacceptable partial voluming, resulting in unreliable quantitation. Having obtained a series of thin slices through the whole length of the hippocampus, the surface area of the hippocampus in each slice can be measured (by drawing around the hippocampus in each slice, and computing the number of voxels enclosed) and the sum of the surface areas is used to calculate the hippocampal volume. The result may be expressed as absolute volumes, ratios, or volumes corrected for total brain/temporal lobe volume. Volumes can be plotted as a volume–length profile, giving an

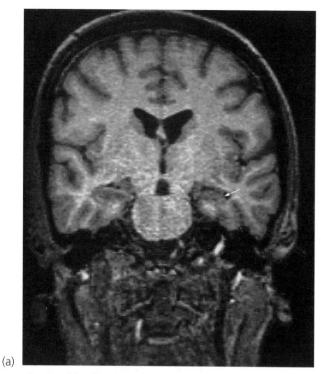

(a)

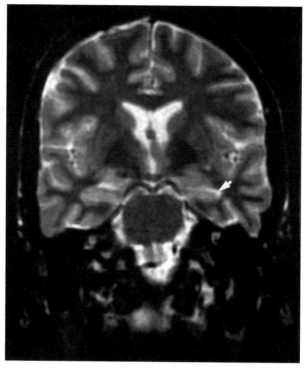

(b)

Fig. 6.1 (a) Left-sided hippocampal atrophy (arrowed), with low intensity within the hippocampus on T$_1$-weighted image. (b) T$_2$-weighted image at same location reveals minor signal-intensity increase of hippocampus on left (arrowed). It is interesting to note that there are only subtle T$_2$ changes despite atrophy of over 50% on volumetry.

impression of the distribution of hippocampal volume loss (Fig. 6.2). Most frequently, this is restricted to the anterior portion of the structure and is the most difficult to detect visually. Severe diffuse atro-phy is also a common pattern, and if severe can be reliably detected by visual analysis. Focal posterior atrophy is relatively rare.

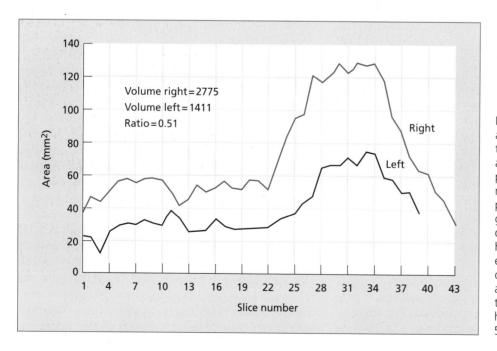

Fig. 6.2 Hippocampal area vs. length curve. In this graph cross-sectional area in each slice is plotted against slice number, progressing from posterior to anterior. This gives an impression of the distribution of hippocampal atrophy. This example shows severe diffuse left hippocampal atrophy, with a ratio of the left:right hippocampal volumes of 51%.

Signal intensity. Hippocampal sclerosis is associated with elevation of the T_2 signal in the hippocampus and less frequently the surrounding temporal lobe (see Fig. 6.1). As with volumetry, this aspect has been quantified with formal T_2 relaxometry and, in experienced hands, is a reliable method for lateralizing hippocampal sclerosis. Numerous imaging artefacts may occur in the mesial temporal region, complicating the assessment of this feature in isolation, and it is best not to rely on signal intensity alone for the detection of sclerosis in surgical candidates.

Care must be taken not to misinterpret the MRI signs. Occasionally, hippocampal atrophy will be the result not the cause of epilepsy (e.g. after status or in lesional cortical epilepsies) or a consequence of trauma (Fig. 6.3). A swollen hippocampus on one side caused by tumour can lead to the mistaken diagnosis of an atrophic contralateral hippocampus. There are also other causes of increased hippocampal T_2 signal, including tumour, vascular or developmental abnormality.

Improved MRI has demonstrated that, in a sizeable proportion of patients with epilepsy, there is more than one potentially causative lesion (dual pathology). For example, about 15% of patients with hippocampal sclerosis exhibit other extrahippocampal dysgenetic lesions (Table 6.2, Fig. 6.4). It is imperative to identify those that are epileptogenic, for hippocampal resection in such cases will clearly not be successful. Recent work has also suggested that quantitative changes in grey and white matter volume, without overt MRI abnormality detectable on visual inspection, occur in other patients with hippocampal sclerosis and these patients have a poorer surgical outcome. If such changes can be reliably detected preoperatively, a quantitative assessment of the neocortex will become an important part of the presurgical work-up; this is an area of active research.

Interictal scalp electroencephalography

The interictal EEG is not a very reliable guide to the extent of the epileptogenic zone. In hippocampal sclerosis, a characteristic finding is an interictal anterior temporal spike discharge, maximal at sphenoidal electrodes but this is only found in a minority of cases (Fig. 6.5). Bitemporal interictal spikes, for instance, are frequently seen in unilateral temporal lobe epilepsy which responds well to surgery and are certainly no contraindication to surgical evaluation.

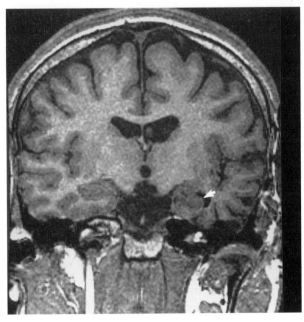

(a)

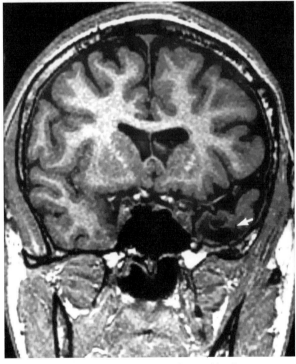

(b)

Fig. 6.3 Post-traumatic changes in a teenager who suffered a closed head injury in a motor accident at age 8 years. He developed complex partial seizures 4 years after trauma. (a) Hippocampal atrophy (arrowed) and reduced signal intensity in left mesial temporal structures. T_2-weighted images showed increased signal in these regions. (b) Anteriorly post-traumatic encephalomalacia is seen involving the cortex of the temporal pole (arrowed).

Table 6.2 Dual pathology: the findings in 100 consecutive patients with MRI-defined hippocampal sclerosis.

Coexistent cortical dysgenesis in 15 patients (15%)	
Subependymal heterotopia	6
Tuberous sclerosis	2
Focal macrogyria	2
Focal cortical dysplasia	1
Band heterotopia	1
Schizencephaly	1
Other gyral abnormalities	2

Dysgenesis often mild: two of the 15 had a history of childhood febrile convulsions.

Ictal scalp electroencephalography and video

An ictal EEG should be recorded using video and EEG telemetry in all patients with hippocampal sclerosis, even in the presence of otherwise concordant investigatory results. Making an exception to this rule can lead occasionally to mistaken operation in inappropriate patients. The presence of a unilateral onset rhythmic discharge of 5 Hz or greater within the first 30 s of the ictal recording is predictive of a seizure focus in about four out of five cases (Fig. 6.6). The absence of any focal features to an epileptic discharge is not uncommon on scalp ictal recordings and is not in itself a contraindication to surgery, although clearly such patients need a particularly careful assessment. A normal EEG during a seizure raises the strong possibility but not the certainty that the seizure was non-epileptic (usually a pseudoseizure). Ictal foci away from the temporal lobe indicate an epileptogenic zone distinct from the hippocampus.

Neuropsychology

Assessments of general intellectual ability and of memory are vital components of the presurgical work-up for several reasons.

● To identify dysfunctioning cortex. If the findings are discordant from those of imaging and neurophysiology, the epileptogenic zone is likely to extend beyond the damaged hippocampus and the outcome of surgery will be generally unfavourable. Broadly speaking, an overall intelligence quotient (IQ) below 70 usually indicates widespread cerebral dysfunction and is a relative contraindication to surgery. A discrepancy between verbal and performance IQ indicates lateralized dysfunction and this should be concordant with the side of the hippocampal sclerosis. Similarly, verbal memory deficits indicate dominant temporal lobe dysfunction and non-verbal deficits non-dominant dysfunction.

● To assess the risk of amnesia as a consequence of

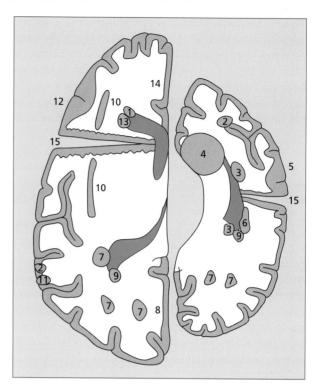

Fig. 6.4 Location of areas of cortical dysgenesis in 15 patients with dual pathology from a series of 100 patients with hippocampal sclerosis.

temporal lobe resection. The better the preoperative verbal memory, the worse will be the memory outcome following dominant temporal lobectomy. Conversely, a poor verbal memory seldom is significantly worse after surgery, as it implies that hippocampal memory function is already damaged by the hippocampal sclerosis. A similar, but less striking pattern is encountered in regard to non-verbal memory and the non-dominant temporal lobe. Bilateral hippocampal dysfunction should be suspected if both verbal and non-verbal memory tests are affected.

● To determine which hemisphere is dominant, where this is in doubt. In a proportion of patients with epilepsy, dominance is bilateral.

The sodium amytal test is a technique required in about 30% of cases. It involves angiography, which carries a small but definite risk of stroke and other complications and so should not be routinely carried out in all cases. This test is indicated in three specific clinical situations. First, if it is not clear which side of the brain language function is located. Second, if there are discordant investigatory findings. Finally, if psychological test findings point to an unexpected or significant risk to memory, either because the hippocampal disease is bilateral or wrongly

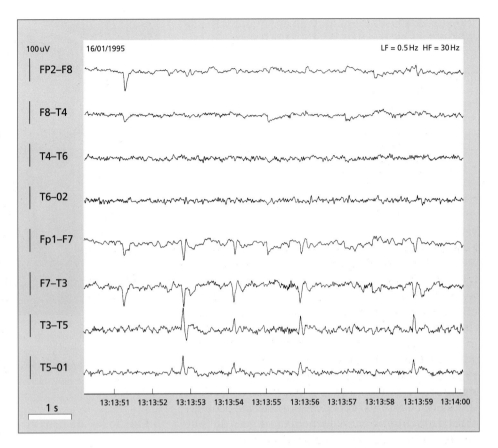

Fig. 6.5 Lateralized temporal sharp waves with phase reversal seen in the left mid-temporal region (T3). This is a common interictal finding in mesial temporal lobe epilepsy.

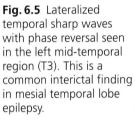

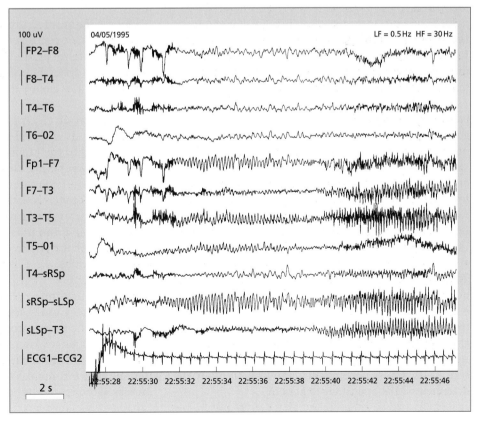

Fig. 6.6 Typical temporal lobe seizures with rhythmic lateralized θ activity.

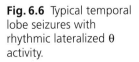

lateralized. The sodium amytal test though is not infallible and a favourable amytal test is not an absolute guarantee of postoperative freedom from memory impairment.

Psychiatric evaluation

A detailed neuropsychiatric evaluation is most appropriate in the early stages of a presurgical assessment. The evaluation has three purposes:

• to establish the risk of psychosis or affective disorder postoperatively;
• to estimate the ability of the person to withstand the long process of surgical evaluation and any adverse consequences of surgery; and
• to estimate the potential for quality of life gains postoperatively, if seizure control is achieved.

Psychiatry is not an exact science, and the predictive value of premorbid psychiatric features is not fully understood. In broad terms, a history of psychosis is a contraindication to surgery, unless the psychosis was entirely confined to a postictal period. Similarly, psychopathy or personality disorder is a relative contraindication as is a history of persistent significant depression. The patient and the family should be counselled about the possible psychological and psychiatric consequences of surgery, so that postoperative psychiatric problems can be swiftly identified.

Intracranial electroencephalography

In some centres, intracranial (depth) EEG recordings used to be frequently carried out to identify the epileptic focus. With the advent of MRI, this practice seems now obsolete in the majority (over 95%) of patients with hippocampal sclerosis being evaluated for temporal lobe surgery. Depth EEG records from otherwise functionally inaccessible cortex. The EEG data, however, come from only small areas of brain (a core < 1 cm), and unless the electrodes are placed logically to address specific questions (Figs 6.7 and 6.8), negative results can be misleading. In the work-up for hippocampal surgery, depth EEG is used in three main areas:

• to determine from which temporal lobe seizures are arising in patients with MRI evidence of bilateral hippocampal sclerosis;
• to determine whether or not seizures are arising from the temporal lobe in patients in whom MRI shows·dual pathology and the scalp EEG is indeterminate; and
• to localize the seizure discharge in patients with discordant MRI and functional data.

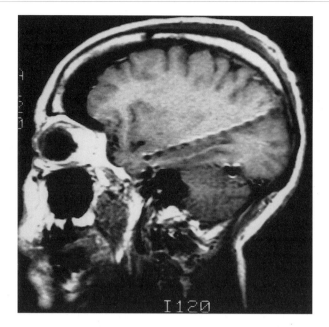

Fig. 6.7 Sagittal magnetic resonance imaging showing posteriorly placed depth electrode targeted to sample hippocampus. Twelve individual contacts can be identified.

Electrodes are usually placed bitemporally, and in other sites as determined by the questions being addressed (Figs 6.8 and 6.9). There is a 1–2% risk of haemorrhage or infection from each electrode placement, and the overall risk of the procedure increases with the number of electrodes inserted. There is no place for insertion of multiple electrodes without a prior idea about the most likely sites of seizure onset.

Foramen ovale electrode placement, in which the electrode tip is inserted through the foramen ovale to lie medial to the hippocampus, is a form of extracerebral intracranial electrode placement. It is a straightforward technique and does not require a craniotomy or stereotactic equipment, but has a significant complication rate, including facial pain, meningitis and vascular damage to the brainstem. There is probably little place for the technique in modern practice.

Functional imaging

Single photon emission computed tomography (SPECT) is the most commonly used functional imaging technique for lateralizing seizure foci. The interictal SPECT shows a decreased tracer uptake in the relevant temporal lobe and the ictal SPECT an increased tracer uptake. In most situations little new

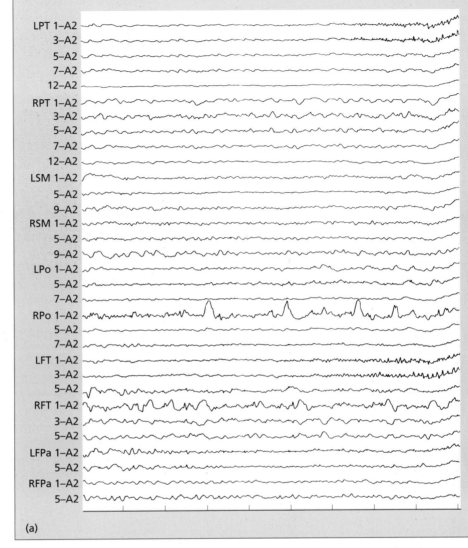

Fig. 6.8 (a,b) One typical mesial temporal seizure onset pattern is seen in these continuous electroencephalogram segments as low-voltage fast discharge in LPT 1,3 (left depth electrode contacts at tip). Electrode placement is seen in Fig. 6.7. Simultaneous seizure onset of similar morphology is identified in distal contacts of left temporal subdural strip (LFT 1,3) overlying entorrhinal cortex. Electrode contacts are labelled from distal (1) to proximal. LPT, RPT, left and right hippocampal depth electrodes; LSM, RSM, supplementary motor subdural strips; LPo, RPo, LFT, RFT, LFPa, RFPa, left and right frontopolar, frontotemporal and frontoparietal subdural strips. Full scale, 1000 μV; each division, 1 s. (continued on p. 204)

information is gained and only a small number of patients require this test as part of a surgical work-up. While positron emission tomography (PET) and functional magnetic resonance imaging (fMRI) do have their proponents, they have no firm place in routine practice in most situations.

Operative procedures and outcome

Temporal lobectomy

The standard temporal lobe resection extends for 4–5 cm behind the temporal pole in the dominant temporal lobe (Fig. 6.10) and up to 6 cm in the non-dominant temporal lobe, sparing the posterior part of the superior temporal gyrus. Most of the hippocampus, the amygdala and some surrounding mesial structures are removed. This operation was introduced in the 1950s and is still a common form of surgery carried out for epilepsy. Recently more selective methods for carrying out a temporal lobectomy have been devised. These all involve the resection of less temporal neocortex. The most common variant involves the removal of about 3 cm of the temporal lobe tip, which provides good access to the amygdala and hippocampus which are then removed in their entirety. This is now probably the most commonly performed operation, its outcome has not been as well studied as that of the standard operation.

The long-term outcome on seizure control of the standard temporal lobectomy has been intensively studied. In units with careful preoperative evaluation, between 60 and 70% of patients are rendered completely seizure-free by a temporal lobectomy and in another 20% the seizures are greatly improved.

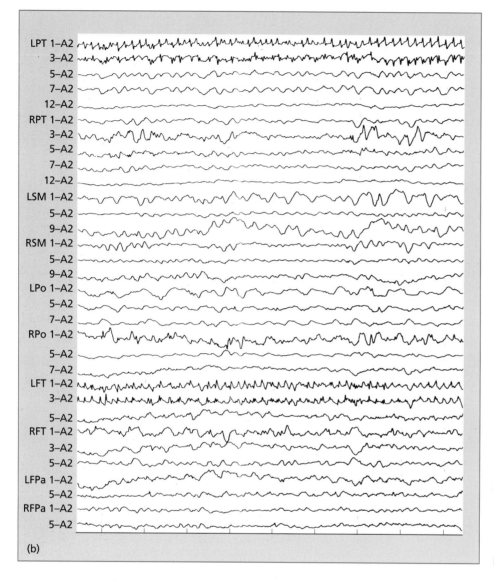

LPT 1–A2
3–A2
5–A2
7–A2
12–A2
RPT 1–A2
3–A2
5–A2
7–A2
12–A2
LSM 1–A2
5–A2
9–A2
RSM 1–A2
5–A2
9–A2
LPo 1–A2
5–A2
7–A2
RPo 1–A2
5–A2
7–A2
LFT 1–A2
3–A2
5–A2
RFT 1–A2
3–A2
5–A2
LFPa 1–A2
5–A2
RFPa 1–A2
5–A2

(b)

Fig. 6.8 (continued.)

In the remaining 10–20% the epilepsy will continue without significant change. The seizure outcome can be predicted with an estimated 90% reliability at 1 year following surgery. If seizures are continuing at this stage, there is only an approximately 10% chance of subsequent remission in the next 5 years. Conversely, there is only a 10% chance of seizures relapsing over the next 5 years in patients seizure-free at one year after surgery.

Generalized tonic–clonic seizures occurring in the first few weeks after surgery are generally considered to be of little prognostic significance to the long-term outcome, and may reflect the acute trauma of surgery. Similarly, partial seizures may continue for a few months and then peter out (run-down seizures). Occasionally, patients develop recurrent convulsive

seizures several years after surgery. These seizures are usually readily controlled medically, but it is important that patients are warned about this prior to surgery. Following successful surgery, drug treatment should be continued unchanged for 12–24 months, and then at a reduced level for at least a further 12 months.

Temporal lobectomy has a number of potential complications. The most common neurological deficit is a superior quadrantanopia, caused by damage to the optic radiation which loops through the posterior temporal lobe. A marked homonymous field defect occurs in about 20% of cases, and in 3% this amounts to a complete hemianopia. If the visual field cut exceeds 15°, it can prevent driving and the patient should be warned about this. The risk of hemi-

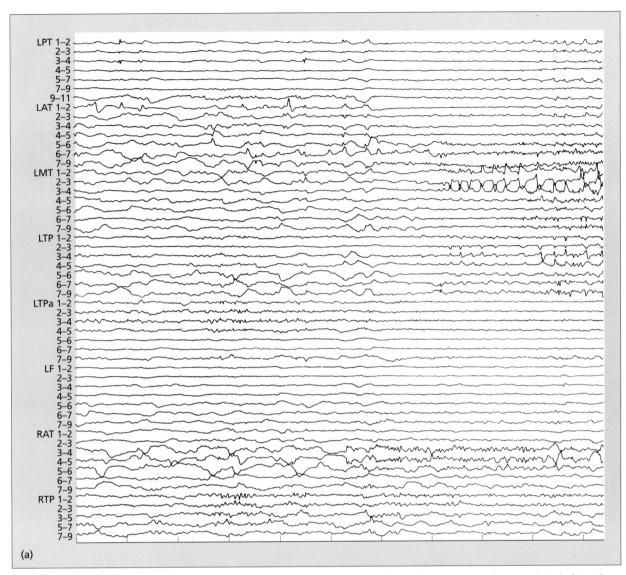

Fig. 6.9 (a,b) Continuous segments of intracranial electroencephalogram during spontaneous seizure activity in lateral temporal lobe. Mixed slow (4 Hz) and low-voltage fast frequencies characterize neocortical seizure onset, seen at LMT 2–3, 3–4 (left mid-temporal subdural strip). LPT, left hippocampal depth electrode; LAT, LMT, LTP, left anterior, mid and posterior temporal subdural strips; LTPa, LF left temporoparietal and frontal strips; RAT, RTP, right anterior and posterior temporal strips. (*continued.*)

plegia is about 1%, caused usually by damage to the anterior choroidal artery and the pial vessels that lie on the surface of the midbrain mesial to the hippocampus. A transient mild dysphasia is not uncommon with dominant temporal lobe resections, and in less than 1% a permanent dysphasia can result. Mild memory deficits detectable only on specialized testing are common, but a noticeable and marked deterioration in memory should be a rare complication if patients are prudently selected. Memory and intellectual function can actually improve after sur-

gery presumably because of better seizure control and the need for fewer antiepileptic drugs. Occasionally, surgery causes a profound amnesia, but this should not occur in a modern unit with satisfactory presurgical neuropsychological assessment. Postoperative psychiatric disturbance occurs in about 15% of patients in the first 6 months after surgery but is usually transient. A severe permanent postoperative psychotic breakdown, not infrequent in the early years of epilepsy surgery, should now occur in less than 5% of appropriately selected cases. Depression

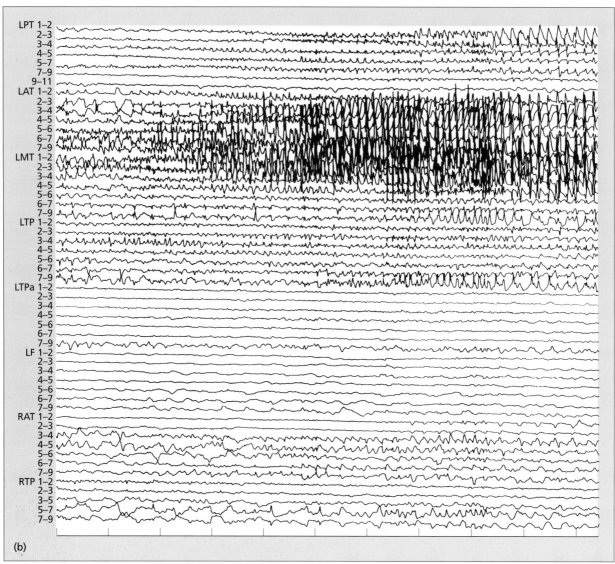

Fig. 6.9 (continued.)

is not uncommon in the first year after surgery, due no doubt to a combination of biological and psychosocial factors. The frequency of cognitive and psychiatric complications is higher in patients whose seizures continue postoperatively.

Other risks of epilepsy surgery include a third nerve palsy, meningitis, bone or scalp infection, vascular spasm, subdural haematoma or empyema, hydrocephalus and pneumocephalus. The overall risk of serious permanent complications of temporal lobectomy in an experienced centre is less than 5%, and the mortality rate of surgery is less than 0.5%. These risks must be carefully explained to the patient prior to surgery, if possible in writing. It should not be forgotten, however, that uncontrolled epilep-

sy carries greater potential risks; the annual mortality rate, for instance, in persons with severe intractable epilepsy is between 5 and 10 per 1000 and is particularly high in patients experiencing convulsive attacks.

Amygdalohippocampectomy

In an attempt to minimize the adverse events, on cognition or memory, a variety of less radical procedures have been devised. These include amygdalohippocampectomies carried out either stereotactically through the middle temporal gyrus or occipital cortex or by an approach along the sylvian fissure.

Whether or not the selective operations actually have a better outcome in regard to memory function

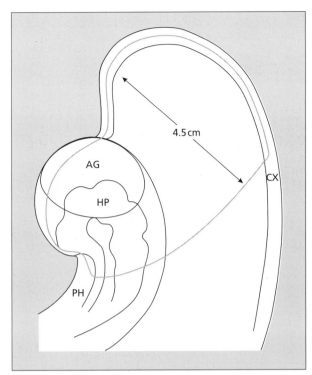

Fig. 6.10 A standard temporal lobectomy. Transverse plane showing the habitual extent of temporal resections (cortical and limbic) in the dominant hemisphere. AG, amygdala; CX, neocortex; HP, hippocampus; PH, parahippocampus; grey line, extent of resection.

and cognition is controversial, although no major differences have been reliably reported. The selective operations are more difficult technically and there is a higher reported risk of vascular disturbance and of hemiplegia, but a lower risk of dysphasia and visual field defect. Furthermore, the rates of long-term freedom from seizure, although not adequately studied, appear at least at an anecdotal level to be less good than after a standard temporal lobe resection. The clinical place of these approaches has not been fully established.

Counselling and rehabilitation

Prior to surgery, detailed counselling on the risks of surgery as well as its potential benefits is mandatory. After successful surgery, most patients experience the need for a major readjustment to a life without epilepsy. This can be difficult and painful, as is the realization that the problems in life are not automatically resolved. There is often a sense of anticlimax, at least in the first 12 months following the operation. Furthermore, if the operation fails, disappointment and depression are almost inevitable. Freedom from seizure will not immediately reverse

years of social isolation, a lack of self-confidence, missed educational or career opportunities. Becoming seizure-free can alter interpersonal relationships, which might have been based on dependence or a sick-role. Appropriate preoperative counselling can help prepare people and in some cases a structured postoperative rehabilitation programme can be helpful.

FOCAL RESECTIONS FOR OTHER LESIONS

Presurgical investigation

The presurgical work-up of lesional epilepsy surgery for small lesions in the temporal lobe is similar to that outlined above for hippocampal sclerosis. In the extratemporal regions, a differing emphasis is required, in relation to neurophysiology, imaging and neuropsychology.

Electroencephalography

The interictal spatial distribution of the scalp EEG focus in extratemporal neocortical lesions is often distant from the site of the lesion, and the interictal scalp EEG has proved to be an unreliable guide to precise localization (Figs 6.11 and 6.12). The ictal EEG is more helpful, but still often shows wide-

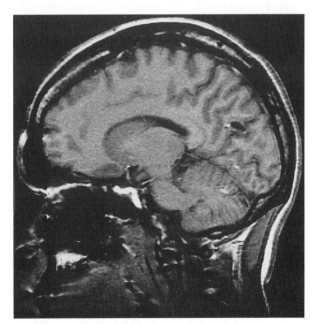

Fig. 6.11 Magnetic resonance image scan showing small parasagittal parieto-occipital lesion (biopsy-proven oligodendroglioma) in a patient with brief complex partial seizures characterized by visual disturbance, arrest of activity and loss of awareness.

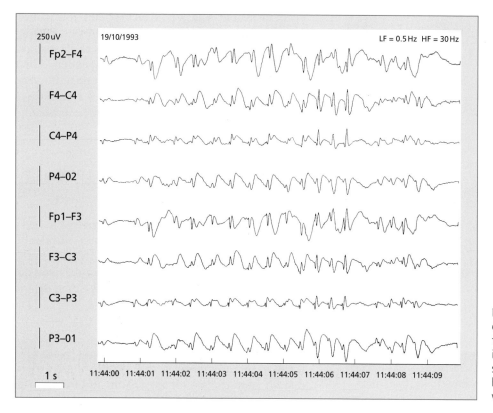

Fig. 6.12 Interictal electroencephalograph from the patient illustrated in Fig. 6.11 showing widespread bilateral slow spike and wave discharges.

spread changes and sometimes discordant changes even in focal lesions (Figs 6.13 and 6.14). Nevertheless, in most patients with intracranial lesions detected by neuroimaging, the additional information gathered by ictal scalp EEG and video recording will

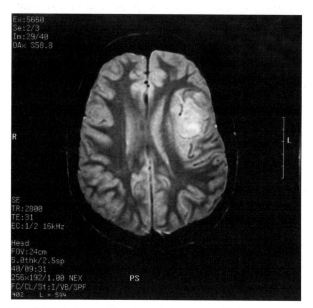

Fig. 6.13 Patient with a large left temporal lobe structural abnormality with apparently discordant ictal electroencephalograph.

be sufficient to allow a decision about surgery to be made without the need for invasive monitoring. In a few cases of extratemporal epilepsies, invasive EEG using either subdural strips or grids or depth electrodes is needed to define the extent of the irritative cortex (cortex with spike discharges) in the vicinity of a lesion. Per-operative corticography can assist the surgeon in deciding the extent of the resection, although the relative value of all these techniques is controversial, and convincing evidence that corticography, for instance, improves outcome is lacking. For instance, neither does the complete resection of all spiking areas identified at corticography always succeed in stopping seizures, nor does incomplete resection of the structural abnormality always fail.

Cortical mapping has an essential role in resections in eloquent areas of the brain, to assess the surgical risks to normal cortical function and thus to plan the extent of the surgical resection. The lesions which cause epilepsy often distort normal cerebral functional anatomy, which only careful mapping can demonstrate. Mapping is usually carried out using chronically implanted subdural grids (Fig. 6.15) or acutely at operation in an awake patient, using cortical stimulation or by recording evoked potentials. Preoperative functional mapping

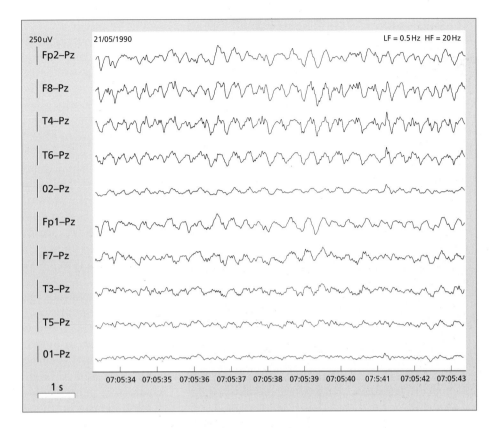

250 uV   21/05/1990   LF = 0.5 Hz   HF = 20 Hz

Fp2–Pz
F8–Pz
T4–Pz
T6–Pz
02–Pz
Fp1–Pz
F7–Pz
T3–Pz
T5–Pz
01–Pz

1 s   07:05:34   07:05:35   07:05:36   07:05:37   07:05:38   07:05:39   07:05:40   07:5:41   07:05:42   07:05:43

Fig. 6.14 Ictal electroencephalograph findings from the patient illustrated in Fig. 6.13 with widespread rhythmic activity over the right hemisphere, and irregular slowing over the left temporal region (the site of the known large structural lesion).

by fMRI is in a stage of rapid development and might possibly replace the need for some types of invasive mapping.

Imaging

Magnetic resonance imaging has greatly improved the sensitivity and specificity of lesion detection. Furthermore, by reformatting a volumetrically acquired dataset in three-dimensional space, the extent of the lesion and its relationship to the surrounding cerebral anatomy can be carefully defined. Magnetic resonance imaging is now routinely used for stereotactic surgical therapy.

HMPAO-SPECT and FDG-PET probably have a more important role in extratemporal epilepsy (lesional or not) than in temporal lobe epilepsy. Their use is mainly in demonstrating large areas of dysfunction, thus excluding surgery, rather than assisting in precise surgical planning. These techniques are used to greatly varying extents in different centres, and no consensus about their role has yet been reached. The same applies to techniques which are currently in research development, such as magnetic resonance spectroscopy, ligand or receptor-based PET and physiological imaging (coregistered fMRI and EEG studies.)

Neuropsychology

The neuropsychological assessment needs to be tailored according to the brain region under consideration for resection. Speech, visual and higher cognitive functions will need to be documented and mapped. In the resection of eloquent cortex the patient should be counselled about the risks of surgery to cortical function.

Underlying pathology

Tumours

Epilepsy occurs in approximately 50% of patients with intracerebral neoplasms. Slow-growing low-grade well-differentiated gliomas are the most epileptogenic lesions. In the Montreal series of 230 patients with gliomas, seizures occurred in 92% of those with oligodendrogliomas, 70% of those with astrocytomas and 37% of those with glioblastomas. Slow-growing or benign tumours account for about 10% of all adult epilepsies, but less in children. The history of epilepsy will often have extended for decades, sometimes even into infancy. In chronic refractory epilepsy caused by tumour, oligodendrogliomas account for between 10 and 30%, dysembryoplastic neuroepithelial tumours for 10–30%, astrocytomas for 10–30%, gangliomas for about 10–20% and

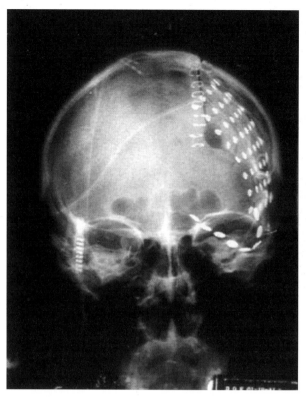

Fig. 6.15 Radiograph demonstrating subdural grid and strip inserted in dominant hemisphere for monitoring and stimulation.

hamartomas for between 10 and 20%. These tumours are sometimes associated with hippocampal sclerosis, particularly if situated in the temporal lobe.

The surgical management of rapidly growing tumours depends on factors other than epilepsy, but in slow-growing or benign tumours the control of epilepsy is usually the main indication for surgery. About 70–90% of patients can expect to become seizure-free or virtually seizure-free after the uncomplicated complete resection of a small neocortical tumour. However, if the lesion is in the temporal lobe and there is coexisting hippocampal sclerosis, seizure control rates are much lower unless the hippocampus is also resected. There is a higher incidence of small benign tumours in the temporal lobe than in other brain areas, and the standard temporal lobectomy (with hippocampal resection) is often the treatment of choice, even if the lesion is neocortical. The complications and outcome are similar to that in hippocampal sclerosis, although the resection of a relatively healthy hippocampus in the dominant temporal lobe is often associated with a significant drop in verbal memory skills. The chances of control of epilepsy are less if the tumour can be only incompletely resected.

Cavernomas

Cavernous haemangiomas (cavernomas) account for about 5–15% of intracranial vascular malformations. They are often not detectable on CT or angiography (because of low flow) but are readily seen on MRI, and their importance as an underlying cause of chronic focal epilepsy has become apparent only since the widespread use of MRI. The epilepsy may be in part because of the leaking of blood from these lesions, resulting in haemosiderin staining in surrounding cortical tissue, and surgical resection should therefore include the surrounding cortex as well as the lesion. There is also a risk of haemorrhage from these lesions which is probably between 0.5 and 1% a year. Complete and uncomplicated resection will control seizures in between 60 and 80% of cases.

Other arteriovenous malformations

Epilepsy is the presenting symptom in 20–40% of cases of cerebral arteriovenous malformation (AVM), and is present in over 60% (Fig. 6.16). The risk of causing epilepsy seems greatest in AVMs in the temporal lobe and in large or superficial AVMs. The chances of controlling the seizures by surgical resection depend on the size of the AVM and its site; resection of small lesions in the temporal lobe results in complete seizure control in over 60% of cases, whereas the resection of a large lesion in other neocortical areas has little chance of rendering the patient seizure-free, although an improvement in seizure control is common. The overall risk of haemorrhage in an AVM is about 2–4% per year, but depends on its size, the presence of aneurysms, the type of feeding and draining vessels, and the anatomy. Some AVMs can also be treated by either endovascular embolization or by focal radiotherapy. Whilst these techniques have been shown to reduce the risk of subsequent haemorrhage from an AVM, there is no controlled evidence that they improve seizure control. These approaches to therapy are usually reserved for inoperable cases or as a prelude to surgery.

Cortical dysgenesis

The introduction of MRI has demonstrated what was previously unsuspected, that cortical dysgenesis is a not uncommon underlying cause of chronic focal epilepsy, accounting for perhaps 15–20% of cases. The abnormalities can be apparently focal, but—except for tumoural forms such as a dysembryoplastic neuroepithelial tumour (DNT) and focal cortical dysplasia in the temporal lobe—there is only limited information about the best surgical approach. The overall progno-

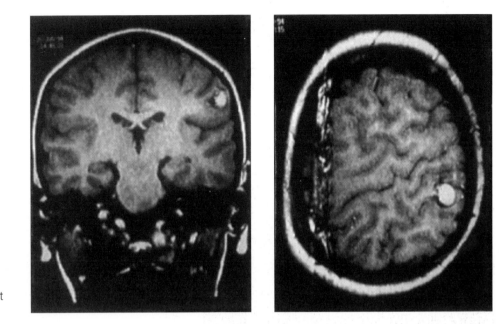

Fig. 6.16 Coronal and axial T$_1$-weighted magnetic resonance imaging scan demonstrating an occult vascular malformation.

sis for resection, even of seemingly well-localized abnormalities is rather poor, and presumably this is because such abnormalities are the only visible sign of what is a much more diffuse process. Quantitative MRI certainly often demonstrates subtle changes in white and grey matter ratios and volumes in distant sites and the scalp or cortical EEG also often shows widespread spiking (Fig. 6.17). This may explain why only a relatively small proportion of patients become seizure-free following epilepsy surgery.

Cerebral infection

In general, surgical therapy for chronic epilepsy following cerebral infection carries a poor outcome. Postmeningitic or postencephalitic epilepsy is often severe and refractory to medical therapy. Even if an apparently single lesion is uncovered on imaging (for instance, hippocampal atrophy following herpes simplex encephalitis), there is usually more subtle widespread diffuse damage in other brain areas and localized resection will fail to control seizures. Even where cortical damage is limited, the boundaries of the destructive process are seldom sharply defined and, as it is the boundary areas which are likely to contribute most to epileptogenesis, surgery is usually ineffective.

There are, however, situations where surgery is successful. Clearly, surgery is mandatory in most cases of acute cerebral abscess, which often presents with epilepsy. This is emergency surgery and can be life-saving. In recent years, human immunodeficiency virus (HIV) infection complicated by opportunis-

tic cerebral infections by bacteria or fungal agents, notably toxoplasmosis, has become common. Blind first-line medical therapy should be initiated, and only occasionally is surgical biopsy or curative resection required. Tuberculoma is the most common lesion causing focal epilepsy in some parts of the developing world, and is common in immunocompromised patients (for instance, with HIV infection). Medical treatment with antituberculous drugs is the therapy of choice, although where tuberculomas are uncommon a stereotactic biopsy is sometimes necessary to establish the diagnosis. Occasionally, excision of the residual cerebral lesion is necessary to control intractable seizures. In India and other parts of the developing world, patients presenting with focal epilepsy not infrequently can have small enhancing lesions on CT without perifocal oedema. Controversy exists about their nature, but most are likely to be tuberculous lesions or cerebral cysticercosis. Biopsy should be delayed for 2–3 months as many resolve spontaneously or on medical treatment. Cysticercosis can frequently present with epilepsy, and is a common cause of epilepsy in endemic regions. Usually the cysts are multiple and surgical resection is not a realistic option. In the occasional case, a single lesion does cause intractable epilepsy and resection of the cyst and surrounding gliosis will alleviate the epilepsy (Fig. 6.18).

Rasmussen's chronic encephalitis is a syndrome of uncertain pathogenesis, but which has the histological appearances of a chronic encephalitis. It presents as intractable focal epilepsy, often with pe-

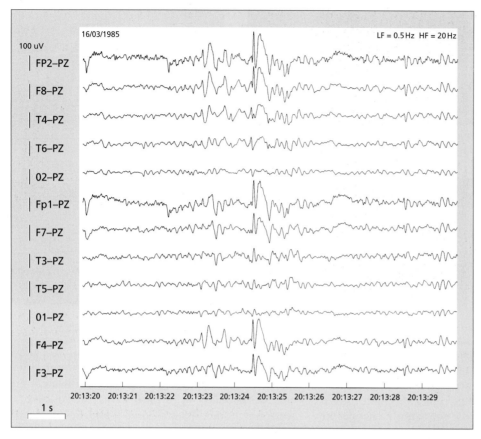

Fig. 6.17 Widespread bilateral anteriorly predominant interictal spikes recorded from a patient with an area of localized macrogyria in the left motor cortex.

riods of epilepsia partialis continua, and progressive neurological deficit, including hemiplegia, aphasia and hemionopia. Wide lobar excision or hemispherectomy can be curative if the lesion is completely excised.

Trauma

As is the case in post-infectious epilepsy, the pathological lesions causing refractory seizures after closed head trauma are often widespread and ill-defined. The MRI lesions do not necessarily correlate well with the extent of the histological changes, and limited surgical resection is often ineffective. In open trauma (including depressed fracture with dural breach), emergency debridement of the lesion will often prevent or reduce the intensity of subsequent epilepsy and should be carried out wherever possible. The wide debridement of established chronic lesions, including the resection of haemosiderin-lined cavities, will also sometimes improve chronic refractory epilepsy, although in general the results of surgery are disappointing even where the damage appears relatively circumscribed.

NON-LESIONAL FOCAL RESECTIONS

Prior to MRI many cases of epilepsy, including virtually all cases of hippocampal sclerosis and cortical dysgenesis, were considered 'non-lesional', in the sense that no lesion could be detected preoperatively. The nature and extent of the surgery in these cases depended heavily on scalp and invasive EEG. It was realized, even then, that if no pathology was found in the operated specimen that the postoperative prognosis for seizure control was poor. Since the advent of MRI, the situation has radically altered. Now many previously occult lesions can be clearly demonstrated preoperatively. The dependency on EEG for localization has been lost, and the requirement for invasive EEG has been greatly reduced. It has also become clear that operating on patients without MRI changes, even in the presence of a clear-cut EEG focus, and even by a wide resection (e.g. a frontal lobectomy for epilepsy originating in anterior frontal regions) has a rather poor postoperative outcome, with less than 10–30% of patients becoming seizure free.

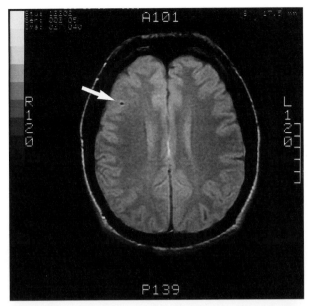

Fig. 6.18 A 36-year-old right-handed male with seizures since age 15 years, including sensations of heat or cold and forced head-turning to the left, with no loss of consciousness or postictal confusion. Axial proton-density magnetic resonance image demonstrates a small lesion with low signal intensity in the right frontal lobe (arrowed). Surgical resection demonstrated a calcified degenerated cysticercal cyst.

HEMISPHERECTOMY AND OTHER MULTILOBAR RESECTIONS

Hemispherectomy, the surgical excision or disconnection of one cerebral hemisphere, is carried out in children or adolescents with severe medically refractory seizures caused by unilateral hemisphere damage. It is nowadays an operation carried out only to improve the control of epilepsy.

Preoperative assessment
The preoperative evaluation should include consideration of the following issues.

Aetiology
The usual aetiologies in patients undergoing hemispherectomy are shown in Table 6.3. It is imperative to ascertain that the cerebral damage is wholly or very largely confined to one hemisphere. Even where the primary pathology is unilateral (for instance, after a vascular or traumatic event), secondary bihemispheric damage can result from prolonged anoxia or coma. The results of surgery where there is bilateral damage are far less good.

Table 6.3 Approximate frequencies of underlying aetiologies treated by hemispherectomy.

Rasmussen's encephalitis	35%
Perinatal insult (usually vascular, leading to unilateral porencephaly)	30%
Hemimegencephaly	10%
Migrational disorder	5%
Sturge–Weber disease	5%
Viral or bacterial infection	5%
Cerebral trauma	5%
Postnatal cerebrovascular event	5%

Seizures
Only patients with severe epilepsy should be considered for this operation. Most patients will have multiple seizure types, with daily seizures. The seizures should be exclusively or predominantly focal and be shown clearly to arise in the affected hemisphere.

Neurological status
To be considered for a hemispherectomy, the great majority of suitable candidates have a preoperative fixed hemiplegia, reflecting the severity of the hemispheric damage. This can be associated with other signs, such as hemionopia or hemisensory loss, and usually the patients have a degree of mental and psychomotor retardation.

The preoperative motor status is important in deciding whether or not surgery is possible. If the patient is unable, preoperatively, to perform individual finger movements or foot-tapping or to open and close their hands beyond a simple pincer motion, then a contralateral hemisphere resection is unlikely markedly to worsen motor performance. Similarly, the preoperative ability to perform gross movements at major joints (e.g. shoulder, elbow, hip, knee) is not usually worsened after a hemispherectomy, nor is a pre-existing spastic gait. If the deficits are progressive, the aggravation of motor deficit postoperatively might not be an unacceptable price for curative surgery. The presence or absence of sensory loss or of a hemionopic field defect influence the decision about surgery less. The degree of psychomotor retardation can be taken as an indication of the integrity of the good hemisphere, and severe retardation should be interpreted as evidence of bilateral cerebral damage and is predictive of less good postoperative seizure control. Finally, if this operation is performed on the language-dominant hemisphere there will be a risk of permanent aphasia, unless language functions can be transferred to the other side of the brain by processes of neuronal plasticity and cortical development. In early-onset damage, language is usually at least partially transferred. However, these processes are age-dependent, and it is possible to operate on the speech-dominant hemisphere safely only in young children. In older children, however, the operation must be largely restricted to the non-dominant hemisphere.

Electroencephalography

Ideally, the EEG should show low-amplitude slow activity and epileptic discharges confined to the affected hemisphere, but this is not always the case. Sometimes the damaged hemisphere is incapable of generating sufficient electrical signals to be detectable on scalp EEG (Figs 6.19 and 6.20). Secondary or independent epileptiform abnormalities can be found ictally and interictally in the unaffected hemisphere and these are not necessarily an adverse prognostic factor. Specialized neurophysiological advice is needed in this situation.

Imaging

This should show unihemispheric atrophy, with increased skull thickness, a smaller hemisphere, enlarged sulci and ventricles and a small cerebral peduncle (Fig. 6.21). Calcification, porencephaly, signal change, dysgenesis or other lesions will be seen, depending on the cause. The contralateral hemisphere should show no major lesions.

Surgical options

The original surgical operation (*anatomical hemispherectomy*) has been shown in recent years to have serious late postoperative complications (see below). For this reason, its use has been largely abandoned and a variety of new surgical techniques have been developed. The *anatomical hemispherectomy* consisted of the complete removal of the affected cerebral hemisphere with or without the basal ganglia, either *en bloc* or in fragments. The *modified hemispherectomy* links this operation with procedures to eliminate communication of cerebrospinal fluid with the hemispherectomy cavity by creating a largely extradural cavity and obstructing the foramen of Monro with a piece of muscle (Fig. 6.22). The operations of *hemidecortication* and *hemicorticectomy* consist of excision of the cortex with the preservation of as much white matter as possible. The *func-*

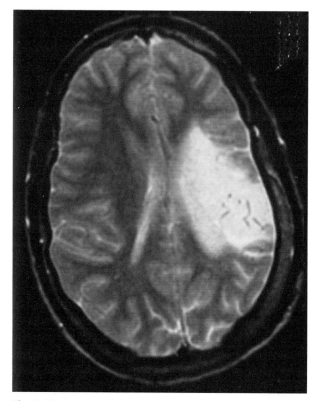

Fig. 6.19 Preoperative magnetic resonance image scan in a patient subsequently undergoing a left hemispherectomy showing cerebral infarction, occurring in early childhood, leading to medically intractable seizures.

tional hemispherectomy consists of a subtotal anatomical hemispherectomy with complete physiological disconnection achieved by undercutting the fibres to and from the cortex left *in situ*. The *hemispherotomy* and *peri-insular hemispherotomy* are variations on this principle, allowing cortical disconnection via alternative operative routes. The choice of surgical method depends on the experience and preference of the surgeon but, generally speaking, the functional hemispherectomies are now preferred to the anatomical hemispherectomies because of the smaller risks of morbidity.

Surgical morbidity

The overall mortality of hemispherectomy, which is often carried out in very young children, is in the region of 2–10%. Early morbidity includes haemorrhage, infection, hydrocephalus and brain herniation. The traditional anatomical hemispherectomy is associated with two specific late complications: superficial cerebral haemosiderosis and late hydrocephalus. Superficial cerebral haemosiderosis results in a gradual neurological deterioration evident at a

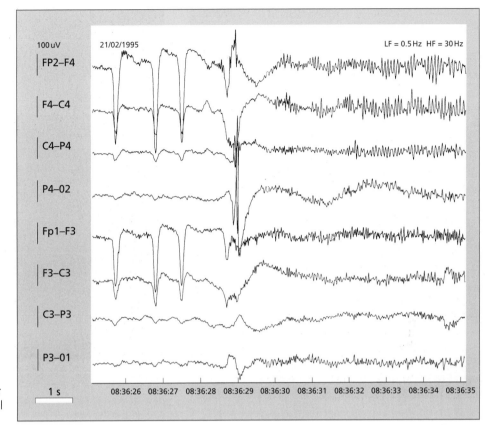

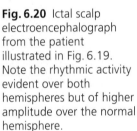

Fig. 6.20 Ictal scalp electroencephalograph from the patient illustrated in Fig. 6.19. Note the rhythmic activity evident over both hemispheres but of higher amplitude over the normal hemisphere.

mean of 8 years after surgery. The pathological findings are obstructive hydrocephalus caused by aqueduct stenosis, gliosis and ependymitis, and the hemispherectomy cavity is lined with a membrane similar to that found in a chronic subdural haematoma. The fluid in the ventricle is brownish and of 'machine oil' appearance. This complication is caused by chronic bleeding into the subdural hemispherectomy cavity, and occurs in about at least 30–50% of cases, leading eventually to disability and death. Late hydrocephalus is presumably produced by a similar mechanism. The newer operations, and in particular the functional operations, are not likely to be followed by these disastrous complications.

Outcome for seizure control and behaviour

Hemispherectomy is a very effective operation in carefully selected patients. A long-term improvement in seizure control is expected in 90–95% of suitably selected and competently operated cases. The chance of complete freedom from seizure is about 70–85%. Only about 5% of operated cases will show no worthwhile benefit.

The primary indication of the operation is to control seizures. Secondary gains in terms of behaviour and psychosocial development usually also occur. Severely abnormal behaviour patterns are common in children with severe epilepsy who undergo surgery, typically taking the form of aggressive or regressive behaviour, these are the results of repeated seizures, subclinical EEG activity and the drug treatment. A remarkable improvement in behaviour can be expected postoperatively in children whose seizures have been controlled, and there are also gains in social development and in intellectual function. Some children will develop to the stage where independent living and work are possible.

OTHER LARGE LOBAR RESECTIONS

A basic principle of surgery of extratemporal neocortical epilepsy is that the wider the excision around an epileptic focus, the more likely is complete seizure control to be achieved. This 'more is better' philosophy has characterized the surgical approach to epilepsy in non-eloquent cortical regions, particularly in

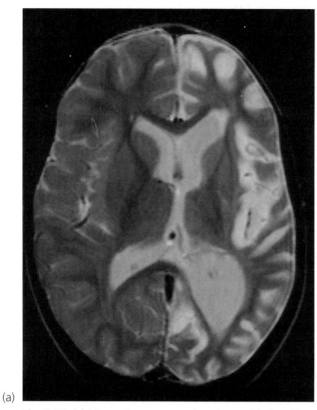

(a)

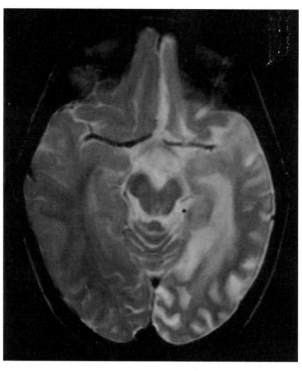

(b)

Fig. 6.21 (a) Magnetic resonance imaging, axial view, T$_2$-weighted, demonstrating left hemispheric atrophy in a patient with chronic encephalitis. (b) Magnetic resonance imaging, axial view, T$_2$-weighted, showing atrophy of the left cerebral peduncle and temporo-occipital lobes.

the pre-MRI era. A large frontal lobectomy for instance, can be carried out with no gross deficit and only an approximately 3% risk of hemiparesis. The inferior central region, over the face area, can be resected without sensory or motor deficit (presumably because of bilateral cortical representation), although resections in the hand or leg areas of the cortex do result in monoplegia. Similarly, a large resection of the non-dominant parietal lobe can be carried out with minor sensory deficit only. Dominant parietal resections carry a risk of profound sensory loss and apraxia. These large lobar resections are less common now because the MRI localization of structural disease has allowed more precise surgical planning.

CORPUS CALLOSECTOMY (CORPUS CALLOSUM SECTION)

This operation, the transection of the corpus callosum, can be carried out in either a one- or two-staged procedure (Fig. 6.23). It was first performed in 1940, yet even now neither the precise physiological ra-

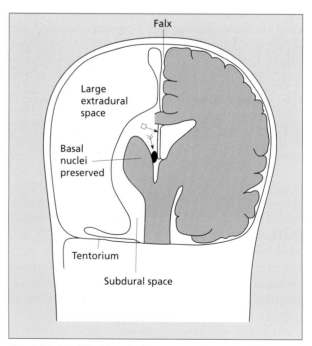

Fig. 6.22 Modified hemispherectomy: diagrammatic representation of the extent of excision. The arrows show the muscle plug and the foramen of Monro.

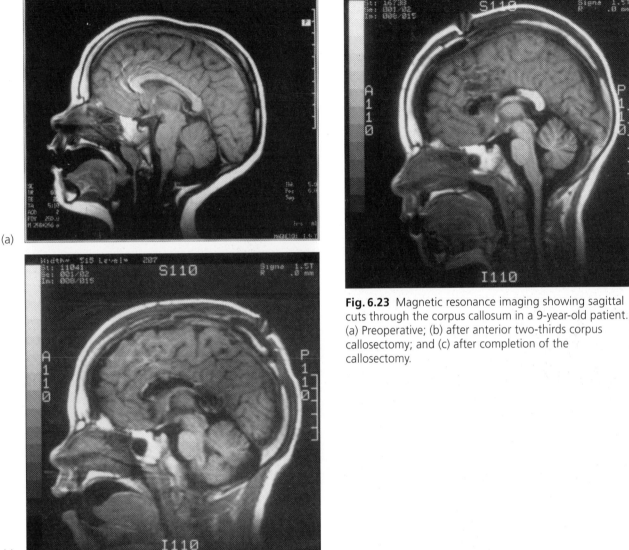

Fig. 6.23 Magnetic resonance imaging showing sagittal cuts through the corpus callosum in a 9-year-old patient. (a) Preoperative; (b) after anterior two-thirds corpus callosectomy; and (c) after completion of the callosectomy.

tionale for the surgery nor its indications are clearly defined.

It was originally proposed that that section of the corpus callosum would prevent the rapid spread of epileptic activity from one hemisphere to the other, but in fact seizure activity can propagate widely via non-callosal pathways. It is simplistic to assume that the operation prevents secondarily generalization, but it does have a desynchronizing effect on epileptic activity, and can inhibit seizures, although exactly how or why is unclear.

Indications

The operation is usually reserved for patients with severe secondarily generalized epilepsy manifest by frequent drop attacks causing injury, in whom medical therapy is ineffective and in whom other surgical procedures are not possible. The procedure should therefore be primarily considered in patients with tonic or atonic seizures, many of whom have other seizure types too and often learning disability (many have the Lennox–Gastaut syndrome). However, it has also been shown to have an effect in complex partial seizures, some myoclonic seizures and in tonic–clonic seizures. It can also be used in combination with resective surgery, and the operation can have a particular role combined with frontal lobe resections in patients with severe frontal lobe damage following trauma or abscess. In any of these indications, there seems little way of differentiating those patients who will do well and those who will not. This lack of specificity combined with its generally disappointing effects and its potential hazards render the corpus callosectomy a last-ditch operation, now only infrequently carried out.

Operative procedure

In most centres, corpus callosectomy is carried out as a two-stage procedure. In the first stage, the anterior two-thirds of the corpus callosum are sectioned. If this is ineffective, the section can be completed at a second operation. The two-stage procedure has a significantly lower morbidity than the one-stage operation.

Outcome

The operation must be considered a palliative procedure, intended to reduce seizure severity and in particular to reduce injuries caused by falls. No patient should undergo the procedure on the assumption that epileptic seizures will stop completely. Short-term freedom from seizure does occur in about 5–10% of cases but there is a strong tendency to relapse over months or years. Nevertheless, the number of generalized seizures or seizures with falls is usually reduced by the operation, albeit sometimes with an increase in the number of partial seizures.

Both the single- and the two-stage operation carry significant risks of neurological deficit. Hemiparesis can be caused by traction per-operatively or by vascular infarction caused by damage to the pericallosal arteries or venous thrombosis. A transient and highly distinctive disconnection syndrome with mutism, urinary incontinence and bilateral leg weakness is a not uncommon consequence of a single-stage complete callosal section. It is present in the immediate postoperative period and resolves usually after a matter of weeks, although in 5% of cases can be permanent; the pathophysiology of this effect is not clear. A posterior disconnection syndrome in which complex motor tasks become impossible occurs in about 5% after a one-stage procedure. After the completed transection, most patients will exhibit elements of a 'split brain' profile on neuropsychological testing although, remarkably, this causes little disability in everyday living. Other recorded complications include extradural haematoma, air embolism, infection and an increase in the frequency or intensity of partial seizures. Callosectomy does not seem to affect overall behaviour or personality. Overall, the risks of permanent severe sequelae after corpus callosal section, either neurological or

neuropsychological, are of the order of 5–10%, and there is a mortality rate of about 1–5%.

MULTIPLE SUBPIAL TRANSECTION

This operation is also referred to as the Morrell procedure. Parallel rows of 4 mm-deep cortical incisions are ploughed perpendicular to the cortical surface, 5 mm apart. The theoretical basis of the operation is that these transections sever horizontal cortical connections and thus disrupt the lateral recruitment of neurones which is essential in producing synchronized epileptic discharges (Figs 6.24 and 6.25). At the same time, normal function is preserved as it is largely supported by vertically orientated afferent and efferent connections. There are many critics of this postulation, and it is not clear whether or not this is a valid explanation of the postoperative consequences. The procedure has, theoretically, one major advantage. It can be used when the epileptogenic zone involves eloquent brain cortex, in which resection would result in significant neurological deficit. It has thus been principally applied to patients with epileptic foci in language, or in sensory or motor cortex. In many cases, it has been combined with a lesion resection in or adjacent to eloquent cortex.

The procedure has been the subject of only a rather limited evaluation, and its true role has yet to be defined. Currently, it should be reserved for use in patients with severe frequent seizures arising from eloquent cortex in whom all alternative strategies have been exhausted. The operation potentially has a particular role in epilepsia partialis continua, in Rasmussen's encephalitis and in the Landau–Kleffner syndrome.

Multiple subpial transection has been successfully carried out in Broca's area, the precentral and postcentral gyrus, and in Wernicke's area without noticeable loss of function (Fig. 6.25). There is a risk of haemorrhage, and a proportion of patients will experience severe motor, sensory and language disturbance following this procedure. The overall morbidity of this operation in routine surgical practice has not been clearly established.

VAGAL NERVE STIMULATION

Left vagus nerve stimulation is a novel therapy which was approved in 1997 in the USA as a treatment for adults with medically refractory partial-onset seizures. The operation entails implantation of a pro-

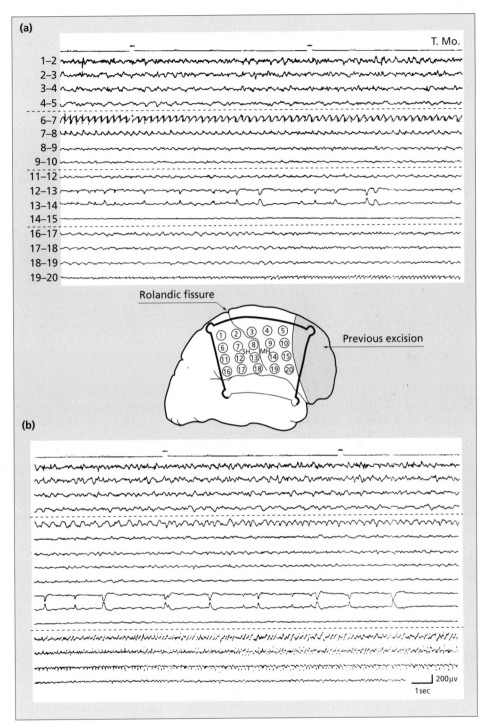

Fig. 6.24 Two samples of an electrocorticographical record from a patient with Rasmussen's encephalitis demonstrating the typical multifocal epileptiform discharges throughout the central region. A previous frontal resection had been unsuccessful.

grammable signal generator into the chest cavity with stimulating electrodes to the left vagus nerve. The stimulator frequency is tailored on an individual basis. The mechanism of action of vagal nerve stimulation is not known, but controlled studies have shown that it will reduce seizure frequency when compared to an active placebo (low-frequency stimulation). One well-conducted multicentre add-on double-blind randomized case–control study has been carried out. Patients receiving high stimulation (94 patients, ages 13–54 years) had an average 28% reduction in total seizure frequency, compared with a 15% reduction in the low-stimulation group (active placebo: 102 patients, ages 15–60 years; $P = 0.04$).

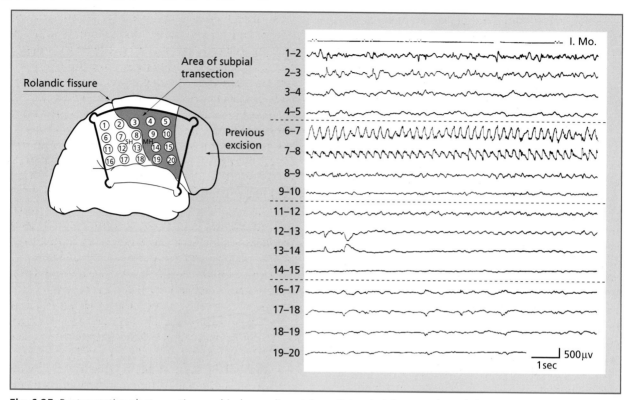

Fig. 6.25 Postoperative electrocorticographical recordings taken after subpial transection of the entire precentral region in the same patient as in Fig. 6.24. Epileptiform activity continued posterior to the rolandic fissure.

The high-stimulation group also had greater improvements on global evaluation scores.

The side-effects of the stimulation include alteration of the voice, dyspnoea and a tingling feeling in the neck every time the stimulator is turned on, but no changes in gastric, cardiac or pulmonary function have been reported. Patients have died suddenly in the months after the insertion of the vagal nerve stimulator, but apparently not at a frequency greater than would be expected in a population of patients with severe epilepsy. The effects on seizure frequency are generally slight and very few patients become seizure-free. In open studies, other seizure types have been treated with sporadic success. The role of this procedure has not yet been fully established.

OTHER FUNCTIONAL SURGICAL PROCEDURES

Stereotactic neurosurgery is a fast-developing technique with various potential applications in epilepsy. Depth electrode implantation is now best carried out using computer-guided stereotaxis. This is currently frame-based, although developments in frame-

less stereotaxy may well make this a safe and a more convenient option. The overall risk of serious complication from each electrode implantation is about 2%. The major risks being haemorrhage and infection. There are recorded cases of transmission of prion disease, but this can be usually avoided by using disposable (but very expensive) electrodes.

Both stereotactic ablation and stimulation have been used for many years, in small numbers of patients, in an attempt to control or modify seizures. Targets have included the amygdala, various thalamic nuclei, the fields of Forel, the anterior commissure, the fornix and the posterior limb of the internal capsule. The results of these operations have been generally poor, and this type of functional surgery had been, until recently, largely abandoned. A recent resurgence of interest has occurred, encouraged by both the improved anatomical precision of stereotaxy made possible by MRI and better surgical instrumentation, and also by the success of these procedures in other conditions, such as Parkinson's disease and in pain. There is also research interest in the possibility of stem cell and neural transplantation and in the possibility of stereotactic drug implantation. None of these procedures is yet at a stage where surgery in human epilepsy is possible, yet all have an exciting potential.

Computer-directed stereotaxy is also used to guide surgical resection, and stereotactic hippocampectomy and amygdalohippocampectomy, for instance, is now in routine use in several centres (Fig. 6.26).

Finally, there is considerable interest in stereotactic radiosurgery, using the gamma knife or the X-knife. These techniques have, not surprisingly, caught the public imagination. The best evaluated techniques have used radiosurgery to obliterate small AVMs or cavernomas. In one series of 160 AVMs, 48 patients had epilepsy. At 2-years follow-up, 38% of these cases were seizure-free, 22% had improved seizure control and 6% were worse. This technique should be currently considered in any inoperable AVM or cavernoma, or as a preference to surgery in small deeply situated AVMs. A recent development has been the use of the gamma knife to irradiate the hippocampal area in mesial temporal sclerosis to control epilepsy. Promising results have been obtained in small numbers of patients, but it is too early to provide any definitive evaluation of this novel approach.

ORGANIZATION OF EPILEPSY SURGERY CARE: EPILEPSY SURGERY CENTRE

It should be clear that epilepsy surgery is a specialized area which requires, for almost every patient, input from specialists in the following non-surgical areas: neurology, neurophysiology, neuroradiology, neuropathology, psychology and psychiatry. The input is needed to select suitable patients for surgery, to counsel patients adequately about the potential risks and benefits of surgery and to follow up patients postoperatively. Furthermore, the surgery itself is often highly specialized, and requires experienced surgeons, good facilities for neuroanaesthesia and the intensive care management of epilepsy. A full range of necessary facilities and expertise is likely to be available only in designated centres, and standards for such centres have been defined.

The International League Against Epilepsy (ILAE) Commission on Neurosurgery has proposed that there should be two levels of epilepsy surgery centre: basic epilepsy surgery centres and reference epilepsy surgery centres. Both should be sited within a comprehensive neuroscience centre with access to all the specialties listed above. The basic centre should have a throughput of at least 25 operated cases per year, and facilities for advanced MRI, amytal testing and video-EEG telemetry. The reference epilepsy surgery centres should have, in addition, access to neuropaediatrics and neurorehabilitation, a throughput of 50–100 operated cases and ancillary operative facilities including electrocorticography, cerebral functional mapping, and for evoked potential studies. Paediatric epilepsy surgery would be likely to be possible only in a reference centre. In the age of clinical governance and audit, it is inevitable as well as desirable that epilepsy surgery services are organized in a formal and regulated fashion.

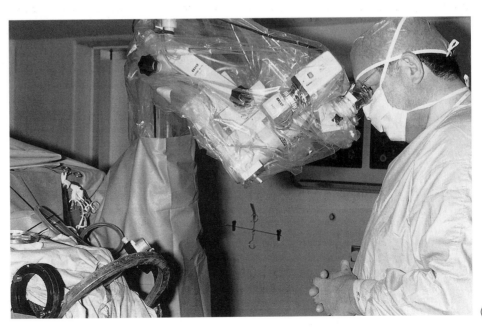

Fig. 6.26 Stereotactic amygdalohippocampectomy. (a) The use of the Compass stereotactic equipment to perform a selective amygdalohippocampectomy. *(Continued on p. 222)*

(a)

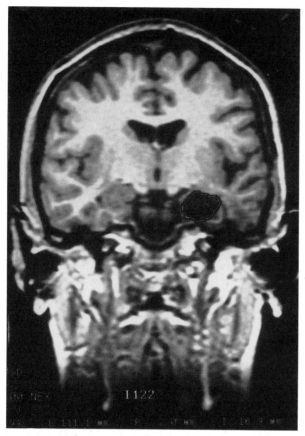

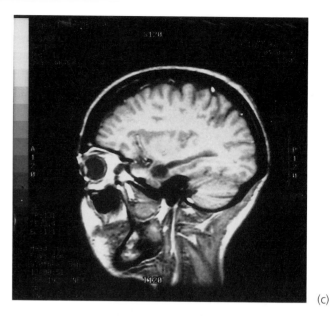

(c)

(b)

Fig. 6.26 (b,c) Postoperative magnetic resonance imaging studies following stereotactic amygdalohippocampectomy via a lateral temporal neocortical approach. Using the Compass stereotactic system, volumetric excisions of epileptogenic areas may be performed, either of foreign tissue lesions or, in this instance, an area of hippocampal sclerosis. It is a frame-based system but may be used under microscopic conditions where the surgeon can view down the cylindrical retractor itself. Computer technology also allows a 'head-up' display, whereby the computer reconstruction of a 'probe's eye' view may be superimposed on the surgeon's eyepiece down the microscope. The coronal (b) and parasagittal (c) postoperative magnetic resonance images demonstrate the focal mesial resection that is possible with this technique, while sacrificing the minimum of temporal lobe neocortex. The parasagittal image demonstrates the core of temporal lobe removed. The coronal image shows complete resection of the mesial temporal structures.

FURTHER READING

Adams, C.B.T. (1983) Hemispherectomy: a modification. *J Neurol Neurosurg Psychiatry*, **46**, 617–19.

Andermann, F. (1992) Clinical indications for hemispherectomy and callosotomy (review). *Epilepsy Res*, **5(189)** (Suppl.), 189–99.

Andermann, F. (ed) (1991) *Chronic encephalitis and epilepsy: Rasmussen's syndrome*. Butterworth Heinemann, Boston.

Andersen, B., Rogvi-Hansen, B., Kruse Larsen, C. & Dam, M. (1996) Corpus callosotomy: seizure and psychosocial outcome. A 39-month follow-up of 20 patients. *Epilepsy Res*, **23**(1), 77–85.

Awad, I., Katz, A., Hahn J. *et al.* (1989) Extent of resection in temporal lobectomy for epilepsy. *Epilepsia*, **30**, 756–62.

Baxendale, S. (1998) Amnesia in temporal lobectomy patients: historical perspective and review. *Seizure*, Feb, **7**(1), 15–24.

Bell, B.D. & Davies, K.G. (1998) Anterior temporal lobectomy, hippocampal sclerosis, and memory: recent neuropsychological findings. *Neuropsychol Rev* Mar; **8**(1), 25–41.

Bergen, D., Morrel, F., Bleck, T.P. & Whisler, W.W. (1984) Predictors of success in surgical treatment of intractable epilepsy. *Epilepsia*, **25**, 656.

Bergin, P.S., Fish, D.R., Shorvon, S.D., Oatridge, A., deSouza, N.M. & Bydder, G. (1995) Magnetic resonance imaging in partial epilepsy: additional abnormalities shown with fluid attenuated inversion recovery (FLAIR) pulse sequence. *J Neurol Neurosurg Psychiatry*, **58**, 439–43.

Blume, W.T. (1984) Corpus callosum section for seizure control: rationale and review of experimental and clinical data. *Cleveland Clin Quart*, **51**, 319–32.

Cascino, G.D., Hulihan, J.F., Sharbrough, F.W. & Kelly, P.J. (1993) Parietal lobe lesional epilepsy: electroclinical correlation and operative outcome. *Epilepsia*, **34**, 522–527.

Cascino, G.D., Jack, C.R. Jr, Parisi, J.E. *et al.* (1991) Magnetic resonance imaging-based volume studies in temporal lobe epilepsy: pathological considerations. *Ann Neurol*, **30**, 31–6.

Cascino, G.D., Jack, C.R. Jr, Parisi, J.E. *et al.* (1993) MRI in the presurgical evaluation of patients with frontal lobe epilepsy and children with temporal lobe epilepsy: pathologic correlation and prognostic importance. *Epilepsy Res*, **11**, 51–9.

Cascino, G.D., Kelly, P.J., Hirschorn, K.A., Marsh, W.R. & Sharborough, F.W. (1990) Stereotactic lesion resection in partial epilepsy. *Mayo Clin Proc*, **65**, 1053–60.

Casey, A.T.H., Kitchen, N.D., Thomas, D.G.T. & Harkness, W. (1994) Stereotactic guided craniotomy for cavernous angiomas presenting with epilepsy. *J Neurol Neurosurg Psychiatry*, **57**, 395.

Cohen, M.S. & Bookheimer, S.Y. (1994) Localization of brain function with magnetic resonance imaging. *Trends Neurosci*, **17**, 268–77.

Cook, M.J., Fish, D.R., Shorvon, S.D., Straughan, K. & Stevens, J.M. (1992) Hippocampal volumetric and morphometric studies in frontal and temporal lobe epilepsy. *Brain*, **115**, 1001–15.

Crawford, M. West,C.R., Chadwick, D.W. *et al.* (1986) Arteriovenous malformation of the brain: natural history in unoperated patients. *J Neurol Neurosurg Psychiatry*, **49**, 1–10.

Crawford, P.M., West, C.R., Shaw, M.D.M. *et al.* (1986b) Cerebral arteriovenous malformations and epilepsy: factors in the development of epilepsy. *Epilepsia*, **27**, 270–75.

Daumas-Duport, C., Scheithauer, B.W., Chodkiewicz, J.P., Laws, E.R. Jr & Vedrenne, C. (1988) Dysembryoplastic neuroepithelial tumor: a surgically curable tumor of young patients with intractable partial seizures. Report of thirty-nine cases. *Neurosurgery*, **23**, 545–56.

Duchowny, M., Levin, B., Jayakar, P. *et al.* (1992) Temporal lobectomy in early childhood. *Epilepsia*, **33**, 298–303.

Duchowny, M., Jayakar, P., Resnick, T. *et al.* (1998) Epilepsy surgery in the first three years of life. *Epilepsia*, Jul; **39**(7), 737–43.

Engel, J. (ed) (1993) *The Surgical Treatment of the Epilepsies*, 2nd edn. Raven Press, New York.

Engel, J., Pedley, T.A. (1997) *Epilepsy: a comprehensive textbook*. Lippincott Raven, Philadelphia.

Fish D, Andermann, F. & Oliver, A. (1991) Complex partial seizures and small posterior temporal or extratemporal structural lesions: surgical management. *Neurology*, **41**, 1781–4.

Fish, D.R., Andermann, F. & Olivier, A. (1991) Complex partial seizures and posterior temporal or extratemporal lesions: surgical strategies. *Neurology*, **41**, 1781–4.

Fish D.R., Smith, S.J., Quesney, L.F., Andermann, F. & Rasmussen, T. (1993) Surgical treatment of children with medically intractable frontal or temporal lobe epilepsy: results and highlights of 40 years' experience. *Epilepsia*, **34**, 244–7.

Gates, J.R., Leppik, I.E., Yap, J. & Gumnit, R.J. (1984) Corpus callosotomy: clinical and electroencephalographic effects. *Epilepsia*, **25**(3), 308–16.

Gates, J.R., Mireles, R., Maxwell, R., Sharbrough, F. & Forbes, G. (1986) Magnetic resonance imaging, electroencephalogram, and selected neuropsychological testing in staged corpus callosotomy. *Arch. Neurol.*, **43**, 1188–91.

Guerrini, R., Dravet, C., Raybaud, C. et al. (1992) Neurological findings and seizure outcome in children with bilateral opercular macrogyric-like changes detected by MRI. *Dev. Med. Child Neurol.*, **34**(8), 694–705.

Handforth, A., DeGiorgio, C.M., Schachter, S.C. *et al.* (1998) Vagus nerve stimulation therapy for partial-onset seizures: A randomized active-control trial. *Neurology*, 5ct 09; 51/1 (48–55).

Hopkins, A., Shorvon, S. & Cascino, G. (1995) *Epilepsy*, 2nd edn.Chapman & Hall, London.

Hufnagel, A., Zentner, J., Fernandez, G. *et al.* (1997) Multiple subpial transection for control of epileptic seizures: effectiveness and safety. *Epilepsia*, Jun; 38(6): 678–88.

Jack, C.R. Jr, Sharbrough, F.W. & Cascino, G.D. (1992) MRI-based hippocampal volumetry: correlation with outcome after temporal lobectomy. *Ann. Neurol.*, **31**, 138–46.

Kelly, P.J. (1986) Computer-assisted stereotaxis: new approaches to the management of intracranial mass lesions. *Neurology*, **36**, 535–41.

Kratimenos, G.P., Pell, M.F., Thomas, D.G.T. *et al.* (1992) Open selective amygdalohippocampectomy for drug resistant epilepsy. *Acta Neurochir.*, **116**, 150–4.

Kratimenos, G.P., Thomas, D.G.T., Shorvon, S.D. & Fish, D.R. (1993) Stereotactic insertion of intracerebral electrodes in the investigation of epilepsy. *Br J Neurosurg*, 7, 45–52.

Kuks, J., Cook, M., Fish, D.R., Shorvon, S.D. & Stevens, J. (1993) Hippocampal sclerosis and febile seizures. *Lancet*, **342**, 1391–94.

Kuzniecky, R., Burgard, S., Faught, E., Morawetz, R. & Bartolucci, A. (1993) Predictive value of magnetic resonance imaging in temporal lobe epilepsy surgery. *Arch Neurol.*, **50**, 65–9.

Levesque, M.F., Nakasato, N., Vinters, H.V. & Babb, T.L. (1991) Surgical treatment of limbic epilepsy associated with extrahippocampal lesions: the problem of dual pathology. *J Neurosurg*, **75**, 364–70.

Levesque, M.F., Sutherling, W.W. & Crandall, P.H. (1992) Surgery of central sensory motor and dorsolateral frontal lobe seizures. *Stereotac Func Neurosurg*, **38(1–4)**, 168–71.

Lindquist, C., Kihlstrom, L. & Hellstrand, E. (1991) Functional neurosurgery—a future for the gamma knife? *Stereotact. Funct Neurosurg*, **57**, 72–81.

Lindsay, J., Ounstead, C. & Richards, P. (1987) Hemispherectomy for childhood epilepsy: a 36 year study. *Dev Med Child Neurol*, **29**, 592–600.

Luders, H. (1992) *Epilepsy Surgery*. Raven Press, New York.

Malla, B.R., O'Brien, T.J., Cascino G.D. *et al.* (1998) Acute postoperative seizures following anterior temporal lobectomy for intractable partial epilepsy. *J Neurosurg* **89**(2), 177–82.

Marks, D.A., Kim, J., Spencer, D.D. & Spencer, S.S. (1992) Characteristics of intractable seizures following meningitis and encephalitis. *Neurology*, **42**(8), 1513–18.

Monteiro, L., Coelho, T. & Stocker, A. (1992) Neurocysticercosis—a review of 231 cases. *Infection*, **20**(2), 61–5.

Moore, J.L., Cascino, G.D., Trenerry, M.R., Kelly, P.J. & Marsh, W.R. (1993) A comparative study of lesionectomy versus corticectomy in patients with temporal lobe lesional epilepsy. *J Epilepsy*, **6**, 239–42.

Morrell, F. & Whisler, W.W. (1982) Multiple subpial transection for epilepsy eliminates seizures without destroying the function of the transected zone. *Epilepsia*, **23**, 440.

Oakes, W.J. (1992) The natural history of patients with the Sturge–Weber syndrome. *Pediatr Neurosurg*, **18**(5–6), 287–90.

Oguni, H., Andermann, F. & Rasmussen, T.B. (1992) The syndrome of chronic encephalitis and epilepsy. A study based on the MNI series of 48 cases. *Adv Neurol*, **57**(419), 419–33.

Oguni, H., Olivier, A., Anderman, F. & Comair, J. (1991) Anterior callosotomy in the treatment of medically intractable epilepsies: a study of 43 patients with a mean follow-up of 39 months. *Ann Neurol*, **30**, 357–64.

Ojemann, G.A. (1992) Different approaches to resective epilepsy surgery: standard and tailored (review). *Epilepsy Res*, **5**(169) (Suppl.), 169–74.

Ojemann, G.A., Crutsfeldt, O., Lettich, E. & Haglund, H. (1988) Neuronal activity in human lateral temporal cortex relates to short-term verbal memory. *Brain*, **111**, 1383–403.

Olivier, A. (1991) Relevance of removal of limbic structures in surgery for temporal lobe epilepsy. *Can J Neurol Sci*, **18**, 628–35.

Oxbury, S., Oxbury, J., Renowden, S, Squier, W. & Carpenter, K. (1997) Severe amnesia: an usual late complication after temporal lobectomy. *Neuropsychologia* **35**(7), 975–88.

Palmini, A., Andermann, F., Olivier, A. *et al.* (1991) Neuronal migration disorders: a contribution of modern neuroimaging to be etiologic diagnosis of epilepsy. *Can J Neurol Sci*, **18**, 580–7.

Palmini, A., Andermann, F., Olivier, A., Tampieri, D. & Robitaille, Y. (1991) Focal neuronal migration disorders: results of surgical treatment. *Ann Neurol*, **30**, 750–7.

Palmini, A., Gambardella, A., Andermann, F. *et al.* (1995) Intrinsic epileptogenicity of human dysplastic cortex as suggested by corticography and surgical results. *Ann Neurol*, **37**, 476–87.

Patrick, S., Berg, A. & Spencer, S.S. (1995) EEG and seizure outcome after epilepsy surgery. *Epilepsia*, **36**, (3), 236–40.

Penfeld, W.J. & Jasper, H.H. (1954) *Epilepsy and the Functional Anatomy of the Human Brain*. Little Brown, Boston.

Plate, K.H., Wieser, H.G., Yasargil, M.G. & Wiestler, O.D. (1993) Neuropathological findings in 224 patients with temporal lobe epilepsy. *Acta Neuropathol (Berl)*, **86**, 433–8.

Radhakrishnan, K., So, E.L., Silbert P.L. *et al.* (1998) Predictors of outcome of anterior temporal lobectomy for intractable epilepsy: a multivariate study. *Neurology*, **51**(2), 465–71.

Ramussen, T. & Villemure, J.G. (1989) Cerebral hemispherectomy for seizures with hemiplegia. *Clev Clin J Med*, **56** (Suppl. 1), S62–S83.

Raymond, A.A., Fish, D.R., Boyd, S.G., Smith, S.J.M., Pitt, M.C. & Kendall, B. (1995). Cortical dysgenesis: serial EEG findings in children and adults. *Electroencephalogr Clin Neurophysiol*, **94**, 389–97.

Raymond, A.A., Fish, D.R., Sisodiya, S. *et al.* (1995) Abnormalities of gyration, heterotopias, tuberous sclerosis, focal cortical dysplasia, microdysgenesis, dysembryoplastic neuroepithelial tumour and dysgenesis of the archicortex in epilepsy. Clinical, EEG and neuroimaging features in 100 adult patients. *Brain*, **118**, 629–60.

Raymond, A.A., Fish, D.R., Stevens, J.M. *et al.* (1994) Association of hippocampal sclerosis with cortical dysgenesis in patients with epilepsy. *Neurology*, **44**, 1841–5.

Raymond, A.A., Fish, D.R., Stevens, J.M., Sisodiya, S.M. & Shorvon, S.D. (1994) Association of hippocampal sclerosis with cortical dysgenesis in patients with epilepsy. *Neurology*, **44**, 1841–4.

Raymond, A.A., Fish, D.R., Stevens, J.M. *et al.* (1994) Subependymal heterotopia: a distinct neuronal migration disorder associated with epilepsy. *J Neurol Neurosurg Psychiatry*, **57**, 1195–202

Raymond, A.A., Halpin, S.F., Alsanjari, N. *et al.* (1994) Dysembryoplastic neuroepithelial tumor: features in 16 patients. *Brain*, **117**, 461–75.

Ring, H.A., Moriarty, J. & Trimble, M.R. (1998) A prospective study of the early postsurgical psychiatric associations of epilepsy surgery. *J Neurol Neurosurg Psychiatry*, **64**(5), 601–4.

Salanova, V., Andermann, F., Olivier, A., Rasmussen, T. & Quesney, L.F. (1992) Occipital lobe epilepsy: electroclinical manifestations, electrocorticography, cortical stimulation and outcome in 42 patients treated between 1930 and 1991. Surgery of occipital lobe epilepsy. *Brain*, **115**, 1655–80.

Salanova, V., Morris, H.H. III, Van Ness, P.C. *et al.* (1993) Comparison of scalp electroencephalogram with subdural electrocorticogram recordings and functional mapping in frontal lobe epilepsy. *Arch Neurol*, **50**, 294–9.

Salanova, V., Quesney, L.F., Rasmussen, T., Andermann, F. & Olivier, A. (1994) Reevaluation of surgical failures and the role of reoperation in 39 patients with frontal lobe epilepsy. *Epilepsia*, **35**, 70–80.

Sandeman, D.R., Sandeman, A.P., Buxton, P. *et al.* (1990) The management of patients with an intrinsic supratentorial brain tumor. *Br J Neurosurg*, **4**, 299–312.

Schachter, S.C., Saper CB (1998) Vagus nerve stimulation. *Epilepsia*, **39**, 677–686.

Shorvon, S.D., Dreifuss, F., Fish, D. & Thomas, D. (eds) (1996) *The Treatment of Epilepsy*. Blackwell Science, London.

Sirven, J.I., Malamut, B.L.; Liporace, J.D., O'Connor, M.J. & Sperling, M.R. (1997) Outcome after temporal lobectomy in bilateral temporal lobe epilepsy. *Ann Neurol*, **42**(6), 873–8.

Smith, D.F., Hutton, J.L., Sandemann, D. *et al.* (1991) The prognosis of primary intracerebral tumors presenting with epilepsy: the outcome of medical and surgical management. *J Neurol Neurosurg Psychiatry*, **54**, 915–20.

So, N., Gloor, P., Quesney, L.F., Jones-Gotman, M., Olivier, A. & Andermann, F. (1989) Depth electrode investigations in patients with bitemporal epileptiform abnormalities. *Ann Neurol*, **25**, 423–31.

So, N., Olivier, A., Andermann, F. *et al.* (1989b) Results of surgical treatment in patients with bitemporal epileptiform abnormalities. *Ann Neurol*, **25**, 432–39.

Spencer, S.S. (1988) Corpus callosum section and other disconnection procedures for medically intractable epilepsy. *Epilepsia*, **29** (Suppl. 2), S85–S99.

Spencer, S.S., McCarthy, G. & Spencer, D.D. (1993) Diagnosis of medial temporal lobe seizure onset: relative sensitivity and specificity of quantitative MRI. *Neurology*, **43**, 2117–24.

Spencer, S.S. & Spencer, D.D. (eds) (1991) *Surgery for Epilepsy*. Blackwell Science, Cambridge, Mass.

Spencer, S.S., Spencer, D.D., Williamson, P.D., Sass, K., Novelly, R.A. & Mattson, R.H. (1988) Corpus callosotomy for epilepsy. I. Seizure effects. *Neurology*, **38**, 19–24.

Spencer, S.S., Williamson, P.D., Bridges, S.L., Mattson, R.H., Cicchetti, D.V. & Spencer D.D. (1985)

Reliability and accuracy of localization by scalp ictal EEG. *Neurology*, **35**, 1567–75.

Spencer, S.S., Williamson, P.D., Spencer, D.D. & Mattson, R.H. (1990) Combined depth and subdural electrode investigation in uncontrolled epilepsy. *Neurology*, **40**, 74–9.

Sperling, M.R., Cahan, L.D. & Brown, W.J. (1989) Relief of seizures from a predominantly posterior temporal tumor with anterior temporal lobectomy. *Epilepsia*, **30**, 559–63.

Theodore, W. (ed) (1992) *Epilepsy Surgery. Epilepsy Research* (suppl).

Tinuper, P., Andermann, F., Villemure, J.G., Rasmussen, T.B. & Quesney, L.F. (1988) Functional hemispherectomy for treatment of epilepsy associated with hemiplegia: rationale, indications, results, and comparison with callosotomy. *Ann Neurol*, **24**, 27–34.

Trenerry, M.R., Jack, C.R. Jr, Ivnik, R.J. *et al.* (1993) MRI hippocampal volumes and memory function before and after temporal lobectomy. *Neurology*, **43**, 1800–05.

Vargha Khadem, F., Carr, L.J., Isaacs, E. *et al.* (1997) Onset of speech after left hemispherectomy in a nine-year-old boy. *Brain*, **120** (Pt 1), 159–82.

Wheelock, I., Peterson, C. & Buchtel, H.A. (1998) Presurgery expectations, postsurgery satisfaction, and psychosocial adjustment after epilepsy surgery. *Epilepsia*. **39**(5), 487–94.

Williamson, P.D., Boon, P.A., Thadani, V.M. *et al.* (1992) Parietal lobe epilepsy: diagnostic considerations and results of surgery. *Ann Neurol*, **31**, 193–201.

Williamson, P.D., French, J.A., Thadani, V.M. *et al.* (1993) Characteristics of medial temporal lobe epilepsy: interictal and ictal scalp electroencephalography, neuropsychological testing, neuroimaging, surgical results and pathology. *Ann. Neurol.*, **34**, 781–7.

Williamson, P.D., Thadani, V.M., Darcey, T.M. *et al.* (1992) Occipital lobe epilepsy: clinical characteristics, seizure spread patterns and results of surgery. *Ann Neurol*, **31**, 3–13.

Wyllie, E., Lüders, H., Morris, H.H. *et al.* (1988) Subdural electrodes in the evaluation for epilepsy surgery in children and adults. *Neuropediatrics*, **19**, 80–6.

Yasargil, M.G., Wieser, H.G., Valavanis, A., von Ammon, K. & Roth, P. (1993) Surgery and results of selective amygdala-hippocampectomy in one hundred patients with nonlesional limbic epilepsy. *Neurosurg Clin N Am*, **4**, 243–61.

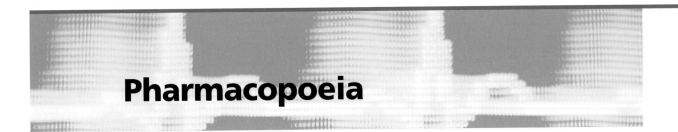

Pharmacopoeia

The tables in this pharmacopoeia (and in Chapters 3 and 4) aim to provide summary data only, and apply to the treatment of adult patients unless otherwise stated. Published pharmacological and pharmacokinetic data are very variable, and the tables attempt to give representative figures or data which reflect the best evidence base. The text of Chapters 3 and 4 expands on areas where conflicting data exist, and the summary tables should be taken in conjunction with the textual comments.

	Carbamazepine	Clobazam	Clonazepam
Primary indications	First-line or adjunctive therapy in partial and generalized seizures (excluding absence and myoclonus). Also in Lennox–Gastaut syndrome and childhood epilepsy syndromes	First-line adjunctive therapy for partial and generalized seizures. Also for intermittent therapy, one-off prophylactic therapy, and non-convulsive status epilepticus	Adjunctive therapy in partial and generalized seizures (including absence and myoclonus). Also, Lennox–Gastaut syndrome and status epilepticus
Usual preparations	Tablets: 100, 200, 400 mg; chewtabs: 100, 200 mg; slow-release formulations; 200, 400 mg; liquid: 100 mg/5 mL; suppositories: 125, 250 mg	Tablet, capsule: 10 mg	Tablets: 0.5, 2 mg; liquid: 1 mg in 1 mL diluent
Usual dosages	Initial: 100 mg at night. Maintenance: 400–1600 mg per day (maximum 2400 mg). (Slow-release formulation, higher dosage.) Children: <1 year, 100–200 mg; 1–5 years, 200–400 mg; 5–10 years, 400–600 mg; 10–15 years, 600–1000 mg	10–30 mg per day (adults); higher doses can be used. Children aged 3–12 years, up to half adult dose	Initial: 0.25 mg. Maintenance: 0.5–4 mg (adults); 1 mg (children under 1 year), 1–2 mg (children 1–5 years), 1–3 mg (children 5–12 years). Higher doses can be used
Dosage intervals	2–3 times per day (2–4 times per day at higher doses or in children)	1–2 times per day	1–2 times per day
Significant drug interactions	Carbamazepine has a large number of interactions with antiepileptic and other drugs	Minor interactions are common, but usually not clinically significant	Minor interactions are common, but usually not clinically significant
Serum level monitoring	Useful	Not useful	Not useful
Target range	20–50 µmol/L	–	–
Common/important side-effects	Drowsiness, fatigue, dizziness, ataxia, diplopia, blurring of vision, sedation, headache, insomnia, gastrointestinal disturbance, tremor, weight gain, impotence, effects on behaviour and mood, hepatic disturbance, rash, and other skin reactions, bone marrow dyscrasias, hyponutraemia, water retention and nephritis	Sedation, dizziness, weakness, blurring of vision, restlessness, ataxia, aggressiveness, behavioural disturbance, withdrawal symptoms	Sedation (common and may be severe), cognitive effects, drowsiness, ataxia, personality and behavioural changes, hyperactivity, restlessness, aggressiveness, psychotic reaction, seizure exacerbations, hypersalivation, leucopenia, withdrawal symptoms

Main advantages	Highly effective and usually well-tolerated therapy	Highly effective in some patients with epilepsy resistant to first-line therapy. Better tolerated than other benzodiazepines	Useful add-on action, especially in children
Main disadvantages	Transient adverse effects on initiating therapy. Occasional severe toxicity	Development of tolerance in as many as 50% of subjects within weeks or months	Side-effects are sometimes prominent, particularly sedation, tolerance and a withdrawal syndrome
Mechanisms of action	Action on neuronal sodium-channel conductance. Also action on monoamine, acetylcholine and NMDA receptors	$GABA_A$ receptor agonist. Also action on ion-channel conductance	$GABA_A$ receptor agonist. Also action on sodium-channel conductance
Oral bioavailability	75–85%	90%	>80%
Time to peak levels	4–8 h	1–4 h	1–4 h
Metabolism and excretion	Hepatic oxidation and then conjugation	Hepatic epoxidation and then conjugation	Hepatic reduction then acetylation
Volume of distribution	0.8–1.2 L/kg	–	2.0 L/kg
Elimination half-life	5–26 h (but very variable)	10–50 h (clobazam); 50 h (N-desmethylclobazam)	20–80 h
Plasma clearance	0.133 L/kg/h (but very variable)	–	0.09 L/kg/h
Protein binding	75%	83%	86%
Active metabolites	Carbamazepine epoxide	N-desmethylclobazam	Nil
Comment	A drug of first choice in tonic–clonic and partial seizures in adults and children	Excellent second-line therapy in some patients with resistant epilepsy	A wide antiepileptic effect, use limited by side-effects, but helpful particularly in children with severe epilepsy

	Ethosuximide	Felbamate	Gabapentin
Primary indications	First-line or adjunctive therapy in generalized absence seizures	Adjunctive therapy in refractory partial and secondarily generalized epilepsy. Also in Lennox–Gastaut syndrome	Adjunctive therapy in adults with partial or secondarily generalized epilepsy
Usual preparations	Capsules: 250 mg; syrup: 250 mg/5 mL	Tablets: 400, 600 mg; syrup: 600 mg/5 mL	Capsules: 100, 300, 400 mg
Usual dosages	Initial: 250 mg (adults); 10–15 mg/kg per day (children). Maintenance: 750–2000 mg per day (adults); 20–40 mg/kg per day (children)	Initial: 1200 mg per day (adults); 15 mg/kg per day (children). Maintenance: 1200–3600 mg per day (adults); 45–80 mg/kg per day (children)	Initial: 300 mg per day Maintenance: 900–3600 mg per day
Dosage intervals	2–3 times per day	3–4 times per day	2–3 times per day
Significant drug interactions	Ethosuximide levels are increased by valproate. Levels reduced by carbamazepine, phenytoin and phenobarbital	Felbamate increases the concentration of phenobarbital, phenytoin, carbamazepine epoxide and valproate. Felbamate lowers the concentration of carbamazepine. Phenytoin, phenobarbital and carbamazepine lower felbamate levels; valproate increases felbamate levels	None
Serum level monitoring	Useful	Value not established	Not useful
Target range	300–700 µmol/L	200–460 µmol/L	–
Common/important side-effects	Gastrointestinal symptoms, drowsiness, ataxia, diplopia, headache, sedation, behavioural disturbances, acute psychotic reactions, extra-pyramidal symptoms, blood dyscrasia, rash, systemic lupus erythematosus	Severe hepatic disturbance and aplastic anaemia are rare but serious side-effects. Insomnia, weight loss, gastrointestinal symptoms, fatigue, dizziness, lethargy, behavioural change, ataxia, visual disturbance, mood change, psychotic reaction, rash, neurological symptoms	Drowsiness, dizziness, seizure exacerbation, ataxia, headache, tremor, diplopia, nausea, vomiting, rhinitis

Main advantages	Well-established treatment for absence epilepsy without the risk of hepatic toxicity carried by valproate	Highly effective novel antiepileptic drug for refractory patients	Lack of side-effects (especially at low doses) and good pharmacokinetic profile
Main disadvantages	Side-effects common	Severe hepatic and aplastic anaemia in occasional patients. Other side-effects also frequent on initial therapy, and in patients on polytherapy	Lack of therapeutic effect in severe cases. Seizure exacerbation
Mechanisms of action	Effects on calcium T-channel conductance	Probably by effect on NMDA receptor (glycine recognition site) and sodium-channel conductance	Not known. Possible action on calcium channels
Oral bioavailability	<100%	90%	<60%
Time to peak levels	<4 h	1–4 h	2–4 h
Metabolism and excretion	Hepatic oxidation then conjugation	Hepatic hydroxylation and then conjugation (60%); renal excretion as unchanged drug (40%)	Renal excretion without metabolism
Volume of distribution	0.65 L/kg	0.75 L/kg	0.9 L/kg
Elimination half-life	30–60 h	20 h (13–30 h; lowest in patients comedicated with enzyme inducers)	5–9 h
Plasma clearance	0.010–0.015 L/kg/h	0.027–0.032 L/kg/h (but variable)	0.120–0.130 L/kg/h
Protein binding	Nil	20–25%	Nil
Active metabolites	Nil	Nil	Nil
Comment	Drug of first choice in absence seizures	Highly effective novel anticonvulsant in severe resistant epilepsy, but use limited by rare but severe hepatic and haematological toxicity	Novel anticonvulsant of uncertain relative efficacy, but easy to use and few side-effects

	Lamotrigine	Levetiracetam	Oxcarbazepine
Primary indications	Adjunctive or monotherapy in partial and generalized epilepsy. Also in Lennox–Gastaut syndrome	Adjunctive therapy in partial seizures with or without secondarily generalized seizures	Adjunctive or monotherapy in partial and secondarily generalized seizures
Usual preparations	Tablets: 25, 50, 100, 200 mg; chewtabs: 5, 25, 100 mg	Tablets: 250, 500, 750, 1000 mg	Tablets: 150, 300, 600 mg
Usual dosages	Initial: 12.5–25 mg per day. Maintenance: 100–200 mg (monotherapy or comedication with valproate); 200–400 mg (comedication with enzyme-inducing drugs)	Initial: 1000 mg per day. Maintenance: 1000–3000 mg per day	Initial starting dose: 600 mg per day. Titration rate of 600 mg per week. The usual maintenance dose is 900–2400 mg per day
Dosage intervals	2 times per day	2 times per day	2 times per day
Significant drug interactions	Autoinduction. Lamotrigine levels are lowered by phenytoin, carbamazepine, phenobarbital and other enzyme-inducing drugs. Lamotrigine levels increased by sodium valproate	None	Fewer than with carbamazepine
Serum level monitoring	Value not established	Value not established	Value not established
Target range	4–60 µmol/L	–	50–125 µmol/L
Common/important side-effects	Rash (sometimes severe), headache, blood dyscrasia, ataxia, asthenia, diplopia, nausea, vomiting, dizziness, somnolence, insomnia, depression, psychosis, tremor, hypersensitivity reactions	Somnolence, asthenia, infection, dizziness, headache	Somnolence, headache, dizziness, rash, hyponatraemia, weight gain, alopecia, nausea, gastrointestinal disturbance

Main advantages	Effective and well tolerated	A recently licensed drug which, on the basis of clinical trial evidence, is well tolerated and highly effective	Better tolerated and fewer interactions than with carbamazepine
Main disadvantages	High instance of rash (occasionally severe), and other side-effects	Limited experience in routine clinical practice, as it is recently licensed	25% cross-sensitivity with carbamazepine. Higher incidence of hyponatraemia than with carbamazepine
Mechanisms of action	Blockage of voltage-dependent sodium conductance	Not known	Sodium-channel blockade. Also affects potassium conductance and modulates high-voltage activated calcium-channel activity
Oral bioavailability	<100%	<100%	<100%
Time to peak levels	1–3 h	0.6–1.3 h	4–5 h
Metabolism and excretion	Hepatic glucuronidation (without phase I reaction)	Partially hydrolysed in the blood to inactive compound	Hydroxylation then conjugation
Volume of distribution	0.9–1.3 L/kg	0.5–0.7 L/kg	0.3–0.8 L/kg
Elimination half-life	29 h (approx. monotherapy); 15 h (enzyme-inducing comedication); 60 h (valproate comedication)	6–8 h	8–10 h (MHD)
Plasma clearance	0.044–0.084 L/kg/h (but variable)	0.6 mL/min/kg	–
Protein binding	55%	Nil	38% (MHD)
Active metabolites	Nil	Nil	MHD
Comment	A useful medication in a wide variety of epilepsies	A novel antiepileptic drug with promise in the therapy of partial-onset seizures (with or without secondarily generalization)	Close structural similarity to carbamazepine but better tolerated and with fewer drug interactions. Licensed in some countries only, and for use for partial and secondarily generalized seizures

	Phenobarbital	Phenytoin	Piracetam
Primary indications	Adjunctive or first-line therapy for partial or generalized seizures (including absence and myoclonus). Also for status epilepticus, Lennox–Gastaut syndrome, benign childhood epilepsy, febrile convulsions and neonatal seizures	First-line or adjunctive therapy for partial and generalized seizures (including myoclonus and absence). Also for status epilepticus, Lennox–Gastaut syndrome and childhood epilepsy syndromes	Adjunctive therapy for myoclonus
Usual preparations	Tablets: 15, 30, 50, 60, 100 mg; elixir: 15 mg/5 mL; injection: 200 mg/mL	Capsules: 25, 50, 100, 200 mg; chewtabs: 50 mg; liquid suspension: 30 mg/5 mL, 125 mg/50 mL; injection: 250 mg/5 mL	Tablets: 800, 1200 mg; sachets: 1.2, 2.4 g; ampoules: 1.3 g; baxter: 12 g; solution: 20, 33%
Usual dosages	Initial: 30 mg per day. Maintenance: 30–180 mg per day (adults); 3–8 mg/kg per day (children); 3–4 mg/kg per day (neonates)	Initial: 100–200 mg per day (adults); 5 mg/kg (children). Maintenance: 100–300 mg per day (adults), higher doses can be used guided by serum level monitoring: 4–8 mg/kg (children)	Initial: 7.2 g per day. Maintenance: up to 24 g per day
Dosage intervals	1–2 times per day	1–2 times per day	2–3 times per day
Significant drug interactions	Phenobarbital has a number of interactions with antiepileptic and other drugs	Phenytoin has a large number of interactions with antiepileptic and other drugs	None
Serum level monitoring	Useful	Useful	Not useful
Target range	40–170 µmol/L	40–80 µmol/L	–
Common/important side-effects	Sedation, ataxia, dizziness, insomnia, hyperkinesis (children), mood changes (especially depression), aggressiveness, cognitive dysfunction, impotence, reduced libido, folate deficiency, vitamin K and vitamin D deficiency, osteomalacia, Dupuytren's contracture, frozen shoulder, connective-tissue abnormalities and rash	Ataxia, dizziness, lethargy, sedation, headaches, dyskinesia, acute encephalopathy. Hypersensitivity, rash, fever, blood dyscrasia, gingival hyperplasia, folate deficiency, megaloblastic anaemia, vitamin K deficiency, thyroid dysfunction, decreased immunoglobulins, mood changes, depression, coarsened facies, hirsutism, peripheral neuropathy, osteomalacia, hypocalcaemia, hormonal dysfunction, loss of libido, connective-tissue alterations, pseudolymphoma, hepatitis, vasculitis, myopathy coagulation defects and bone marrow hypoplasia	Dizziness, insomnia, nausea, gastro-intestinal discomfort, hyperkinesis, weight gain, tremulousness, agitation, drowsiness, rash

Main advantages	Highly effective and cheap antiepileptic drug	Highly effective and cheap antiepileptic drug	Well tolerated and very effective in some resistant cases
Main disadvantages	CNS side-effects	CNS and systemic side-effects	Not effective in many cases
Mechanisms of action	Enhances activity of GABA$_A$ receptor, depresses glutamate excitability, affects sodium, potassium and calcium conductance	Blockade of sodium channels and action on calcium and chloride conductance and voltage-dependent neurotransmission	Unclear
Oral bioavailability	80–100%	95%	<100%
Time to peak levels	1–3 h (but variable)	4–12 h	30–40 min
Metabolism and excretion	Hepatic oxidation, glucosidation and hydroxylation, then conjugation	Hepatic oxidation and hydroxylation, then conjugation	Renal excretion without metabolism
Volume of distribution	0.42–0.75 L/kg	0.5–0.8 L/kg	0.6 L/kg
Elimination half-life	75–120 h	7–42 h (mean, 20 h: dependent on plasma level)	5–6 h
Plasma clearance	0.006–0.009 L/kg/h	0.003–0.02 L/kg/h (dependent on plasma level)	–
Protein binding	45–60%	70–95%	Nil
Active metabolites	Nil	Nil	Nil
Comment	Highly effective antiepileptic, now not used as a first-line therapy because of potential CNS toxicity, especially in children	Well-established first-line therapy whose use is limited by side-effects	Useful drug for some patients with refractory myoclonus

	Primidone	Tiagabine	Topiramate
Primary indications	Adjunctive therapy in partial and secondarily generalized seizures (including absence and myoclonus). Also Lennox–Gastaut syndrome	Adjunctive therapy or monotherapy in partial and secondarily generalized seizures	Adjunctive therapy or monotherapy in partial and secondarily generalized seizures. Also for Lennox–Gastaut syndrome and primary generalized tonic–clonic seizures
Usual preparations	Tablets: 250 mg; oral suspension: 250 mg/5 mL	Tablets: 5, 10 and 15 mg	Tablets: 25, 50, 100, 200 mg; sprinkle: 15, 25 mg
Usual dosages	Initial: 125 mg per day. Maintenance: 500–1500 mg per day (adults), 250–500 mg (under 2 years), 500–750 mg (2–5 years), 750–1000 mg (6–9 years)	Initial: 15 mg per day. Maintenance 30–45 mg per day (combination with enzyme-inducing drugs), 15–30 mg per day (comedication with non-enzyme inducing drugs)	Initial: 25–50 mg per day (adults), 0.5–1 mg/kg per day (children). Maintenance: 200–600 mg per day (adults), 9–11 mg/kg per day (children)
Dosage intervals	1–2 times per day	2–3 times per day	2 times per day
Significant drug interactions	Primidone has a large number of interactions with antiepileptic and other drugs	Tiagabine levels are lowered by comedication with hepatic enzyme-inducing drugs	Topiramate levels are lowered by carbamazepine, phenobarbital and phenytoin
Serum level monitoring	Primidone, not generally useful. Derived phenobarbital, useful	Not useful	Not generally useful
Target range	<60 µmol/L primidone, 40–70 µmol/L derived phenobarbital	6–74 µmol/L	–
Common/important side-effects	Acute dizziness and nausea on initiation of therapy. Other side-effects as for phenobarbital	Dizziness, tiredness, nervousness, tremor, diarrhoea, headache, confusion, psychosis, flu-like symptoms, ataxia, depression	Dizziness, ataxia, headache, parasthesia, tremor, somnolence, cognitive dysfunction, confusion, agitation, amnesia, depression, emotional lability, nausea, diarrhoea, diplopia, weight loss

	Primidone	Tiagabine	
Main advantages	Highly effective and cheap antiepileptic drug	Clinical experience is too limited to define the place of tiagabine in clinical practice, but initial experience is favourable	Highly effective, recently introduced antiepileptic drugs
Main disadvantages	CNS side-effects. Also acute reaction on initiation of therapy	CNS side-effects	CNS side-effects
Mechanisms of action	Enhances activity of $GABA_A$ receptor, depresses glutamate excitability and affects sodium, potassium and calcium conductance	Inhibits GABA reuptake	Blockade of sodium channels, enhancement of GABA-mediated chloride influx and modulatory effects of the $GABA_A$ receptor and actions at the AMPA receptor
Oral bioavailability	<100%	96%	<100%
Time to peak levels	3 h	1 h	2 h
Metabolism and excretion	Metabolized to phenobarbital and phenylmenlymalonamide	Hepatic oxidation then conjugation	Mainly renal excretion without metabolism (majority of the drug dose)
Volume of distribution	0.6–1.0 L/kg (derived phenobarbital)	1.0 L/kg	0.6–1.0 L/kg
Elimination half-life	5–18 h primidone; 75–120 h derived phenobarbital	3.8–4.9 h	18–23 h (but varies with comedication)
Plasma clearance	0.006–0.009 L/kg/h (derived phenobarbital)	12.8 L/h	0.022–0.036 L/kg/h
Protein binding	25% primidone; 45–60% derived phenobarbital	96%	15%
Active metabolites	Phenobarbital	Nil	Nil
Comment	Primidone is converted in the body to phenobarbital, and its antiepileptic effect is due to phenobarbital. It is therefore doubtful whether primidone carries any antiepileptic advantages over phenobarbital, but in many countries it is not subject to controlled drug restrictions which apply to phenobarbital	Newly licensed antiepileptic drug with promise for use in therapy of refractory partial seizures	Highly effective recently introduced antiepileptic

	Valproate	Vigabatrin
Primary indications	First-line adjunctive therapy in generalized seizures (including myoclonus and absence and also partial seizures), Lennox–Gastaut syndrome and drug of first choice in the syndrome of primary generalized epilepsy. Also for childhood epilepsy syndromes and febrile convulsions	Adjunctive therapy in partial and secondarily generalized epilepsy. Also infantile spasm and Lennox–Gastaut syndrome
Usual preparations	Enteric-coated tablets: 200, 500 mg; crushable tablets; 100 mg; capsules: 150, 300, 500 mg; syrup: 200 mg/5 mL; liquid: 200 mg/5 mL; slow release tablets: 200, 300, 500 mg; Divalproex tablets: 125, 300 and 500 mg; sprinkle	Tablets: 500 mg; powder sachet: 500 mg
Usual dosages	Initial: 400–500 mg per day (adults); 20 mg/kg per day (children under 20 kg); 40 mg/kg per day (children over 20 kg). Maintenance: 500–2500 mg per day (adults); 20–40 mg/kg per day (children under 20 kg); 20–30 mg/kg per day (children over 20 kg). (Slow-release formulation not suitable for children)	Initial: 1000 mg per day (adults). Maintenance: 1000–3000 mg (adults), 40 mg/kg per day (children) or 500–1000 mg per day (body weight 10–15 kg), 1000–1500 mg (body weight 15–30 kg), 1500–3000 mg (body weight over 30 kg)
Dosage intervals	2–3 times per day	2 times per day
Significant drug interactions	Valproate has a number of complex interactions with antiepileptic and other drugs	Vigabatrin may lower phenytoin levels
Serum level monitoring	Not generally useful	Not useful
Target range	300–600 μmol/L	–
Common/important side-effects	Nausea, vomiting, metabolic effects, endocrine effects, severe hepatic toxicity, pancreatitis, drowsiness, cognitive disturbance, aggressiveness, tremor, weakness, encephalopathy, thrombo-cytopenia, neutropenia, aplastic anaemia, hair thinning and hair loss, weight gain	Sedation, dizziness, headache, ataxia, paraesthesia, agitation, amnesia, mood change, depression, psychosis, aggression, confusion, weight gain, tremor, diplopia, severe visual field constriction, diarrhoea
Main advantages	Drug of choice in primary generalized epilepsy and a wide spectrum of activity	Highly effective recently introduced antiepileptic drug
Main disadvantages	Cognitive effects, weight gain, tremor and hair loss. Potential for severe hepatic and pancreatic disturbance in children	CNS side-effects and visual field constriction
Mechanisms of action	Uncertain but may affect GABA glutaminergic activity, calcium (T) conductance and potassium conductance	Inhibition of GABA transaminase activity
Oral bioavailability	<100%	<100%
Time to peak levels	1–8 h (dependent on formulation)	2 h
Metabolism and excretion	Hepatic oxidation and then conjugation	Renal excretion without metabolism
Volume of distribution	0.1–0.4 L/kg	0.8 L/kg
Elimination half-life	4–12 h	4–7 h
Plasma clearance	0.010–0.115 L/kg/h	0.102–0.114 L/kg/h
Protein binding	85–95%	Nil
Active metabolites	Nil	Nil
Comment	Drug of choice in primary generalized epilepsy and useful in a wide spectrum of other epilepsies	Highly effective recently introduced antiepileptic drug whose usage is limited by potential for neuropsychiatric side-effects and effects on visual field

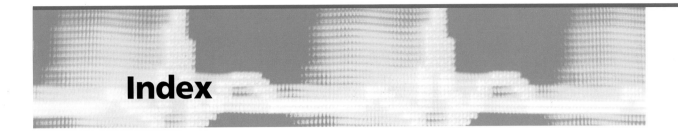

Index